Rehabilitation of the Older Person

Rehabilitation of the Older Person

A *handbook for the interdisciplinary team*

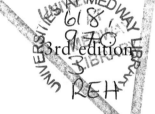

3rd edition

Edited by Amanda J. Squires
Clinical Governance Review Manager,
Commission for Health Improvement

and

Margaret B. Hastings
Head of Physiotherapy, Lomond Physiotherapy Service,
Alexandria, UK

First published in 1988 by:
Chapman & Hall
Second edition 1996

Published in 2002 by:
Nelson Thornes Ltd
Delta Place
27 Bath Road
CHELTENHAM
GL53 7TH
United Kingdom

06 / 10 9 8 7 6 5 4 3

A catalogue record for this book is available from the British Library

ISBN 0 7487 5470 9

Page make-up by Florence Production Ltd

Printed and bound in Spain by GraphyCems

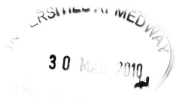

Contents

CONTRIBUTORS

Helen Alaszewski BA, RGN
Research Assistant, School of Community and Health Studies, University of Hull

Elizabeth Baikie MPhil, MA(Hons), CPsychol
Head of Clinical Psychology, Royal Victoria Hospital, Edinburgh

Kirsten Beining BSc (Hons), MRCSLT
Senior Speech and Language Therapist, Western Community Hospital, Southampton

Fiona Bevan BPharm (Hons), MRPharmS
Clinical Pharmacy Manager, Countess of Chester Hospital, Chester

Norman F. Button PhD, BSc (Hons), F.C.Optom, DCLP
Eye Clinic Director, Department of Vision Sciences, Glasgow Caledonian University

Marie Donaghy PhD, BA(Hons), MCSP, SRP
Senior Lecturer, Department of Physiotherapy, Queen Margaret University College, Edinburgh

Chris Drinkwater CBE, FRCGP, FFPHM
Head of Centre for Primary and Comunity Care Learning, University of Northumbria, Newcastle upon Tyne

Olwen E. Finlay MBE, FCSP, HT, SRP, DMS
International Co-ordinator, Physiotherapists working with older people, Bath

Colin J. Fullerton M.Med.Sci, F.Pod.A
Senior Podiatrist, Centre for Podiatric Medicine, The Queens University of Belfast

James George MB, FRCP
Consultant in Medicine for the Elderly and Director of Rehabilitation, Carlisle Hospitals

Margaret B. Hastings MBA, BA, FCSP, SRP
Head of Physiotherapy, Lomond Physiotherapy Service, Vale of Leven District General Hospital, Alexandria

Susan A.R. Hawkins MPH, BSc (Hons), MCSP, SRP
Superintendent Physiotherapist, Rehabilitation Team, Royal Cornwall Hospitals Trust (Treliske), Truro

Suzanne Hogg MCSP, SRP
Superintendent Physiotherapist, Department of Medicine for Elderly People, Portsmouth Healthcare NHS Trust

Jill Manthorpe MA
Reader in Community Care, Department of Social Work, University of Hull

Jill Mantle BA, FCSP, DipTP, SRP
Research Physiotherapist, Urogynaecology Department, King's College Hospital, London

Jane Maxim PhD, MA, MRCSLT, FRCSLT
Head of Department, Human Communication Science, University College, London

Ronnie McGovern BA, RMN, RGN
Clinical Nurse Manager, Ravenscraig Hospital, Greenock

Helen McGrath MRCP
Specialist Registrar in Geriatric and General Medicine, Cumberland Infirmary, Carlisle

Tali Mendelsohn BA
Audiology Policy Officer, The Royal National Institute for Deaf People, London

Rowena D. Plant, PhD, MSc, PGCED, MCSP, SRP
Professor of Rehabilitation Therapy, Institute of Rehabilitation, University of Northumbria, Newcastle upon Tyne

Kiran Shukla BSc, BEd, SRD, DMS
Head of Nutrition and Dietetics, South Essex Mental Health and Community Care NHS Trust

Joyce M. Smith PhD, BDS, M.Med.Sci., MCCCD, RCS
Consultant in Dental Public Health, Barking & Havering and Redbridge & Waltham Forest Health Authorities, London/Essex

Amanda J. Squires PhD, MSc, FCSP, SRP
Clinical Governance Review Manager, Commission for Health Improvement

Cameron G. Swift PhD, FRCP
Professor of Health Care of the Elderly, King's College London and Consultant Physician, King's College Hospital, London

Jennifer Wenborn MSc, DipCOT, SROT
Independent Occupational Therapist, London

Jayne Whitaker DipCS, MRCSLTT
Principal Speech-Language Therapist, Southampton University Hospital Trust

Brian Owen Williams MD, FRCP
Consultant Geriatrician, Gartnavel General Hospital, Glasgow

John Young MB MSc FRCP
Consultant in Medicine for the Elderly, St Lukes Hospital, Bradford

ACKNOWLEDGEMENTS

We would like to thank all other contributors to the first and second editions whose work stimulated the need for further editions:
Alison Blenkinsopp, Penelope Fenn Clark, Katherine Coombes, Alison Froggatt, Anne Gale, Jane Gayland, Rosemary Gravell, Linda Haldane, Jean Hall, Thelma Harvey, Marion Judd, Denise Keir, Judith Kemp, Rosemary Oddy, Janet Pierce, Anna Smith, Adrienne Little, Jane Milligan, Jane Stephenson, Madeline Taylor, Linda Thomas, Charles Twining, Patricia Wardle, Fiona Watts and Lindsay Winterton.

We are also grateful to the following people and organizations for granting permision to use material in this edition:
HMSO for Figure 1.1 on page 11 and Table 3.1 on page 34; the Parkinson's Disease Society for Figure 15.1 on page 237; and *Physiotherapy* for Table 15.1 on page 240.

Preface to the Third Edition

Attitudes to rehabilitation of older people, particularly among specialist health and social care practitioners, have become increasingly personally positive in recent years. A growing number of professionals see the specialty as a rewarding and necessary career experience. This needs encouragement if the professions are to be prepared for the increasing numbers and expectations of older people who will require help from their members.

The purpose of this book is to bring together the skills and experience of experts in several fields of rehabilitation to provide a primer for those needing knowledge of how to manage older people in whatever environment or specialty they present. Readers will be able to enhance their own knowledge already gained in a variety of fields, and play an immediate part in the team. The information will also be of value to interested carers, agencies contributing to the widened provision of service to older people, and service commissioners.

The continuing transformation of health and social care delivery worldwide, resulting from changing user and provider expectations influencing government policies, is altering approaches to and delivery of rehabilitation services. These current and envisaged future changes are addressed by each discipline, using the UK as an example.

This third edition, entitled *Rehabilitation of the Older Person: A handbook for the interdisciplinary team,* builds on the first, entitled *Rehabilitation of the Older Patient* (1988), and the second, entitled *Rehabilitation of Older People* (1996), both intended as a handbook for the multidisciplinary team. The change in emphasis from patient, to people, to person, and from multidisciplinary to interdisciplinary reflects the change in status of older people in their rehabilitation from paternalism to partnership; the change in the style of rehabilitation from standardised to personalised; and the change in the way of working from many different professionals to those professionals working together. Other key changes include a leading chapter on primary care (from a mention in 1988 and end chapter in 1994), reflecting the growing importance of this contribution; a dedicated chapter on carers included for the first time, reflecting not only the growing contribution of this group but also their increasing involvement and assertiveness in the care process; and new chapters on stakeholders' expectations and rehabilitation settings, reflecting the growing plural approach outlined in the new NHS Plan and National Service Framework for Older People, which are also considered.

Currently many of the clinical judgements made by team members are based on 'experience' or 'intuition', seldom available to the student, newly qualified practitioner, or recent returner. In addition, the multiple facets of management of the older person can quickly overwhelm and deter the unprepared. The 'team' concept should no longer be new, having started within the field of geriatric medicine, but the links between disciplines and the services each provides can easily confuse the new participant, come as a revelation to interested observers and can be a potential minefield. A case study is used in this edition to demonstrate how successful co-ordination of individual approaches to assessment, goal setting, intervention and outcome measurement differentiates the successful team from others.

Devolution has had particular consequences for health care. The National Health Service in Scotland, Wales and Northern Ireland is a devolved responsibility. England and Wales continue to be linked, and Northern Ireland has for some time been a unified provision. This has meant that crossing the line between statutory providers as either patient or professional may result in service differences. Contributors to this edition are well placed to explain these changes relevant to rehabilitation of the older person.

We hope, in this revised edition, to have clarified these issues, both existing and emerging.

Amanda Squires and Margaret Hastings, 2001

PART One _____

THE
OPPORTUNITY
FOR
REHABILITATION

1 THE REHABILITATION OF THE OLDER PERSON – PAST, PRESENT AND FUTURE

Amanda J. Squires

AIMS OF THE CHAPTER

Since the first and second editions of this book, health and social care in the UK, like many such services worldwide, have undergone repeated and fundamental change. To understand the consequences for rehabilitation of older people and to put the chapters that follow in this third edition into perspective, this chapter presents a review of the history, current changes and the possible future.

The key issues that emerge are that rehabilitation has moved from a paternalistic to a partnership approach, in line with an increase in the numbers of older people with chronic conditions amenable to rehabilitation; an increasing complexity of multi-agency provision; increased expectations of older service users and their carers; and service reforms which have been aimed at improving efficiency, effectiveness, responsiveness and accountability. Progress from a multi-disciplinary approach, where a number of disciplines are involved, to an interdisciplinary approach, where those disciplines provide an integrated service, is proposed as a solution to balance supply and demand. The chapter concludes by suggesting that rehabilitation of older people increasingly requires new and positive attitudes, an expanded evidence base and access to a wide range of competent skills.

THE PAST – EVOLUTION OF GERIATRICS AS A SPECIALITY

Traditional practice in the rehabilitation of older people is inextricably linked with the development of medicine for old age. A variety of institutions, and particularly the family, have supported and at times neglected the poor, sick and disabled across the centuries in the UK. The Middle Ages saw the religious institutions providing hospitals and hospices as houses of rest and entertainment for travellers or strangers, gradually changing to care centres for the sick, destitute or dying (Williams, 1999). The dissolution of the monasteries in the sixteenth century affected such provision. In 1601 the Poor Law introduced the idea of each parish caring for and controlling its own poor, and a poor rate was levied from parishioners – the forerunner of the council tax of today. The Gilbert Act of 1782 promoted the principle that parishes should combine to construct workhouses for the poor. With the new pressures of industrialisation, the Poor Law was amended in 1834 centralising relief for the poor. Parishes were grouped together and the number and size of the workhouses increased. While workhouses accommodated paupers, their purpose was to deter the poor, rather than provide care. This resulted in large, grim, prison-like institutions to discourage admission. The sick poor were generally accommodated in adjacent infirmaries.

Britain was the first country in the world to industrialise as a consequence of a range of factors (Duggan and Duggan, 2000). With changes in working practices from home-based agricultural and cottage industries to large-scale factories, the Industrial Revolution, which began during the nineteenth century, changed the nature of poverty and unemployment. It also promoted the need for more worker mobility and decreased the availability of home-based family help.

The mixing of different categories of paupers (disabled, old, mentally ill and non-disabled poor) in institutions was not altogether changed until the end of the nineteenth century. Some specific separate categories did develop, for instance, those who were blind or deaf from birth were often treated separately (French, 1994). The health needs of older people, unfortunate enough to have to enter such institutions, were not considered separately from the poor in general, although basic poor relief was more likely to be given to them in their own homes.

By the 1930s custodial care for sick older people without resources or family was still generally the norm, often in workhouses or infirmaries. Brocklehurst (1975) suggests that it was not until the state took responsibility for the large number of chronic beds in the public hospital system that the health needs of older people began to be officially realised. This occurred largely as a result of the need to relocate 'chronic' patients from hospitals to make way for 'acute' injuries predicted or admitted during the Second World War. The transfer of such large numbers of patients from hospitals to the only large institutions available to take them, workhouse infirmaries, resulted firstly in appalling overcrowding, and secondly in their accompaniment by 'hospital' staff. One such junior doctor was Marjorie Warren, and accounts of what she found and subsequently began to change form a priceless social record (Williams, 1999).

Four groups of patients were described as being found on the chronic sick wards; 'the recovered', comprising a few active patients who, due to their perceived social inadequacy, were kept on by hospitals as staff; second, 'homeless' people; the third and biggest group were the long-stay invalids; and the last and smallest group were those considered to be capable of some response to treatment (Adams and McIlwraith, 1963).

At this time a problem-solving approach to disability, and the concepts of progressive patient care and team work were added to the acute model of care (accurate diagnosis, classification, prognosis, treatment, cure and discharge). 'Geriatric medicine' as a speciality was born, but has continued to struggle for both recognition and resources in competition with long-established, more media attractive and dramatically curative specialities.

The UK National Health Service (NHS) was established in 1948 to meet the medical needs of such ill and disabled people, as well as providing aids and home nursing equipment. The principle of free access to health care has largely remained, with only dental, pharmaceutical and optical services requiring a nominal fee. In a separate arena, the 1947 National Assistance Act provided financial and (in Part III in England and Wales, Part IV in Scotland) residential support for disabled and needy older people, under local authority control.

Under the NHS, rehabilitation departments developed to meet the needs of war veterans and also those affected by the polio epidemic of the early 1950s. Both of these events resulted in a great increase in the number of young disabled people. Rehabilitation units were largely staffed by the surplus of health-care and physical training staff leaving the armed forces (Stewart and Hawker, 1999). Rehabilitation began to replace convalescence as a means of recovery and its proponents instituted the idea of active treatment involving the patient. The 1950s also saw expansion in all industries, including health care, and the need to recruit labour from outside the UK – particularly countries with previous 'colonial' connections. These first generation migrants are now themselves reaching old age (Squires, 1991).

The structure of the rehabilitation team of the 1950s comprised a core group of health-care professionals – doctors, nurses, physiotherapists and occupational therapists, possibly with some untrained or volunteer support workers. Social work input continued to form a link between hospital and local government support services, but did not develop significantly until the 1970s.

Thus the process of rehabilitation was one of 'hands on' work by professionals, and although 'active', this was paternalistic in terms of activity decided by the team for the patient to undertake towards meeting team-set goals. The process of rehabilitation looked at restoring optimum function following impairment due to illness or injury and took place over many weeks, months or even years within a single institutional setting. Equipment used for physical rehabilitation was generally adapted from traditional gymnastic apparatus or was innovative, forming the origin of much that is used today (for example, the walking frame).

THE PRESENT – AN AGEING POPULATION

Demographers consider a population to be aged if 7 per cent of its number are 65 years or older (Hendricks and Hendricks, 1977) and for consistency this age is used in this book to define an 'older person'. At present in the UK there are approximately 10.5 million people who are over the age of 65, and by 2010 this is likely to increase to 11.8 million (Age Concern, 1998), both exceeding the 7 per cent criterion. However, it is the steadily continuing growth in the numbers of those aged 85 years or over that is changing the distribution of age in the population.

A combination of factors has led to changes in supply and demand for a number of services, including health and social care. These include the following:

- the need for health care increases with age (people over 65 years of age use half the NHS resources)
- acute health disorders become superimposed on existing chronic conditions
- the health and social care needs of older people are likely to be complex and multi-system
- the need for redirection of capital resources to provide more cost-effective care in people's own homes

- fewer adults available for full-time informal or paid care
- increased expectations of all products and services – we all expect more and complain more.

Reform of health care

To respond to all these demands, the NHS has undergone continuous and major reform, particularly over the last decade. The 1990 reforms (Department of Health [DoH], 1989a) were based on the purchaser/provider market principle in an effort to improve cost effectiveness through competition. Health Authorities held the total budget responsibility for their defined population. Following an assessment of the health needs of the population, services were defined, purchased and monitored.

The need both to reduce the incidence of disease and encourage a more positive approach by the population to its own health resulted in the publication of *The Health of a Nation* (DoH, 1992), *Our Healthier Nation* (DoH, 1998a), and *Better Health, Better Wales* (Welsh Office, 1999). These focused on a small number of specific conditions which, it was anticipated, would decline in incidence and prevalence and therefore reduce the need for health-care resources. Older people have benefited from an increased focus on stroke and prevention of falls, and there is evidence that attention to smoking, diet and exercise can be effective in advanced age, but in some cases preventive approaches need to be 'lifelong' for effect, decreasing the opportunity specifically to benefit older people.

The Patients' Charter (DoH, 1991) specified service requirements for England easily recognised by patient, provider and purchaser, but failed to address the more complex issues around 'clinical autonomy', necessary to enable clinicians to respond to unique conditions but also providing an escape route for those not willing or able to respond to emerging evidence based clinical practice. Politicians had to accept that this might only be reviewed competently and credibly by peers, and so the requirement for medical audit was also incorporated into the reforms, later becoming, more appropriately, multidisciplinary 'clinical' audit, interdisciplinary audit being the ultimate goal.

Simultaneous reform of community care

Social care has also been reformed in conjunction with health care to meet the apparent capital and social advantage of increasing home-based care, as well as the cost benefits of reducing physical dependency levels. Social care is now largely means tested, causing some confusion to users and friction between providers of health and social care, as users, quite naturally, seek the cheapest option, for example a non-means tested 'health bath' rather than a means tested 'social bath'.

Many aspects of social care have parallels with health provision. Indeed the Poor Law legacy is arguably more evident in social or community care. Briefly the Poor Law provided institutional but also cash support to the deserving poor up to the Second World War. Victorian ideals and philanthropy were critical of such harsh responses and developed a number of charitable alternatives. Many of these exist today in the voluntary sector: often as a result of work with discrete groups, such as ex-servicemen or occupational groups, such as ex-railwaymen or fishermen or those with disabilities such as blindness. Charitable relief was localised and variable, even though some attempts were made to provide fair and 'efficient' systems through local Charity Organisation Society schemes.

Social administrators in the Second World War drew together a number of emerging functions taken up by local authorities in the inter-war years to cope with demand and to reduce reliance on charity. Beveridge's aims for a welfare state envisaged older people escaping the dreaded Poor Law into a more dignified old age through the provision of pensions or national assistance. Local authorities were given a range of discretionary powers to set up welfare services for older people, which over the years developed into services we now see as central to community care – the provision of home-based care around activities of daily living and social relations, and the provision of equipment for home independence.

Pressure on social services arising from increasing demand from an ageing population and the emphasis within health care on treatment and discharge back to social service support, resulted in the 1980s in a series of fundamental reviews of community care for adults – but particularly around older people's services. The White Paper *Caring for People* (DoH, 1989b) set in motion a series of changes, which, while giving local authorities the lead role in community care, shifted their priorities. New policy demands included a shift to targeting support on those in most need and using the independent sector as much as possible. Under the NHS and Community Care Act 1990, new rights to assessment were introduced but more formal and restrictive eligibility criteria meant that low-level preventive or rehabilitative provision were often lost. Social care reform has also been a response to public concerns about the effects of institutionalisation on both residents and staff revealed in damning reports (Martin, 1984; Stanley *et al.*, 1999).

Social care, then, is mostly undertaken by older people themselves – and their families. Formal arrangements are, so far, under the responsibility of social services but will increasingly be arranged by older people themselves. Tying this to the rehabilitation agenda will be an early challenge.

To facilitate cost-effective health care, improved arrangements for care in the community were implemented as part of the NHS reforms (DoH, 1989b). Those for whom hospital discharge is being planned and who are felt to need ongoing care, as well as those already in the community, can be assessed for their needs. This process is the responsibility of local authority social services or social work departments, but other members of the health and social care team should be involved to ensure a comprehensive picture is drawn and therefore requires interdisciplinary communication.

The result of the assessment is a 'statement of need', developed with and agreed by the user and their carer. The ensuing package of care can be implemented by care managers using their departments' allocated budgets and making use of local, perhaps non-traditional, services or informal supports. Again, this may reveal a range of differing values which need to be considered. Individuals and their carers are now considered major partners in the social care and rehabilitation process, and are expected to take more responsibility for the programme and its outcome. In return they may expect to be consulted. Access to appropriate short break or respite care can be essential to retain the goodwill of informal carers shouldering the responsibility of community care. Even where care at home is not envisaged as possible by the team, the older person may still insist on returning home along with expectations of the support they feel is necessary. Where care at home is agreed as not possible, arrangements can be made for residential or nursing home care. This may attract financial support from local authorities or may be paid for by the individual out of income and capital.

Further structural change (DoH, 2001) could have a positive impact on services for older people. Thirty Strategic Health Authorities will replace the 99 currently in place in England. They will be co-located with regional Government Offices, with the appointment of a Regional Director of Health *and* Social Care. This will facilitate joint working across the two agencies whose coordinated services are crucial for maintaining independence for many older people. The *Community Care: A Joint Future* report (Scottish Executive Health and Comunity Care Department, 2000) requires joint resourcing and management of services for older people in Scotland by April 2002 (Scottish Executive, 2001). It is anticipated that there will be some reorganisation to allow co-terminus boundaries between health and local authorities to facilitate partnership working throughout the lifetime of this book.

What consequently emerges is the existence of a number of teams along the patient's pathway of care, which, depending on need, may include primary, acute, rehabilitation, continuing care and specialist teams, for example in mental health. Although some professionals may be members of more than one team, each team has its specialist contribution to make, along with responsibility for timely and informed handover to the next team to ensure efficient and effective health and social care.

Devolution

Devolution for Scotland, Wales and Northern Ireland has resulted in health being a devolved power. While there has always been variety in the delivery of Social Services under local authority control, we now see changes in the structures and delivery of health care in the different countries. We recommend that people working in these countries remember that their own system may be different and that documents referred to throughout the text have probably been produced within the Scottish, Welsh and Northern Ireland Health/Social Services with distinct differences reflecting these countries' needs.

Working in the community

Professionals from statutory, voluntary and private sectors whose work is included in the user's care plan, will need to agree the plan to enable appropriate (joint where possible) intervention and regularly review progress. Where the resulting care is of a routine nature and not needing professional intervention, support workers can make a cost-effective contribution, especially if trained and supervised and supported by professional(s) on a regular basis.

Primary versus secondary care

The increasing focus on community-based health and social care, the rising cost of secondary care and the need for greater coordination, all contributed to the 1997 NHS reforms (NHS Executive, 1997). These firmly locate responsibility for commissioning secondary care within developing Primary Care Groups (PCGs) or Trusts (PCTs) – local Health Groups in Wales. Over time it is intended that this will shift power, financial resources and services from secondary to primary care. Traditionally, the rehabilitation team has been medically led, but this is also changing with the professional most appropriate to the case, whether in hospital or community, taking the lead and sharing responsibility.

In addition to creating PCGs and PCTs, the 1997 White Paper also proposed a number of other significant policy changes. These included making Health Authorities responsible for drawing up a strategy for meeting the needs of the local population, in the form of a Health Improvement Programme (HimP) in England and Health Improvement Plans (HIP) in Scotland, developed in partnership with all local interests. More specifically, in terms of rehabilitation, the HimP was given responsibility for ensuring that patients with continuing health and social care needs get access to more integrated services through Joint Investment Plans (JIPs), and for continuing and community care services, which all Health Authorities are expected to produce with partner agencies. Other policy developments in the document included:

- a 'clinical governance' framework to make service quality both the responsibility of NHS organisations and individual professionals; and
- the production of National Service Frameworks (NSFs) for major care areas and disease groups, with that for older people being among the first tranche.

The 1997 NHS reform proposals have been reinforced in a number of areas by more detailed guidance. This includes a 1998 consultative document *Partnership in Action: new opportunities for joint working between health and social services* (NHS Executive, 1998). This document proposes three ways of facilitating partnerships between the NHS and local authority social service or social work departments:

- pooled budgets
- delegation to a lead commissioning agency; and
- integrated provider organisations.

Clinical governance

The two key themes of clinical governance are the progressive improvement of services and the provision of systematic evidence of quality of service based on:

- clear lines of responsibility and accountability for the overall quality of clinical care
- a comprehensive programme of quality improvement, including
  - clinical audit
  - evidence based practice

- – national guidelines
- – workforce planning and development
- – continuing professional development
- – adequate clinical record keeping
- clear policies aimed at managing risks
- procedures to identify and remedy poor performance, including
  - – critical incident reporting
  - – complaints procedures
  - – performance reviews.

A culture that facilitates quality improvement will be the key to success of clinical governance. This can be likened to the culture established as necessary for Total Quality Management, initially for manufacturing and subsequently for the service sector:

- **Quality** is a primary organisational goal in every activity.
- **Internal and external customers** determine what quality is.
- **Customer satisfaction** drives the organisation.
- **Variation** in processes must be measured, understood and reduced.
- **Change** is continuous and accomplished by teams and team work.
- **Top management commitment exists,** promoting a culture of quality, employee empowerment, team working and a long-term perspective.
- **Organisational commitment exists to change the culture.**
- **Consistency** of message exists.

(Martin, 1993; Morgan and Murgatroyd, 1994)

To this should be added for health care an **open and fair culture** where errors can be revealed for process improvement to prevent recurrence; and **performance management** arrangements that aim to enable individuals to improve their practice against clear and agreed objectives within an agreed time frame, which includes review and revision.

Quality in the new NHS

The publication of *A First Class Service* (DoH, 1998b), *Quality Care and Clinical Excellence* (Welsh Office, 1998) and *Designed to Care* (DoH, 1998c) in Scotland, pulled together the numerous initiatives involved in quality improvement through setting, delivering and monitoring standards (Figure 1.1).

Standard setting is to be through the National Institute for Clinical Excellence (NICE) in England, set up to produce and disseminate clinical guidelines, and National Service Frameworks (NSFs) to reduce variation in services across the country through the development of national standards, a service model, implementation support and performance measures of progress.

Delivery of quality standards is to be assured through open, responsive and publicly accountable self-regulation by the professions; continuous professional development of staff based on an assessment of personalised learning needs; and clinical governance by organisational accountability for quality improvement.

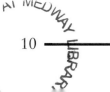

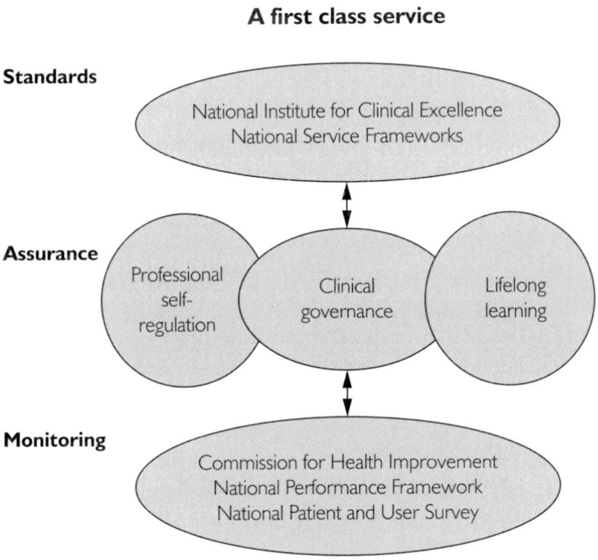

A first class service

Standards

National Institute for Clinical Excellence
National Service Frameworks

Assurance

Professional
self-
regulation

Clinical
governance

Lifelong
learning

Monitoring

Commission for Health Improvement
National Performance Framework
National Patient and User Survey

Figure 1.1   Setting, delivering and monitoring standards
(*DoH, 1998b*)

Monitoring of standards is to be accomplished by the Commission for Health Improvement (CHI) set up to support implementation and ensure clinical governance arrangements are in place, as well as identify, investigate and propose recommendations for problem areas; the National Performance Framework against which local services would be monitored; and a National Survey of Patient and User Experience to enable the service to measure itself against the aspirations and experience of its users.

The need to collaborate with other statutory services was further reinforced by the NHS Act 1999. The most obvious example of this joined-up approach is that, instead of having annual priorities and planning guidance for the NHS, we now have *Modernising Health and Social Services: national priorities guidance 2000/01–2002/03* with four key priorities relating to older people's services:

1 a multidisciplinary audit of existing services in preparation to implement the NSF for Older People
2 joint local charters for long-term care in line with Better Care, Higher Standards, to be completed by June 2000
3 jointly agreed preventative strategy by March 2002
4 provide more diverse and flexible opportunities for carers to have a break, by March 2002, in line with Caring about Carers.

While high media attention is given to the General Medical Council (GMC) as the regulatory body for doctors, similar bodies exist for other professions, for example the UK Central Council (UKCC) for nurses and the Council for the Professions Supplementary to Medicine (CPSM) for allied health professionals.

The new Health Professions Council will replace the UKCC and CPSM as the regulatory body for nurses and allied health professionals. In social work, the new General Social Care Council, and General Social Work Council in Scotland, looks set to establish a regulatory body, initially for qualified social workers. For all health-care professionals, evidence of continuous professional development will be a requirement for maintenance of professional registration for work in the public sector. For all sectors and professions, the extent to which non-qualified staff can or should be regulated remains a major issue.

The NHS Plan

The NHS Plan (DoH, 2000) is described as a plan for investment and reform to provide a health service fit for the twenty-first century. Key features are that there will be:

- investment in capital and staff
- a Modernisation Agency to spread best practice
- reward for achievement
- Care Trusts to commission health and social care in a single organisation
- new contracts for doctors
- role extension opportunities for other staff
- a Leadership Centre to develop management and clinical leadership and
- a concordat with private providers for NHS patients.

Care for older people is particularly singled out for improvement. A similar document has been published for Wales (National Assembly for Wales, 2001).

For a quality rehabilitation service, the issues that will require consideration will be the practical implementation of plans to overcome unnecessary boundaries between professions and agencies, and expansion of 5,000 beds and 1,700 non-residential places for intermediate care. These are in addition to 7,000 extra NHS beds. While the reduction in boundaries and extension of roles should release some staffing capacity, much has already been achieved in rehabilitation of older people, as outlined in this book. Measures of performance and resources for investment will need to take established change into account and reward rather than penalise this pro-active position.

From a rehabilitation viewpoint, the development of nurse and therapist consultant roles offer almost limitless opportunities for personal and service development. Although the detail of the more recently proposed therapist consultant role has yet to be published, an indication can be gained from that established for medicine and emerging for nursing. Phipps (2000) explains that a key function of nurse consultants will be working across professional and organisational boundaries to progress clinical governance. Consultants will demonstrate expert practice, undertake research and service development, ensure education and training supports practice development, and provide supervision and leadership.

So, how does all this fit together? Our conclusion is – with difficulty, and successful integration of policies and roles is what will distinguish the effective health and social care team from the rest. What seems to be emerging is a model (Figure 1.2), equally applicable in both hospital and community settings, where the following occurs:

- All participants will be making personal assessments of perceived needs based on their own values.
- A doctor has the key role in diagnosis of disease, to which the patient/carer and some members of the team will contribute; assessing mental status; deciding on the medication needs; and overall coordination of the team.
- A named nurse has the key role in ensuring the provision of generic care in hospital and at home in conjunction with the patient/carer and some members of the team forming the essential foundation on which others will build; overall communication and continuity between team and patient/carer; and continuity of routine activities.

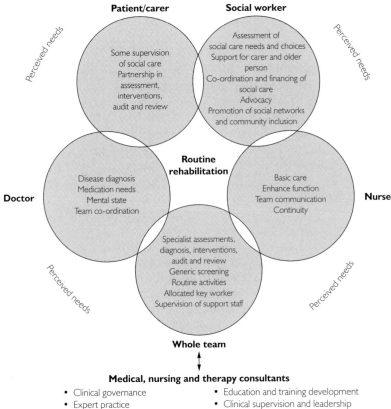

Figure 1.2 Responsibilities and integration of the interdisciplinary health and social care team

- The whole team, including the doctor and nurse, then provide *specialist* assessments and interventions unique to its discipline, while training each other and the patient/carer to carry out the *routine* practice of different skills and endurance activities (rehabilitation) and the ability of team members to undertake simple screening to know when specialist intervention is required to appropriately refer on to each other and elsewhere.

- A key worker for the plan of a specific patient is appointed from the team depending on the needs of the patient and skills within the team.
- The medical, nurse and therapist consultants will incorporate expert practice, quality improvement, research and service development, education and training development, and supervision and leadership. Most importantly they will work across boundaries on new approaches to patient care.
- Supervision of unqualified staff is split between the team with health professionals having accountability for their assistants, social services having some direct accountability for domiciliary or residential staff, and older people themselves having some control over their care providers, particularly if they directly or indirectly pay for services themselves.

THE FUTURE – THE INFLUENCE OF THE OLDER CONSUMER

There can be no doubt about the continuing drive for cost-effective, high quality, responsive, seamless health and social care, intended to focus on more flexible community-based care and multi-agency prevention strategies. Reorganisation and additional resources will be needed to meet the costs entailed through reduced caseload and new ways of working. The assessors of, and providers of, care may be different, and although the former is necessarily the province of the trained professional, the latter may not need to be. The role of the professional as a 'teacher' and/or 'treater' of those in need requires consideration by both providers, patients and commissioners.

Those planning services for future generations of older people will need to be aware of cohort differences. Those receiving old age pensions in 2000 will have been born prior to the creation of the NHS, remembering the fear of being unable to afford 'the doctor', and remaining grateful for relief from such fear. Falkingham (1997) paints a picture of two distinct, subsequent cohorts, commonly described as the post war 'baby boomers'. Those born between 1946 and 1950 entered an austere post war world, grew up in a culture of collectivism, entered an expanding labour market, and experienced an era of social freedom. Those born between 1961 and 1965 grew up in a prosperous world, entered a labour market in recession and contributed towards a culture of individualism. For both groups the divide between prosperity and poverty will widen; they will be likely to have their parents alive as they themselves enter old age; and information technology (IT) and assistive technology have the potential to transform their lives.

Dalley (1997) considers the health and health-care experience of these cohorts born into an improving health service. They will age in better health than their predecessors although the divide between prosperity and poverty affecting their health will be apparent. The delivery of care will be demanded in a style more conducive to the recipient than convenient to the provider. Time of day and goal of the intervention will be more 'user led', which may conflict with provider responsibilities for efficiency, risk avoidance and clinical effectiveness. There can also be no doubt of the drive for accountability. Evidence based access criteria, validated assessment tools, rationale for the choice of pathways of care, audit of processes, comparison of outcomes, subsequent change as part of a learning culture and confirmation of staff competence will be the expected norm, and confirmed through regular internal and external reviews. Such information on the various services will be sought and compared by funders, potential users and staff seeking to commission, use and work in areas of excellence. Funders and staff will seek quantitative evidence, and while potential users may initially employ softer quality measures as proxy for competence, they too may gradually share quantitative measures. As part of this drive for 'contracts of care', users too will be expected to take greater responsibility. Not meeting evidence based access criteria, non-adherence to a programme, non-attendance at an appointment, and so on, may be objective grounds for discharge from the programme.

Professional providers will also undergo change. The 'job for life' expectation has ended, and so a range of skills will need to be developed to meet innovative requirements for time-limited and part-time contracts. New approaches to training for all staff, both professionals and others, will require constant revision to keep pace with the times.

Rehabilitation will take place within many settings for user convenience, not just the specialist centre. This multiplication of venues will have its own consequences for staffing levels, supervision, development, professional fragmentation, loss of clinical leadership, continuity and travel. With it come opportunities for recognition of greater responsibility, enhanced professional autonomy and innovative ways of working.

Current and upcoming generations of older people are already showing their numeric, economic and political power (Vincent, 1999). For example, on 24 May 2000, pensions were discussed in the House of Commons with both major parties competing to be the 'pensioner's friend' and gain the crucial 'grey vote' (18 per cent of those eligible to vote and 25 per cent of active voters), with older people being particularly prolific in marginal constituencies in the general election of 2001. As the largest users of the NHS, the writing is on the wall for a similar response in health care. What is apparent is that rehabilitation of older people requires different attitudes, an expanded evidence base and access to a wide range of competent skills.

SUMMARY

To meet these health and social care challenges in rehabilitation of the older person, an appreciation by all stakeholders of the following seemed prudent and comprises the contents of this book:

- the need for a specialist response (Chapter 2)
- the different needs of minority groups (Chapter 3)
- the concept of rehabilitation (Chapter 4)

- the different needs held by stakeholders (Chapter 5)
- implications of the National Service Framework for Older People (Chapter 6)
- the skills for successful team working (Chapter 7)
- the need for effective assessment as the prelude to successful care (Chapter 8)
- psychology and the rehabilitation of older people (Chapter 9)
- the different settings in which rehabilitation may occur (Chapter 10)
- the growing emphasis on primary care-led rehabilitation (Chapter 11)
- the needs of carers as individuals (Chapter 12)
- the perspectives, skills and influence of different disciplines (Chapters 13–20)
- an overview and future of rehabilitation with the older person (Chapter 21).

References

Adams, G.F. and McIlwraith, P.L. (1963) *Geriatric Nursing: A study of the work of geriatric ward staff*, Oxford University Press, Oxford.

Age Concern (1998) *Older People in the UK: Some basic facts*, Age Concern England, London.

Brocklehurst, J.C. (ed.) (1975) *Geriatric Care in Advanced Societies*, MTP Press, Lancaster.

Dalley, G. (1997) Health and healthcare. In: *Baby Boomers: Ageing in the 21st Century* (ed. Evandrou, M.), Age Concern England, London.

Department of Health [DoH](1989a) *Working for Patients*, HMSO, London.

DoH (1989b) *Caring for People*, HMSO, London.

DoH (1991) *The Patients' Charter*, HMSO, London.

DoH (1992) *The Health of a Nation. A Strategy for Health in England*, HMSO, London.

DoH (1998a) *Our Healthier Nation*, HMSO, London.

DoH (1998b) *A First Class Service*, HMSO, London.

DoH (1998c) *Designed to Care. Scottish Office*, HMSO, Edinburgh.

DoH (2000) *The NHS Plan*, The Stationery Office, London.

DoH (2001) *Shifting the Balance of Power within the NHS*, The Stationery Office, London.

Duggan, S. and Duggan, D. (2000) *The Day the World Took Off: The roots of the industrial revolution*, Macmillan, London.

Falkingham, J. (1997) Who are the baby boomers? A demographic profile. In: *Baby Boomers: Ageing in the 21st Century* (ed. Evandrou, M.), Age Concern England, London.

French, S. (1994) In whose service? A review of the development of services for disabled people in Great Britain. *Physiotherapy*, 89(4), 200–204.

Hendricks, J. and Hendricks, C.D. (1977) *Ageing in Mass Society: Myths and realities*, Winthrop, Cambridge, MA.

Martin, J.P. (1984) *Hospitals in Trouble*, Blackwell, Oxford.

Martin, L.L. (1993) *Total Quality Management in Human Service Organisations*, Sage, London.

Morgan, C. and Murgatroyd, S. (1994) *Total Quality Management in the Public Sector*, Open University Press, Buckinghamshire.

National Assembly for Wales (2001) *Improving Health in Wales*, National Assembly for Wales, Cardiff.

NHS Executive (1997) *The New NHS: Modern and Dependable*, NHS Executive, London.

NHS Executive (1998) *Partnership in Action: new opportunities for joint working between health and social services*, National Health Service Executive, London.

Phipps, K. (2000) Nursing and clinical governance. *British Journal of Clinical Governance*, 5(2), 69–70.

Scottish Executive (2001) *Changing for the Future – Social Work Services for the 21st Century*, The Scottish Stationery Office, Edinburgh *http://www.scotland.gov.uk/library3/social/swor-05.asp*

Scottish Executive Health and Comunity Care Department [SECC] (2000) *Community Care: A Joint Future – report of the Joint Future Group*, SECC, Edinburgh.

Squires, A. (ed.) (1991) *Multi-cultural Health Care and Rehabilitation of Older People*, Age Concern England and Edward Arnold, London.

Stanley, N., Manthorpe, J. and Penhale, B. (eds) (1999) *Institutional Abuse: Perspectives across the lifecourse*, Routledge, London.

Stewart, M. and Hawker, M. (1999) *Early Rehabilitation. AGILITY – Commemorative 21st Anniversary issue. AGILE – Physiotherapy with Older People*, Chartered Society of Physiotherapy, London.

Vincent, J.A. (1999) *Politics, Power and Old Age*, Open University Press, Buckingham.

Welsh Office (1998) *Quality Care and Clinical Excellence*, Welsh Office, London.

Welsh Office (1999) *Better Health, Better Wales*, Welsh Office, London.

Williams, B. (1999) *History of Geriatric Medicine in the United Kingdom. AGILITY – Commemorative 21st Anniversary issue, AGILE – Physiotherapy with Older People*, Chartered Society of Physiotherapy, London.

2 DISEASE AND DISABILITY IN OLDER PEOPLE — THE EFFECTIVENESS OF SPECIALIST INTERDISCIPLINARY HEALTH-CARE SERVICES

Cameron G. Swift

AIMS OF THE CHAPTER

In spite of much progress, the provision of health care for older people is still often perceived as a problem rather than as a stimulating challenge awaiting professional application. Overriding considerations of a rapidly expanding dependent elderly population, confronting a fixed system of supply and demand for services, have often led to negative and defensive strategies, which stifle innovation and engender professional reluctance towards the old and their particular health-care needs.

This chapter will argue the case against such an approach by tracing the principles that have emerged from the evolution of specialist health-care services for older people, especially comprehensive interdisciplinary assessment and outcome-focused management in partnership with the patient. Documented achievements from such an approach include specialist departments, measurable standards and improved student and staff education. Tangible and positive service objectives are now identifiable, opening the way to further progress. Without these, the older members of our society, particularly the more vulnerable, are at risk of continued disservice. While resource provision is an obvious and critical factor, many perceived problems have their origin in concept rather than quantity, in professional practice rather than in structures.

PRINCIPLES OF SPECIALIST PRACTICE

Foundation principles

The emergence of the medicine of old age as a defined discipline has been based on a composite foundation of principles, including the following:

- 'Normal' ageing may be compatible with good health.
- Care and skill in the diagnosis and treatment of disease in older people are both appropriate and fundamental to sound management.
- Assessment of function – physical, mental and social – should always occur in parallel with medical diagnosis and treatment.
- Difficulties in diagnosis and assessment commonly occur because of atypical disease presentation and concurrent disorder. Access to the full investigational and treatment facilities of mainstream hospitals is therefore essential.
- Organised professional team work, shared responsibility and efficient linkage across statutory agencies and the informal sector are necessary at all stages.

- Training, skill and experience in problem identification and interdisciplinary management of objectives developed and agreed with the patient and carer are fundamental alongside those of standard medical diagnostic and treatment regimens.
- The capacity of older people to recover from illness and regain complete or partial independence should not be underestimated.
- The organisation of care should be so structured as to eliminate delay, minimise personal disruption and ensure consistency of information and continuity of professional contact.

The extent to which these interdependent concepts have been developed and given organised expression has largely governed the 'success' or otherwise of health-care services for older people in any locality. The cardinal achievement has been the shift in emphasis from custodial care to successful therapeutic intervention (see Chapter 1), an investment in the capacity of the older person to respond to treatment and in the willingness of a caring community network to stay involved in helping him or her with the practical problems of independent daily living.

Measurement of efficacy and effectiveness

Quantitative measurement of efficacy and effectiveness has often been somewhat crude, focusing on hospital activity (such as waiting times, numbers of admissions and discharges and duration of stay), rather than results for patients themselves. There is an ongoing need to refine and standardise clinically oriented measures of therapeutic performance in the care of older people. To some extent this is because 'need' in service terms can only be defined by means of a range of possible outcomes. Such measures should be sensitive and specific to the variables required, and also amenable to documentation by professionals involved in the busy task of day-to-day service provision (see Chapter 8).

Some standards of service delivery have, nevertheless, been set. These have involved elimination of delay in intervention, access to high quality care and treatment, and prospects for successful restoration to community living after significant illness. The performance and efficiency of any future initiatives should be assessed with reference to these if the clock is not to be turned back (see 'Achievements in the delivery of care' below).

A common conflict affecting professionals involved in rehabilitation is between (1) the entirely appropriate drive to develop, refine and document new techniques and interventions on the one hand; (2) the pressure to ensure the continuation of a service to individuals in need within finite resource constraints on the other; and (3) the need to discontinue techniques and interventions enjoyed by both practitioner, patient and public on the basis of emerging evidence. This should be perceived as an exciting challenge requiring the closest possible co-operation between the research community, the public and media, and those responsible for day-to-day service provision. It should also direct government funding strategies for research and development.

The population as a starting point

Such standards should also govern the type and amount of resource provision in order to address the challenges posed by demographic trends. The latter have been the subject of a number of reports (for example, Muir-Gray; 1991, Age Concern Institute of Gerontology, 1992; Grundy, 1992; Warnes, 1993). The overall projections for Britain may be summarised as follows:

- 20 per cent of the population is currently over 60, compared with 7.5 per cent at the beginning of the century. By 2021 it is expected to rise to 24.3 per cent.
- The elderly population is itself ageing. Over the last 25 years the proportion of over 60s who are older than 75 has risen from a quarter to a third. By 2021, those aged 75 are projected to account for 8 per cent of the total population.

The male:female ratio in old age is broadly about 1:3, probably because of the protective effects of oestrogens against atheroma and the hitherto more hazardous lifestyle pursued by men (including the First and Second World Wars, smoking, alcohol, reckless driving and homicide).

In determining service provision, other demographic characteristics, such as the relative numbers of supporting adults, migration patterns of elderly people and their families, changes in family structure, economic status and availability of adequate housing all require proper scrutiny. Of particular significance is the traditional role played by women of working age in caring for older relatives. This is likely to change with current patterns of increased employment and careers for women. Migration is another issue of importance. In the UK, for example, large numbers of indigenous older people migrate to certain coastal or rural retirement communities, while the families of many remaining in deprived inner city areas have moved away to the suburbs or beyond. Migration of non-indigenous elderly may follow a quite different pattern (see Chapter 3). It is important to recognise that these factors may influence not only social structure, but also health, and that a corresponding provision of health and social care resource will therefore be required.

The size of the wage-earning workforce has generally decreased and the numbers of older people themselves in employment have also fallen. The net effect of this is to give rise to an increase in the 'dependency ratio', a source of major anxiety to political economists. Against this backdrop, it is, however, important to recognise the substantial role played by older people themselves as carers. Investment in this major resource will clearly be a prudent focus of health policy, but is also a key element for day-to-day clinical practice affecting the professions concerned with rehabilitation (see also Chapter 12).

The interrelationship of disease and disability, illness and 'function' in older people

It is well known that a number of diseases that cause disability become more common with advancing age, although this is clearly not always the case, as with (for instance) the demyelinating diseases, for example multiple sclerosis. Examples include cerebrovascular disease, Parkinson's disease, dementia, the commoner forms of arthritis and osteoporosis. In addition, some diseases encountered in older people are often at an advanced stage of progress, for example, chronic airflow obstruction or ischaemic heart disease. Other conditions, such as normal pressure hydrocephalus and pseudo-gout are more particularly 'old-age disorders'.

These and a range of other disorders, together with a reduction in physiological and functional 'reserve' resulting from the normal ageing process, constitute the backdrop against which modern acute and preventive medicine of old age is practised.

The level of function achieved by an older person with one or more such conditions may remain remarkably stable (if sub-optimal) for long periods. When, however, an acute intercurrent disease (such as infection) or exacerbation of one of the underlying pathologies (such as cerebral or myocardial infarction) occurs, the immediate effect on function is often dramatic, so that the whole range of disorders presents in the form of a functional or social crisis, with or without clear-cut signs of the acute disease itself.

Successful management of such complex clinical situations requires an immediate response, skilled interdisciplinary assessment and highly organised team work if the risk of long-term dependency is to be avoided (see Chapters 7 and 8). It is very difficult, as a rule, to predict in advance the range and scale of problems from an initial presumptive diagnosis. The likelihood that these will be considerable does, however, increase exponentially with age. This is apparent from cohort population studies, such as the OPCS Disability Survey (Martin et al., 1988), which identifies an approximate doubling of the prevalence of disability with each successive decade over the age of 50 years. Forty-one per cent of those aged 70 to 79 were found to have some level of disability, with 4 per cent in the severest category. In a longitudinal four-year follow-up study in the US of changes in the mobility status of 6,981 men and women aged 65 and older, 36.2 per cent suffered mobility loss. Increasing age and lower income levels were strongly associated with this, even after controlling for the presence of chronic conditions at baseline. Furthermore, the occurrence during the study of a new heart attack, stroke, cancer or hip fracture was associated with a substantially greater risk of mobility loss than was the presence of these conditions at baseline. An important subset of this analysis showed additionally a major concentration of disability during the three years prior to death (Guralnik et al., 1991, 1993).

Analysis of UK hospital inpatient data, which characteristically shows an exponential increase with age in the predicted duration of stay (particularly over the age of 75), further emphasises the importance of this perception for both service policy-makers and clinicians. Mainstream services (including acute care) should be planned on the basis that episodes of illness increasingly go hand in hand with short, medium and long-term disability as day-to-day practice reflects the ageing of populations.

ACHIEVEMENTS IN THE DELIVERY OF CARE

Measuring progress in the health care of older people will never be easy. Few indicators of 'success' enjoy universal acceptance, and there is at times heated controversy amongst the general public, health and social services professionals, informal carers, managers and even older people themselves as to what is desirable. While some of this debate may be useful in focusing attention on the needs of older people, lack of consensus can also be a major barrier to concerted action, and it is important to identify common objectives.

Developments in the UK

Under the umbrella of the NHS, the early lessons of rehabilitation of older people (see Chapter 1) were cumulatively applied to a greater or lesser extent across the health districts of the UK, with increasing recognition of the eight principles outlined earlier. The value of specialist departments based in mainstream district general hospitals, offering immediate access for medically ill old people to the full range of diagnostic, assessment, treatment and remedial facilities, and staffed by physicians and professional co-workers with specific accountability for their care, was set out in several early published studies (Hodkinson and Jefferys, 1972; Bagnall *et al.*, 1977; Evans, 1983; Rai *et al.*, 1985; Horrocks, 1986; Mitchell *et al.*, 1987).

Measurable standards of Health Service performance in specialist units

As stated above, the reported outcome has commonly been in terms of hospital activity. Total numbers of hospital beds per head of the older population have been dramatically reduced, waiting lists and bed blockage are under attack, the throughput of patients has been greatly increased (typically 12 or more patients per bed per year, some 10 to 15 per cent only of beds at any one time being occupied by patients staying in hospital more than six months and overall average duration of stay reduced to 20 to 30 days. Such departments have been characterised by a clearly defined role in the acute medical care of older patients, by operational policies promoting continuity of care, by efficient liaison with the community and with other hospital services (usually by means of a central information/liaison office) and by positive policies of rehabilitation and discharge, with well-developed multidisciplinary (Horrocks, 1986), and more recently interdiscipinary team work (see Chapter 7).

The contribution to 'community care' (see 'The community dimension' below) made by this hospital-oriented model has consisted, to some extent, in its accessibility to, and dialogue with, general practitioners, community nurses and allied health professions, social services staff, informal carers and other community-based agencies. Day hospital, intermediate care and outreach services have developed from this model, with links with day centres and resource centres awaiting universal action (see Chapter 10). Other important consequences have included the successful recruitment of high-quality professional staff, the obvious scope for training and research, and clear-cut departmental 'identity'.

Viewed in the historical context, it can be demonstrated that clear benefits for patients have been achieved, notably removal of the problems of access to hospital treatment without delay and of the fear of waiting to 'go into hospital to die'. Relatives and other carers retain an involvement, sustained by organised support and the confidence that rescue in a crisis or planned relief is available without delay. These are important criteria of progress with which few would disagree. They constitute documented evidence of a workable balance between community and hospital care, based on professional commitment within the framework of a defragmented service. Such a framework is critical, since fragmentation of care is a particular hazard faced by older people if their multiple or recurring problems are addressed solely by the various agencies of a system-specialised medical service, with disjointed community support, and no planned coordination or focused staff development.

Rehabilitation of the older person after illness must also be perceived and evaluated in the context of such a comprehensive service. It may otherwise run the risk of becoming a self-perpetuating activity concerned more with the role of its practitioners than the service needs of its recipients.

The methodology for measuring clinical outcome shows some evidence of progress, particularly with the advent of a small number of controlled intervention studies using clinical outcome criteria and avoiding confounding factors within the framework of a randomised prospective design.

Developments in education

The logical movement of specialist departments into mainstream hospitals has provided the foundation for medical education in the care of older people. Organised teaching of undergraduate medical students in this discipline now takes place in all UK medical schools and, to a varying extent, in many medical schools in the US, Canada, Australasia and Europe. Academic Departments of Geriatric Medicine or Health Care of the Elderly have expanded, providing a focus for research into the medicine of old age, the processes of ageing and the delivery of care. The involvement of a wide range of professions, including nurses, therapists and social workers, in the formal education of medical students and staff is increasingly promoted in most modern departments. Specific training in the special needs of older people is represented to a varying degree in the undergraduate curricula of these professions themselves, the majority being post-graduate.

The community dimension

Much of the above discussion has centred on the historical development of hospital-based services. It is well known, however, that care of the elderly is undertaken predominantly outside hospitals or institutions, although the hospital constitutes a focus of concentrated acute need and high dependency. Since most older people are likely to experience some hospital contact at some stage, the role of hospital care and its relationship to the community is a major determinant of the long-term outcome they obtain. Prospects for community living, particularly if there is disability, depend fundamentally on the range of accommodation and services available. These services include primary medical care, community nursing and health visiting, physiotherapy, occupational, and speech and language therapy, clinical psychology, chiropody, dietetic, dental, ophthalmic and audiological services, social work, residential care, home-care and day-care provision (Horrocks, 1986) to which we would now add pharmacy and continence services. They also depend on a strong partnership between hospital and community care, and between health and social services. Recent legislation (see Chapter 1) has sought to reverse justifiable concern about the outcome of previous government policies, which have strengthened the distinction, and to some extent division, between these key agencies (for example, Department of Health [DoH], 1989a, b). While in theory providing a basis to identify the needs of a greatly under-resourced community care sector, the concept of 'substitution' of one sector for the other is almost certainly fallacious and may be prompted by the wish to reduce the overall costs of hospital care. There may, however, be further opportunities for substitution between disciplines where although specialist staff will continue to provide specialist assessments and interventions within their professional and legal responsibilities, all members of the team can carry out the routine practice of different skills and endurance activities, and particularly simple screening to refer on appropriately. A model is provided in Chapter 1.

There is at present a major drive in the UK to establish and expand 'intermediate care' as a concept with the intention of accelerating the discharge of older people from acute hospital beds and in some cases diverting their admission there in the first place (see also Chapters 1, 6 and 10 for more on this). While this may provide a focus for good practice development outside mainstream general hospitals, it may not succeed in achieving the foundation principles stated above, except as one part of a larger, revitalised, integrated specialist service for older people (covering acute general hospital care and rehabilitation), and may risk disadvantaging their access to mainstream diagnostic and treatment facilities.

A proposal in the NHS Plan (DoH, 2000) is the use of private sector nursing homes for rehabilitation of older people. Again, not only will this only succeed where provision is part of an integrated service, but also the different space, equipment, philosophy and specialist personnel requirements that have evolved over many years in the NHS will need to be in place (see Chapter 10). There are particular concerns that the proposed relocation of rehabilitation together with the expansion of 5,000 beds and 1,700 non-residential places for intermediate care in addition to 7,000 extra NHS beds, will risk dilution of specialist services during the time lag until the proposed expansion of training places has an effect on the workforce.

In reality, the truly cost-effective goal is to ensure the free flow of older people across the divide between sectors as determined by clinical and personal need. Service strategies based on demarcation or substitution are more likely to result in the recrudescence, demographically driven growth and escalating cost of a continuing inappropriately high demand for institutional care.

An important point is that older people are often unaware themselves of their entitlement, a problem that the voluntary organisation Age Concern (1982) has sought to address over the years. Housing may be a critical factor, and its poor standard often reflects the low economic status of many older people, especially in large urban areas. Very elderly people often decline rehousing at a later stage, so that forward-looking policies are necessary for the future, while a responsive and flexible approach to adaptations is needed now.

Sheltered housing with warden cover is a potential growth industry, but where such resources are limited there are difficulties in rationing their use according to need.

Relatives and informal carers continue to constitute the mainstay of community and long-term care. The importance of the enabling role of health and social services by providing adequate training, support, advice and relief has already been mentioned and cannot be over-stressed. Rejection by relatives is the exception rather than the rule, and is usually the result of too little support too late. Voluntary bodies, including Age Concern and the Association of Carers, have done much to highlight the importance of their critical contribution and their needs have also received greater recognition in research (for example, Homer and Gilleard, 1990, 1994; Williams and Fitton, 1991; Jones and Peters, 1992; Jones and Lester, 1994).

Effective liaison between social services and health service provision is vital for several reasons, but particularly to ensure that scarce community resources are used economically to meet genuine need, and that health problems presenting as social crises do not go unrecognised and untreated. The hospital-based social worker, as a member of the interdisciplinary health care of the elderly team, has historically played a vital role in this respect, not only in casework with older people and their carers, but also in providing the operational link with social care services or the long-term care sector (see Chapter 19).

The critical challenge ahead is to mimimise fragmentation of care in the community as well as in the hospital and between the two. The activities of any one discipline, whether it be medicine, nursing, allied health professions, social work or voluntary agencies, may at best be wasted or at worst harmful, if they are not related to an assessment and planned programme of care, agreed with the patient and carer, and involving an integrated team and integrated services.

PROSPECTS FOR THE FUTURE

Improving the measurement of service and clinical outcome

The medicine of old age incorporates a shift in emphasis from the reduction of mortality to the prevention and management of morbidity, a goal that is difficult to quantify.

A common error is to deduce the type and quantity of service provision required from single time-point prevalence studies. The assumption is made, for example, that the amount of perceived disability in a community at any one point in time indicates the need for 'support' and 'accommodation', when in fact the need may be for better and earlier intervention. Such an approach fails to recognise that health problems in old age, and their functional and social consequences, commonly follow an acute, rapidly-changing, recovering and relapsing pattern, a pattern that may be profoundly affected by the availability or otherwise of skilled diagnosis and properly organised management.

What is absolutely clear is the central importance of measuring function as a component of well-being or ill health in older people, an exercise that has been conspicuously neglected by doctors in the past, but has been the bread and butter of therapists and nurses working within the team. Recent studies of stroke (which is in some respects an excellent model for rehabilitation of older patients in general) have highlighted the usefulness of functional prognostic indicators as predictors of medium and longer term outcome, focusing on their superiority over neuro-anatomical and other, more conventional diagnostic categories, as well as their applicability to typical populations of older patients (Kalra and Crome, 1993).

In the development of functional assessment scales, physiotherapists have led the way and there is much excellent published work (Asburn, 1982; Collen et al., 1991; Squires, et al., 1991; Smith, 1994). The subject of functional assessment is explored in detail later in this book (see Chapters 8, 15 and 16–18).

To date, none of the many rating scales and 'quality of life' measures devised has been shown to have optimal sensitivity or specificity, nor achieved universal acceptance in any one domain of clinical outcome assessment or cost-effectiveness. The necessary experimental studies are often overwhelmed by the drive to achieve quick-fix audit criteria. On the other hand, operational evaluation studies commonly require very large numbers in multiple centres to produce a study of adequate power. Under these circumstances, the selection of outcome criteria may be a compromise based on consensus and pragmatism – without which the study could not be undertaken at all. In research terms, it all depends on the precise question being asked. Ideally, the two approaches – the first, developing sensitive outcome measures and the second, measuring broad service effectiveness – need to go hand in hand, with a balance to be struck by research grant-giving bodies.

A third, but absolutely crucial, research method is the smaller or intermediate scale controlled intervention study. This is analogous to a Phase 2 or 3 clinical trial in drug development, characterised by a tightly defined study population sample, a degree of standardisation of both the intervention and the measures of outcome, and a prospective randomised protocol with some element of blinding. These studies are difficult to mount, but are often the only way to reach anything like a firm conclusion about a form of treatment. They are gradually beginning to permeate health service research literature, historically peppered with descriptive data, confounding variables and inferences unsupported by hard evidence.

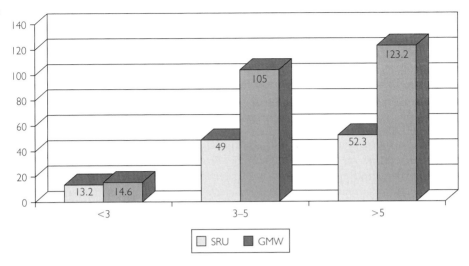

Figure 2.1 The effect of treatment setting (Stroke Rehabilitation Unit [SRU] v Geriatric Medical Wards [GMW]) on duration of inpatient stay in a prospective randomised controlled comparative study. The difference between control and intervention groups was significant for those stratified into intermediate (3–5) and poor (>5) prognostic categories using a validated scale (the Orpington Prognostic Scale, OPS). *(Kalra* et al., *1993)*

Figure 2.1 shows some data from such a controlled study of stroke rehabilitation in a specialised unit compared with existing rehabilitation practice dispersed across more general wards. In this randomised, prospective evaluation, the patient populations were unselected, but stratified into three prognostic categories, the patient characteristics and therapy interventions were clearly documented and comparable between control and intervention groups, and the results showed the benefit of tightly focused interdisciplinary practice (i.e. the stroke unit) on a number of key indicators of clinical and service outcome. Had a retrospective comparison been undertaken, say between two different centres, no firm conclusion could have been drawn because of the possibility of a whole range of confounding variables. There is an urgent need for more experimental work of this kind.

Prevention

So far we have concentrated on how health problems are managed and treated when they present, typically as some form of acute crisis or breakdown in function, and have emphasised that the skill or otherwise of such management may profoundly influence the subsequent prospects for independent living of older people and the numbers requiring long-term institutional care. In other words, good treatment of illness in old age has, to some extent, a preventive function.

A common reaction, however, is to say 'if only this particular problem had been dealt with earlier, it might have been much less serious or prevented altogether; irreversible damage might have been averted'. Primary prevention in the sense of dealing with the known cause of the condition and so completely preventing its occurrence has been largely, hitherto, an exercise for the medicine of earlier life. Examples would include the common immunisations, elimination of asbestos exposure and perhaps the reduction of tobacco consumption. Secondary prevention is concerned with the early detection of disease or its precursors in patients who are asymptomatic and consider themselves fit, and constitutes the rationale for screening programmes.

This can be distinguished from case finding, in which established disease and its consequences are present but for a variety of reasons unreported by the sufferer. Case finding, with a view to earlier diagnosis and the prospect for better results from treatment, has been described as a form of tertiary prevention (Williamson, 1981).

Although universal screening of the older population (defined by a given chronological age) has become statutory in some developed countries, it has so far met with little favour among practitioners and researchers, not least because of the unrealistic time required of professional staff (whether general practitioners or other members of the health-care team) and the apparently low returns achieved in such a blanket approach. Attention has instead been focused more on attempting to define categories of older people who are arguably at risk of health problems and to target case-finding initiatives at these groups, as in an early survey conducted in Aberdeen (Age Concern Research Unit, 1983). The latter, expanding an earlier World Health Organisation (WHO) list, selected the very old (80 years and over), socially isolated (not necessarily living alone), those without children, those in poor economic circumstances, those recently discharged from hospital, those who had recently changed their dwelling, the divorced/separated and those in social class V (Registrar General's classification). Interestingly, many of these 'conventional' risk factors proved rather inefficient as markers for case finding. An alternative two-stage approach, based on an initial postal screening questionnaire, followed, where appropriate, by a comprehensive health visitor assessment, was also described (Age Concern Research Unit, 1983). This proved somewhat more efficient, and the analysis of findings suggested further economies based on selecting the most discriminating questions identified. The main benefits overall consisted of determining and addressing a number of unmet needs (mainly contact with available services and treatment of active health symptoms). These benefits were clearly demonstrable, and could also be shown to be achievable with feasible changes in doctor, health visitor and community nurse workload.

A number of further studies have been published over the previous decade, unfortunately with wide variations in methodology (for example, in the choice of professionals and health assessments employed and in the outcome measures) (for example, Hendriksen et al., 1984; Vetter et al., 1984; Carpenter and Demopoulos, 1990; McEwan et al., 1990; Pathy et al., 1992; Fabacher et al., 1994). An important and positive shift in the thinking underlying screening studies has been towards functional and disability-related outcome criteria rather than medical and pathological outcomes. To date, however, it remains impossible to draw firm conclusions about the possible benefits of screening programmes for older people. A variety of positive outcomes has included a rise in morale among those screened, an increase in referrals to all agencies, a reduced duration of inpatient stay in some studies and (interestingly) a reduction in mortality. No trial has demonstrated an improvement in functional ability, and the workload of general practitioners appears only to be reduced where alternative services are provided (Iliffe, 1993).

By contrast, targeted interdisciplinary secondary prevention initiatives focusing on specific health needs in high-risk groups have been shown to yield substantial dividends. In a bi-disciplinary model of multi-dimensional assessment of older people attending an accident and emergency department after falling, careful medical and occupational therapy assessment of those who fell and of their living environment reduced subsequent falls in the intervention group (versus controls) by approximately two-thirds (Figure 2.2) and the number of those who subsequently fell by nearly 50 per cent (Close *et al.*, 1999) (see also Chapters 15 and 16).

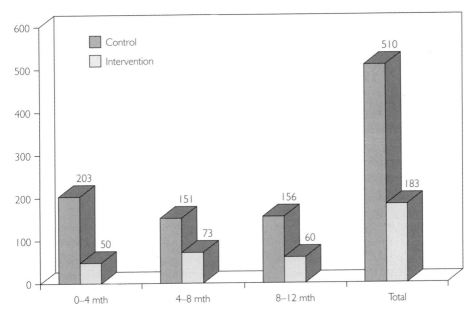

Figure 2.2 The effect of a structured interdisciplinary assessment on the incidence of subsequent falls at 4, 8 and 12 months in older people attending Accident and Emergency
(*Close* et al., 1999)

There is an ongoing need for further research on screening. New studies are under way (for example those supported by the MRC and the European Union 5th Framework Programme). Prevention studies should preferably be undertaken as a joint initiative with viable and well-organised secondary care services whose positive impact in reducing long-term bed occupancy is well attested. There seems little point in embarking on a study of preventive approaches when there is a fundamental deficiency in the ability of services to meet those unmet needs that are identified. The opportunities for general practitioners, physicians in geriatric medicine and the professionals with whom they work to combine their respective skills in further research with an accent on prevention are clearly most exciting. Some cautionary points, however, emerge from the projects already undertaken, in particular:

- It is a major necessity to refine both markers of need and measures of outcome in the health care of older people. This requires careful research and observation, since our current perception of health and ill-health determinants, however 'logical', may easily be mistaken.
- Prevention may well (in time) result in much benefit to many older people, but there is no guarantee that it will make their health care cheaper. Indeed, available evidence, in so far as it points up major areas of unmet need, suggests that the opposite may be the case. Thus naive planning assumptions about prevention and 'community care' as economical alternatives to current medical practice are seriously ill founded.
- It follows, therefore, that policy-makers and planners should not divert funds wholesale from existing services to new initiatives, unless the latter have been thoroughly validated and shown to be of measurable value to the large majority of older people.
- Resources for well-designed, controlled, prospective intervention studies constitute sound investment (while ensuring that existing services that are evidence based and working well remain adequately supported and are made more uniformly available).

SUMMARY

Disease and disability go hand-in-hand with increasing frequency, the older the sufferer. For many decades, while medical science has advanced technically, the disabilities of the old have met with a passive and negative acceptance by some medical practitioners, some health-care providers and many of the population at large. It is now clear, however, that a positive, organised, professional and to some extent specialised, approach to diagnosis, assessment, intervention and management can have a major and positive impact on the prospects for continued autonomy of a large majority of ill older people, and on the responsibilities carried by relatives and caring communities. The collaboration and coordination of several professionals and other agencies is a central factor in achieving results. Successful models of health care have been developed and described. These require consolidation and wider application. At the same time research into new patterns of intervention with an accent on preventive health care is now a clear requirement. It presents a challenge to the commitment and skill of all those concerned to ensure a better future for older people.

REFERENCES

Age Concern (1982) *Your Rights*, Age Concern, Mitcham, London.

Age Concern Institute of Gerontology (1992) *Life After 60: A profile of Britain's older population*, Age Concern Institute of Gerontology, King's College, London.

Age Concern Research Unit (1983) *Research Perspectives on Ageing, 6; The elderly at risk*, Age Concern, Mitcham, London.

Ashburn, A. (1982) Assessment of motor function in stroke patients. *Physiotherapy*, 68, 109–113.

Bagnall, W.E., Datta, S.R., Knox, J. and Horrocks, P. (1977) Geriatric medicine in Hull: A comprehensive service. *British Medical Journal*, 2, 102–104.

Carpenter, G.I. and Demopoulos, G.R. (1990) Screening the elderly in the community: controlled trial of dependency surveillance using a questionnaire administered by volunteers. *British Medical Journal*, 300, 1253–1256.

Close, J., Ellis, M., Hooper, R., Glucksman, E., Jackson, S. and Swift, C. (1999) Prevention of falls in the elderly trial (PROFET). A randomised controlled trial. *Lancet*, 353, 93–97.

Collen, F.M., Wade, D.T., Robb, G.F. and Bradshaw, C.M. (1991) The Rivermead Mobility Index: a further development of the Rivermead Motor Assessment. *International Disability Studies*, 13, 50–54.

Department of Health [DoH] (1989a) *Caring for People*, HMSO, London.

DoH (1989b) *Working for Patients*, HMSO, London.

DoH (2000) *The NHS Plan*, The Stationery Office, London.

Evans, J.G. (1983) Integration of geriatric with general medical services in Newcastle. *Lancet*, I, 1430–1433.

Fabacher, D., Josephson, K. Pietruszka, F., Linderborn, K., Morley, J.E. and Rubenstein, L.Z. (1994) An in-home preventive assessment program for independent older adults. *Journal of the American Geriatrics Society*, 42(6), 630–638.

Grundy, E. (1992) The epidemiology of ageing. In: *Textbook of Geriatric Medicine and Gerontology*, 4th edn (eds Brocklehurst, J.C., Tallis, R. and Fillit, H.), Churchill Livingstone, Edinburgh.

Guralnik, J.M., LaCroix, A.Z., Branch, L.G., Kasl, S.V. and Wallace, R.V. (1991) Morbidity and disability in older persons in the years prior to death. *American Journal of Public Health*, 81(4), 443–447.

Guralnik, J.M., LaCroix, A.Z., Abbott, R.D., Berkman, L.F., Satterfield, S., Evans, D.A. et al. (1993) Maintaining mobility in late life. I. Demographic characteristics and chronic conditions. *American Journal of Epidemiology*, 137(8), 845–857.

Hendriksen, C., Lund, E. and Stromgard, E. (1984) Consequences of assessment and intervention among elderly people: a three year randomised controlled trial. *British Medical Journal*, 289, 1522–1524.

Hodkinson, H.M. and Jefferys, P.M. (1972) Making hospital geriatrics work. *British Medical Journal*, 4, 536–539.

Homer, A.C. and Gilleard, C. (1990) Abuse of elderly people by their carers. *British Medical Journal*, 301, 1359–1362.

Homer, A.C. and Gilleard, C. (1994) The effect of inpatient respite care on elderly patients and their carers. *Age and Ageing*, 23(4), 274–276.

Horrocks, P. (1986) The components of a comprehensive District Health Service for elderly people – a personal view. *Age and Ageing*, 15, 321–342.

Iliffe, S. (1993) Screening the elderly – two steps forward, one step back? In: *The Medical Annual* (ed. Fry, J.), Bristol.

Jones, D. and Lester, C. (1994) Hospital care and discharge: patients' and carers' opinions. *Age and Ageing*, **23(2)**, 91–96.

Jones, D.A. and Peters, T.J. (1992). Caring for elderly dependants: effects on the carers' quality of life. *Age and Ageing*, **21(6)**, 421–428.

Kalra, L. and Crome, P. (1993) The role of prognostic scores in targeting stroke rehabilitation in elderly patients. *Journal of the American Geriatrics Society*, **41**, 396.

Kalra, L., Dale, P. and Crome, P. (1993) Improving stroke rehabilitation: a controlled study. *Stroke*, **24**, 1462.

Martin, J., Meltzer, H. and Elliot, D. (1988) *OPCS Surveys of Disability in Great Britain, Report 1*, HMSO, London.

McEwan, R.T., Davison, N., Forster, D.P., Pearson, P., Sterling, E. and Perkins, E.R. (1990) Screening elderly people in primary care: a randomised controlled trial. *British Journal of General Practice*, **40**, 94–97.

Mitchell, J., Kafetz, K. and Rossiter, B. (1987) Benefits of effective hospital services for elderly people. *British Medical Journal*, **295**, 980–983.

Muir-Gray, J.A. (1991) Social and community aspects of ageing. In: *Principles and Practice of Geriatric Medicine*, 2nd edn (ed. Pathy, M.S.J.), Wiley, Chichester.

Pathy, M.S., Bayer, A., Harding, K. and Dibble, A. (1992) Randomised trial of case-finding and surveillance of elderly people at home. *Lancet*, **340**, 890–893.

Rai, G.S., Murphy, P. and Pluck, R.A. (1985) Who should provide hospital care of elderly people? *Lancet*, **I**, 683–685.

Smith, R. (1994) Validation and reliability of the Elderly Mobility Scale. *Physiotherapy*, **80(11)**, 744–747.

Squires, A., Rumgay, B., and Perombelon, M. (1991) Audit of contract goal setting by physiotherapists working with elderly patients. *Physiotherapy*, **99(12)**, 790–795.

Vetter, N.J., Jones, D.A. and Victor, C.R. (1984) Effect of health visitors working with elderly patients in general practice. *British Medical Journal*, **288**, 369–372.

Warnes, A.M. (1993) *The Demography of Ageing in the United Kingdom of Great Britain and Northern Ireland*, International Institute on Ageing, Malta.

Williams, E.I. and Fitton, F. (1991) Survey of carers of elderly patients discharged from hospital. *British Journal of General Practice*, **41(344)**, 105–108.

Williamson, J. (1981) Screening, surveillance and case-finding. In: *Health Care of the Elderly* (ed. Arie, T.), Croom Helm, London.

3 THE REHABILITATION OF OLDER PEOPLE FROM ETHNIC MINORITIES

Helen McGrath, James George and John Young

AIMS OF THE CHAPTER

The elders of ethnic minorities face a potential triple jeopardy: at risk through old age; through discrimination; and through lack of access to health and social services (Norman, 1985). In this chapter the authors review the reasons for settlement in the UK through either the push of desperation or the pull of betterment of first generation migrants, family links or birthright of subsequent generations. The health and social consequences for older people, particularly of first generation migrants and those joining younger family members, include poverty, isolation, communication, expectations and different health and social needs. Knowledge of these differences will enable more appropriate and effective service provision.

MULTICULTURAL BRITAIN

Historically, Britain has always accepted a variety of ethnic minority groups within its population so that many different races and cultures are represented in the elderly population profile. This has occurred through a number of reasons, summarised as 'pull/push' factors (Young and George, 1991). Pull factors operate when individuals are attracted to the UK for self-betterment. Usually the family or village (male) protégé migrates to be followed later by his family. While such pioneers may have prepared for the move through learning language and skills, their dependants may have not and all retain strong cultural links with their mother country. These links tend to weaken in second and third generations, sometimes causing inter-generational conflict. The UK actively attracted workers from the South Asian continent and Caribbean islands in the 1950s (see also Chapter 1). These groups were attracted to specific geographic areas for employment, gradually establishing communities in areas vacated through growing affluence of previous inhabitants. Unlike the indigenous elderly, migration to coastal resorts in retirement is rare. In general, ethnic minority communities tend to be concentrated in urban areas and in low cost housing.

The 'push' factor typifies refugees seeking to escape intolerable political and/or economic circumstances within their own country. They frequently arrive desperate, impoverished, in poor health, separated (sometimes permanently) from their family and frequently unprepared through lack of learning, language and other skills to thrive in the new, not necessarily chosen, culture. Allocation of accommodation may lead to dislocated communities and loss of mutual support. Ethnic minority elderly people are at a disadvantage in obtaining community care services in the UK, nor are they necessarily able to compensate by 'looking after their own' (Carlisle, 1998).

The numbers of ethnic minority elders are increasing with the ageing of the resident population and the arrival of older dependants. The current position is shown in Table 3.1. In order to provide appropriate health and social care, we need to be aware of the background, specific health problems and requirements of ethnic minority groups, and to be able to communicate effectively with them.

Table 3.1   Population: by ethnic group and age, 1998–99, Great Britain (percentages)[1]

	Under 16	16–34	35–64	65+	All Ages (= 100%) (millions)
White	20	26	38	16	53.1
Black					
Black Caribbean	23	29	38	9	0.5
Black African	37	37	29	2	0.4
Other Black groups	43	37	18	–	0.1
All Black groups	29	33	33	6	0.9
Indian	24	32	38	7	0.9
Pakistani/Bangladeshi					
Pakistani	35	36	25	3	0.6
Bangladeshi	43	32	22	3	0.2
All Pakistani/Bangladeshi	37	35	24	3	1.0
Other Groups					
Chinese	15	40	39	6	0.2
None of the above	43	30	24	2	0.8
All other groups[2]	38	32	27	3	1.0
All ethnic groups[3]	21	26	38	15	56.8

[1] Population living in private households. Combined quarters: Spring 1998–99.
[2] Includes those of mixed origin.
[3] Includes those who did not state their ethnic group.
(Social Trends, 2000)

DEFINITION

The term 'ethnic minority group' is used to refer to any group that sees itself as sharing a common culture, which is distinct from that of the majority of the population as a whole.

Since April 1995 collecting data on ethnic groups from all patients admitted to NHS hospitals has been routine. Such data is intended to be used in planning, access, take up and development of action plans on deficiencies in relevant services. Patients are required to indicate their 'felt ethnicity', which can prove confusing to some older people and the reliability of such data, particularly for this age group, is a cause for concern.

Health Services are required to base their questions on the major census groups: White; Black; Black African; Black other; Indian; Pakistani; Bangladeshi; Chinese; and Other. This may need to be supplemented by adding other locally significant groups.

BACKGROUND OF SOME ETHNIC MINORITY GROUPS

The brief background of some common ethnic minority groups will now be described.

Elderly people of Jewish origin

Jewish people have been in Britain for many centuries but the main Jewish immigration occurred during the Second World War, following Jewish persecution in mainland Europe. Jewish people have successfully integrated into British society and have had immense influence in the world of finance. There are large differences between various British groups and individuals. There are strictly orthodox Jews who live within their own community and non-religious Jews who still feel culturally Jewish. Jews who originate from Eastern and Central Europe are called Ashkenazi; Jews from the Middle East, North Africa and Spain are Sephardic Jews. It is estimated that there are over 400,000 people of Jewish origin living in Britain.

Elderly people of Polish origin

At the turn of the twentieth century many Polish Jews came to the UK fleeing persecution. They settled mainly in the East End of London, together with Manchester and Leeds, and tend to speak Polish or Yiddish. After the Second World War 100,000 members of the Polish forces stayed in Britain and there were also many wartime refugees. Most of these Poles settled in London, Manchester, Birmingham and Bradford, with smaller populations in Wolverhampton, Leeds, Nottingham, Sheffield, Coventry, Leicester, Slough and the West of Scotland, after they were released from internment camps. The post-war Polish settlers are mostly Roman Catholic, although some are Jewish. Many of the original Polish settlers could speak little English and they built up their own self-supporting networks with their families.

Elderly people of Indian origin

People came to the UK from two main Indian states; Punjab and Gujarat. The men came in the 1950s and early 1960s and were joined by their families, often many years later. People from the Indian Punjab speak Punjabi and are mostly Sikh by religion. There are large Punjabi Sikh communities in the West Midlands, Glasgow, West London and Leeds. People of Gujarati origin from India and East Africa live mainly in North and South London, Coventry, Leicester and Manchester. Most are Hindus. Although the national language of India is Hindi, relatively few people of Indian origin speak it as their first language, speaking instead languages specific to their district of origin; many may speak it as a second language.

Elderly people of Pakistani origin

Many people from Pakistan came to Britain during the late 1950s and early 1960s. They came from three main areas: Mirpur in Azad (Free) Kashmir; Punjab Province; and North West Frontier Province. As well as their regional language, they will probably speak Urdu. Most people of Pakistani origin live in Yorkshire, Lancashire, Greater Manchester, West Midlands, Cardiff and Glasgow. The majority of Pakistanis are Muslim.

Elderly people of Bangladeshi origin

Most people from Bangladesh came to the UK in the 1950s and 1960s, and settled throughout the country, but especially in the East End of London. Almost all are Muslim and come from the rural Sylhet district of Bangladesh and speak a Sylheti dialect.

Elderly people of Vietnamese origin

Vietnamese refugees are fairly recent migrants, mainly arriving in the 1970s. Many were forced to leave Vietnam after the fall of Saigon, because they had been associated with the Americans. Several thousand Vietnamese now live in Britain and many have come via refugee camps in Hong Kong. The majority came from North Vietnam and most are ethnic Chinese who speak both Cantonese and Vietnamese. They may be culturally isolated as placement policies initially resulted in housing allocations throughout the UK in rural areas, far from other Vietnamese and Chinese families.

Elderly people of Afro-Caribbean origin

The great majority of people from the then named West Indies came to the UK in the 'boom' period after the Second World War (see also Chapter 1). Many intended originally to return home. Over half of the West Indians who came to Britain came from Jamaica; others came from Guyana, Barbados, Trinidad and Tobago. As with other groups, they tend to be concentrated in inner city areas.

It is important to remember that there are very distinct differences in culture and previous experience between people from different islands in the Caribbean. Many Afro-Caribbeans are Christians; the largest group are Pentecostalists, some are Anglicans or Baptists and a few are Methodists or Roman Catholics. The departure of a male 'village protégé' to Britain after the war in the anticipation of prosperous return and marriage was often not achieved as a result of the menial and poorly paid employment that was found on arrival. Consequently, the delay in return has meant that many protégés stayed single and are now lonely and isolated in old age (Schweitzer, 1991).

Elderly people of Ugandan Asian origin

In 1972 the military dictator Idi Amin expelled Asians from Uganda *en masse*. Many came to Britain and were forced to start a new life in the wake of being expelled from their previous adopted homeland.

Recent refugees

Recent years have seen many asylum seekers, some of them elderly, come to Britain from many parts of the world including Afghanistan, former Yugoslavia, former Soviet Union, Somalia, China and Turkey (Jones and Gill, 1998). They arrive as a result of the 'push' factor described above. Around half of these refugees live in London but are also concentrated in areas where local authorities have given refugee housing a high priority. Refugees are particularly vulnerable to mental health problems because of high stress levels and communication may be difficult because of language barriers. Refugees are entitled to the full range of NHS services free of charge, including registration with a general practitioner. Asylum applications to the UK number around 80,000 per year of which 75 per cent are rejected (*Daily Telegraph*, 2001).

RELIGIOUS AND CULTURAL ATTITUDES

To assist rehabilitation staff and service planners, some main points concerning the Muslim, Hindu, Sikh and Jewish religions are briefly described below.

Islam

Older male Muslim patients may be unaccustomed to dealing with women of professional status. Muslim women may not agree to being examined by a male member of staff and may prefer to have a female chaperone. In adversity, a Muslim is forbidden to despair, seeking help through prayers. Ramadan is a month-long period, which forms part of the Islamic calendar and is a basic tenet of the Islamic faith. During Ramadan, Muslims are required to abstain from food, tobacco and liquids (including water) between the hours of dawn and sunset. However, those who are ill and/or elderly are usually excused.

Hinduism

Hinduism is the religion of 80 per cent of the people in India. It involves a strong sense of personal responsibility, and the concept that actions and thoughts in the present life determine the circumstances of the next. Hence, illness may engender feelings of passivity and acceptance.

Sikhism

The Sikh religion stresses an individual personal relationship with God, and involves helping and serving others. All Sikhs should wear the five signs of Sikhism (the five k's): *kesh* (uncut hair); *kanga* (the comb); *kara* (the steel bangle); *kirpan* (a short sword); and *kaccha* (white shorts). The turban is also a visible symbol for Sikh men and has the same importance as the five k's. The religious significance of these symbols needs to be appreciated by doctors, nurses and allied health profesionals. Religious symbols worn by patients should be afforded the same respect as the Western wedding ring and not be unnecessarily removed (Karseras, 1991).

Judaism

Judaisim has been in existence for five-and-a-half thousand years. It is based on the worshipping of one God, obedience to the ten Commandments, and the need to practise charity and tolerance towards one's fellow human beings. Jewish religion and culture are inextricably mixed. Jews eat only meat, which has been killed by their own religious trained personnel. Jews are not allowed to eat pork. If a Jewish patient dies in hospital then it is usual for burial to be arranged for as soon as possible.

HOUSING AND SOCIAL ASPECTS OF ETHNIC MINORITIES

Within Britain there are marked ethnic differences in housing tenure. Most ethnic minority elders are concentrated in the inner and middle centres of cities where environmental problems are most acute; consequently Asian and Afro-Caribbean households are more likely to live in poorer quality housing and to suffer overcrowding (Baxter, 1997).

Ethnic minority elders still tend to have backgrounds in unskilled and semi-skilled occupations and are therefore more vulnerable to unemployment; this in turn means reliance on minimum state pensions and poverty. Furthermore, language difficulties may make it difficult for ethnic minority elders to receive appropriate housing benefits (see Further Reading list at the end of this chapter).

Some commentators have pointed to racial discrimination and employment dis-advantage as being responsible for the concentration of ethnic minorities in poor housing in specific areas; others suggest that the disadvantages are compensated for by a close network of support among extended families in the context of the wider 'community'. Unfortunately, this does not seem to be so, and the pattern of elderly parents living with their children appears to be changing. Over one-third of Afro-Caribbean elders live alone; 30 per cent of elderly Asians live alone or with a spouse (Karseras, 1991). Similarly, all departments involved in the care of the ethnic minority elder should be aware of the specific housing problems faced, and should be able to provide information about help and benefits.

In all cultures, comfort is derived from common association, and cultural communities have developed, providing social and retail facilities, making it unnecessary to use mainstream facilities or to learn English. This mirrors the British ex-patriot communities in some Mediterranean countries. The main difference in Britain is that the ethnic minority migrants are generally in the lower socio-economic groups and have consequently settled in areas of poorer housing stock and other deprived facilities and high unemployment, from which other groups ascending the ladder of prosperity have willingly moved away. It is only when reliance on 'majority' facilities is needed – such as emergency health or social care – that communication problems are exposed, a common fear for the British abroad.

COMMUNICATION ACROSS LANGUAGE AND CULTURAL BARRIERS

Rehabilitation is a highly active process in which the onus of responsibility for recovery is transferred from the rehabilitation staff to the individual and their carers. It involves the patient relearning old tasks or making adjustments to allow a new way of life. Two factors are essential. Firstly, the patient and their family should gain an understanding of the disabling condition and its consequences. This is essentially an education and communication process. Secondly, the patient and family will need to be actively involved in a set of often alien, complex and progressive manoeuvres to maximise recovery of the damaged body system. Adequate communication, taking into account not only language, but also cultural values, is fundamental to the success of both.

The 'language barrier' is more likely to be a problem in rehabilitation of the older person. Studies have shown that among ethnic minority elders, levels of spoken English are generally lower than among younger migrants (Henley and Schott, 1999).

Language issues in communication

There are several practical ways in which rehabilitation staff can improve communication with people who speak little or no English. Successful communication across a language barrier requires forethought and planning. Attention should be paid to the use of non-verbal communication (gesture, body language, etc.), although these may not be consistent between cultures and may be misinterpreted. Attention should also be paid to the pace and intonation of the conversation, as well as to the use of simple, clear English and to the avoidance of medical 'jargon'.

Conversations across a language barrier are wearing and may become stressful; simple measures such as allowing extra time for consultations and taking time to build a relationship with the patient may reduce this stress and may even serve to improve the patient's ability in English by creating a more relaxed atmosphere. This of course conflicts with quantitative measures of caseloads and throughput performance, but would score high on qualitative measures of performance (see also Chapters 1 and 2).

Where possible, simple written instructions may help to reinforce verbal communication and symbols may also be of assistance. Even when words are not understood by the patient, relatives or friends may be able to help with translation. Many advice leaflets are available in various languages (see Resources) and may be helpful. However, literacy in the patient's first language should not be assumed. The use of alternatives to the written word, such as video, may be more useful. Ideally, it should be possible to use a qualified **interpreter** who has had training and is skilled in the nuances of the technique; every hospital and comunity health service should have a list of locally available interpreters. This should be in preference to sole reliance on a list of staff who can only **translate** from other languages, but may be a useful resource in an emergency situation. More than just a 'translator', a good interpreter can bring his or her experience of both language and culture of both parties, providing a 'bridge' between patient and health-care professional. Such resources are probably undervalued and underused.

The use of relatives or friends as interpreters has the potential advantage of family and friends becoming closely involved with the rehabilitation programme and therefore being in a better position to maintain recovery following discharge from hospital. However, such informal interpreters are unlikely to be familiar with clinical procedures and language, and may have a personal interest in the content of the conversation, making translation more likely to be inaccurate and unreliable. Further, the patient him- or herself may be unwilling to communicate personal information through someone he or she knows. Despite these well-developed warnings concerning unsuitability of friends and relatives as interpreters, they are still widely used even in districts with established interpreting services (Phelan and Parkman, 1995). This implies inconsistent satisfaction by both patients and professionals with such services. There is a view that even good interpreters are no substitute for the presence of bilingual staff (Westermeyer, 1990). Ensuring the rehabilitation staff are drawn from the full diversity of the local community should be an important strategic human resource policy objective.

Cultural issues in communication

Good communication in a multi-ethnic society requires not only the use of language and other aids to convey information, but also an understanding of, and respect for, differences in background, culture and experience of different ethnic groups (see also Chapter 17). Evidence suggests that such understanding is often lacking in professionals' relationships with ethnic minority populations, especially in relation to chronic disease (Will, 1993). There are cultural differences in health and illness suggesting that effective communication requires recognition of the patients' and their families' social and cultural context. Communication is thus far more than a technical and linguistic activity. Differences may occur in attitudes towards decision-making; male and female roles; the preservation of modesty; and attitudes to specific medical interventions. Religious and cultural differences may exist between patient and health professional, for example, in activities of daily living, hygiene and the provision of food. Sociological literature differentiates between abstract and embodied knowledge (Anderson and Bury, 1988). The former is cognitively understood but remains distant, the latter becomes a resource of daily living.

Successful communication depends upon the establishment of mutual respect, careful explanation of specific rehabilitation and medical procedures, awareness of potential concerns, and asking effective questions to elucidate these concerns and work in a way appropriate to the needs of the individual (Table 3.2).

GENERAL APPROACH TO HEALTH CARE OF ETHNIC MINORITY PATIENTS

The National Survey of NHS Patients accessing general practice (Department of Health [DoH], 1998) found that in virtually all sections of its research questionnaire minority ethnic respondents presented views and reported experiences distinct from those of the general population. They reported a less favourable view of treatment received by GPs and were less satisfied with the extent of effective communication. Pakistani (26 per cent) and Bangladeshi (28 per cent) respondents were more likely to have requested out-of-house calls during the preceeding 12 months than the national average (14 per cent). Irrespective of cultural background, illness brings anxiety and distress for individuals and their families. However, for some ethnic minority patients admitted to hospital, unfamiliarity with the system, fear of 'government' buildings, separation from family, home and culture and potential language difficulties may exaggerate the upset involved with illness. This may be magnified further by staff who have insufficient knowledge to modify their approach to suit the differing needs of the individual patient. The need for staff to appreciate such cultural differences is particularly evident in community health care where staff are visitors in the patient's domain – and culture.

Table 3.2   Ways to improve communication

• Get the patient's name right and pronounce it correctly.	• Check back – check instructions by asking the patient to explain back to you what he or she is going to do.
• Use a qualified interpreter if possible.	
• Simplify your English.	• Try to avoid questions in which the answer is simply 'yes'.
• Speak slowly and be patient.	
• Give non-verbal reassurance.	• Avoid idioms (e.g. 'spend a penny').
• Keep comprehensive notes to avoid repetition.	• Write down important points on a piece of paper for the patient to take away.

The cultural differences described above apply equally to patients and to staff, and conflicts within the team may occur over plans for treatment, whatever the culture of the recipient, and will need to be handled sensitively. Religious and cultural attitudes towards activities of daily living, such as hygiene and food provision, as well as the preservation of modesty, may have far-reaching effects in rehabilitation, when a good ongoing relationship between health care professional, patient and family is vital to a successful outcome, and where the restoration of function needs to be planned in a way acceptable to the individual.

Modesty

Modesty should always be maintained as far as possible during nursing procedures and therapy sessions, especially in open treatment areas and mixed ward environments. Health-care services do not always take into account the greater value some minority groups, and almost all older women, place on personal modesty. For example, many Hindu, Muslim and Sikh women are embarrassed at having to expose areas of their body. Legs and upper arms should remain covered at all times.

Careful explanation, if necessary through an interpreter, tact and negotiation of the most appropriate and acceptable method of performing a task, should be the aim. This also fosters a spirit of understanding and concern, which helps minimise feelings of isolation and distress engendered by the hospital admission.

This is particularly valuable if the patient has a disabling condition, as the framework will be laid for the necessary close co-operation (often for a long period) between staff and patient. Irritation, impatience and intolerance will be counter-productive and ultimately undermine the rehabilitation process. It should be borne in mind that the feelings of modesty are deeply ingrained and cannot be overcome by simple willpower. Empathy and understanding are required.

Hygiene

Similar respect should be paid to hygiene requirements. For example, Asian patients may prefer to wash in free-flowing water rather than sit in a bath. After using the lavatory, people from the Indian subcontinent usually wash themselves with their left hand. Lavatory paper is not traditionally used in the Indian subcontinent and may be regarded with distaste. Since the left hand is used to wash the private parts of the body, the right is usually used for eating and other tasks. Thus, when fixing an intravenous infusion, the right hand should be kept free if possible. Objects should be handed to a patient so that the right hand can be used, for example when placing food where a patient can reach it.

The particular consequences for a patient from the Indian subcontinent having a stroke affecting either upper limb will be obvious, and poses challenges for the rehabilitation team and the patient as they work to restore function. Again, the presence of a mutually respectful relationship may facilitate open and useful communication to overcome such hurdles.

Food

Some ethnic minority patients will have specific food requirements. For example, restrictions on what may be eaten by Muslims are clearly laid down in the Holy Koran and are regarded as a direct command from God. Elderly Muslim patients in hospital or receiving meals delivered at home will probably need help in working out which foods on the menu are acceptable, although community meal services are often more responsive. Most will stick to a vegetarian diet, since the meat provided is unlikely to be 'halal' (i.e. killed according to Islamic law). Muslims should not eat pork or anything made from pork products, such as sausage, bacon and ham. Alcohol in all forms is forbidden in the Koran, and the composition of medication should be checked and may not be taken by the patient if they are suspicious of the content (see also Chapter 20c).

Care

Hospitals in many developing countries expect the family to undertake much of the basic care. Illness is shared and generally one family member will always be present at the bedside – night and day. The British practice of restricted hospital visiting by relatives (but expecting their considerable input on discharge) may need to be reviewed, and this would benefit all relatives. It is essential to use the correct name for all patients, including the personal name (e.g. 'Mr Rajinder Singh', not just 'Mr Singh') for all treatments, particularly pharmaceutical, when a large section of the population shares a small number of family names. This will also aid more general record keeping.

Expectations

Attitudes to ill health also differ. Illness is sometimes regarded as something to be suffered, and it is the expected behaviour to remain 'ill' and in bed until full recovery has occurred. Thus, illnesses in which full recovery may not occur without effort (e.g. stroke, arthritis) may need particularly careful management. The concept of active rehabilitation may therefore be unfamiliar to many ethnic minority patients, not least due to their experience of the scarcity of therapy resources in their homeland, often limited by geography to a community based service (Leavitt, 1999), or even survival to an age at risk of such morbidity when life expectancy in their homeland may be much lower.

Sometimes there may be conflict in the family between the elders with traditional views and the children who have become 'Westernised' and may expect the state to provide much of the care. Occasionally, residential care may be regarded with suspicion by the older person and, in line with generic best practice, arrangements should be made for a visit to a residential home before deciding whether this is an option. The issue of combination/segregation of ethnic groups in such homes is complex and many factors may need to be considered, not least of which are religious and cultural requirements, but also the rich social gain from ethnic mix (Table 3.3).

Table 3.3 Checklist for rehabilitation staff

Communication: Have the following been explained? (Use an interpreter if necessary.)
- Instructions about medication
- Implications of illness and likely recovery
- Need for further tests
- Roles of various therapists
- Aims of rehabilitation therapy
- Follow-up arrangements

Religion: Are there particular religious requirements?
- Formal prayer
- Fasting

Diet: Are there particular dietary requirements?
- Vegetarian
- Halal meat

Hygiene: Are there any particular hygiene requirements?
- Running water for washing
- Ritual washing
- Use of left hand for toilet and right for eating

Social: Is the patient receiving appropriate social benefits?
- State or private pension
- Attendance allowance
- Housing benefit

Repatriation may be sought by first generation older migrants who retain strong links with their homeland and wish to be buried there rather than in a country where they have not always felt welcome. Although central funds may be available for such a journey, staff have a responsibility for ensuring that the consequences of the current economic, political, social and health-care framework that exists in the country of origin are fully appreciated before such a momentous and usually irreversible move is contemplated.

Medical aspects of the care of ethnic minority patients

It is now well documented that ethnic minority populations in Britain have poorer health status than the general population at a national level (Will, 1993). However, there has been comparatively little research on the specific medical problems of ethnic minority patients, and on the potential inequalities in patient care caused by the lack of understanding of these problems, difficulty in communicating symptoms and cultural differences in coping with illness. Such problems may prevent realisation of the NHS principles of 'equal access to available care, equal treatment for equal cases and equal quality of care'. Lack of familiarity with the system and distrust of Western medicine may lead ethnic minority elders to consult traditional healers and use folk remedies, which are becoming more widely accessible and are highly acceptable through their responsive approach. There is as yet little evidence of the effects of traditional medicine, a similar situation to some frequently used Western medicine, and an open mind may prove beneficial.

Ischaemic heart disease

Myocardial infarction is roughly twice as common in Asian patients presenting to hospital but only half as common in Afro-Caribbean patients compared to British rates (Rawaf and Bahl, 1998). Coronary atheroma seems to occur prematurely in Asian patients and its progress is accelerated. Furthermore, there may be more delay in their being transferred to the coronary care unit from casualty, presumably because of language difficulties (Lawrence and Littler, 1985). Use of outside interpreters and resources such as the *Red Cross Multilingual Phrase Book* (British Red Cross, 1988) can assist in such emergencies. Health promotion in appropriate languages should be particularly directed at this group.

Hypertension

Hypertension is more frequent in Black African and Afro-Caribbean populations than in Asian or White groups – a trend also seen in the US (Beevers and Beevers, 1993). These differences in blood pressure partially explain the high incidence of strokes and renal failure in black people, but not why coronary artery disease is relatively uncommon. Treatment of hypertension may need to be modified as beta-blockers and ACE-inhibitors may not be as effective in these groups (Beevers and Beevers, 1993).

Tuberculosis

Notification of tuberculosis has been undertaken since 1978. Groups who have their origin in the Indian subcontinent have notification rates 25 times that of the white population, while rates among people of West Indian origin are four times as high (Rawaf and Bahl, 1998).

Diabetes

In both Afro-Caribbean and Asian populations non-insulin dependent diabetes is more common than in the indigenous UK population. One in five South Asian men and women will develop diabetes by the age of 55 years compared to one in 20 of the general population. Complications of diabetes including renal damage, cataracts and ischaemic heart disease are also more common. Interestingly, Asian diabetics are less prone to foot ulcers, possibly due to regular and ritual foot washing; conversely, lateral foot ulceration, thought to be due to sitting cross-legged, is more common in Sikhs (Burden, 1993) (see also Chapter 18). Because of the higher prevalence of diabetes and hypertension in Asians and African-Caribbeans, there is a three to fourfold higher acceptance rate on renal replacement therapy programmes than white people and in some districts they comprise up to half of all patients receiving such treatment (Raleigh, 1997).

Amputation

Leg amputations may be very much more difficult to accept in some ethnic minority groups. This is because it implies disfigurement and potential loss of income. Patients may not be aware of the possibilities of achieving independence and a good quality of life following the operation, given the appropriate help and support. Effective counselling, peer support and a positive approach may help to overcome these problems.

Osteomalacia

Osteomalacia or rickets is considerably more common in Asian patients; the reason for this is not entirely clear but is probably due to a combination of factors, including lack of exposure to sunlight, consumption of chapattis (chappati flour is high in phytic acid, which reduces the absorption of vitamin D (Rawaf and Bahl, 1998)), a diet low in vitamin D and genetic differences. Osteomalacia is an easily overlooked coexisting condition. The main symptoms are generalised musculo-skeletal pain and muscle weakness. Osteomalacia is easily treatable with vitamin D and appropriate lifestyle advice, possibly through Indian and Pakistani social organisations or specifically directed health promotion campaigns (Rawaf and Bahl, 1998).

Cerebrovascular disease/stroke

Risk factors for stroke are more common in some ethnic minority groups (e.g. hypertension in Afro-Caribbeans, diabetes in Asians), resulting in increased frequency of stroke. For example, the recorded mortality from cerebrovascular disease (a proxy marker for incidence) among migrants from India, Pakistan and Bangladeshi is one-and-a-half times higher compared to the indigenous white population (Wild and McKeigue, 1997). Recent research in South Asians suggests clustering of risk factors occurs (hyperinsulinaemia, increased insulin resistance and increased tissue plasminogen activator levels) that might explain the susceptibility (Kain *et al.*, 2001).

A difficult multidisciplinary challenge in any situation, such as language and cultural barriers, may make the rehabilitation process and long-term plans more difficult for the ethnic minority patient, demanding greater awareness of potential difficulties and innovative use of available resources by all staff involved in their care. Both patients and relatives will be required to play an active part and should be encouraged to do so from the outset. There are many common and universal misapprehensions about stroke (Table 3.4), which may hamper recovery and need to be tackled. More leaflets and videos about stroke, in appropriate languages, are required. The establishment of more 'stroke clubs' to cater for ethnic minorities may also help. 'Segregation' here may be beneficial due to language and perceptual difficulties often encountered after a stroke.

Table 3.4 False beliefs about stroke

• Strokes are the same as heart attacks.
• Strokes are a punishment.
• Patients can get better as quickly as they became ill.
• Exercise is bad for the affected side.
• Patients need plenty of rest until complete recovery occurs.
• Physiotherapists, occupational therapists and speech therapists are types of nurse.
• Treatment of strokes is mainly tablets from the doctor.
• Relatives and friends can't help with treatment.

Depression and dementia

Depression may be undertreated in all elderly populations, since it is often difficult to diagnose and may present with predominantly physical symptoms. This is particularly true of the ethnic minority patient. It may prevent a patient reaching his or her full potential, and may be more readily detected by nurses, therapists and social workers who spend longer periods in close contact and intimate discussion with the individual patient than do doctors. Indeed, a recently described mood rating instrument designed for observers, rather than a self-assessment questionnaire, may be particularly relevant for people with low literacy skills (Hammond *et al.*, 2000).

Likewise, dementia is less easily diagnosed, as the family may be less forthcoming with the symptoms of personality change and memory impairment. Psychological tests can be misleading as they are dependent on language ability and education and cultural background. Instruments have now been described that aim to overcome these limitations (Jitapunkel *et al.*, 1996). Transcultural psychiatry is becoming an accepted specialist branch of practice (Burke, 1989).

Skin and hair care

People of Afro-Caribbean origin often use moisturising cream on the skin and this will need to be continued. Hair care is also a specialised task and should be appropriately undertaken.

A multi-cultural workforce that reflects the cultural make up of the local population can be seen to be advantageous in understanding a number of the above culture specific issues. Culture should not however be assumed by proxy measures of race or colour; the age difference may reflect quite different values – as in the indigenous population; and social standing between individuals from minority groups may be significant and difficult for staff from the indigenous society to appreciate.

RECOMMENDATIONS TO IMPROVE THE CARE OF ELDERLY ETHNIC MINORITY PATIENTS

The many ethnic minority groups have widely differing needs and it is, therefore, difficult to make general recommendations. However, the following four points should be considered:

1 Teaching about the special needs of ethnic minority populations should be included in the training of all health and social care practitioners.
2 More health education and social service leaflets, books and videos should be available in different languages to help explain the facilities already available, their accessibility and purpose.
3 More stroke clubs and day centres, where specific health and social needs can be met, should be established for ethnic minority groups, with the facility for cross-cultural exchange to feed interest and alleviate widespread ignorance.
4 More research, at both local and national level, should be undertaken into the needs of ethnic minority elderly patients and into ways of helping them make use of available help and resources.

ETHNIC MINORITIES AND THE HEALTH REFORMS

Recent reforms in the National Health Service (see Chapter 1) present opportunities for commissioners to improve health-care provision. Historically, the NHS was not organised to cater for a multi-ethnic population, which barely existed in 1948. The low uptake of health and social services by members of minority cultures is well documented (Karseras, 1991). The Department of Health has responded to this by emphasising six key themes that should be incorporated in the development of health policies (Bahl, 1993):

• Elimination of racial discrimination
• Availability of data on black and ethnic minority groups

- Delivery of appropriate quality services
- Training of health professionals
- Information for black and ethnic minority groups on health and health services
- Recognition of differing patterns of health and disease.

These six themes should be incorporated in local needs assessment and service development plans. However, it is believed by many that the needs of ethnic minorities are far too complex to leave safely to local plans and that there needs to be direct intervention from the centre (Karmi, 1993). The challenge for the future is to ensure that the six themes are acted upon by all health and social care providers, not just incorporated into strategic plans. This could be achieved in health care by such standards being incorporated into the National Service Frameworks; implemented by staff working in a learning culture; and monitored through the Commission for Health Improvement, National Performance Framework and National Survey of Patient and User Experience. Within social care, commissioning of such services should again reflect such principles or themes. Provision and good access to appropriate services for ethnic minority communities is emphasised in the recent National Service Framework for Older People (see also Chapter 6). There is also an excellent guide published by the King's Fund for Primary Care Groups and Trusts to help formulate a strategy to improve health for minority ethnic groups (Arora *et al.*, 2000).

Summary

Elderly ethnic minority patients come from widely diverse backgrounds and have a wide variety of needs. Successful rehabilitation will require not only attention to the individual clinical condition, but also an understanding of the various backgrounds, religions and cultures of the ethnic minority patient.

Fundamentally the same empathic concern, attention to detail, perseverance and patience are needed as are required for the care of all older people. Further research is required into the needs of this important and expanding group of elderly people.

References

Anderson, R. and Bury, M. (1988) *Living with Chronic Illness*, Unwin & Hyman, London.

Arora, S., Coker, N., Gillam, S. and Ismail, H. (2000) *Improving the Health of Black and Minority Ethnic Groups. A Guide for PCGs*, The King's Fund, London.

Bahl, V. (1993) Development of a black and ethnic minority health policy at the Department of Health. In: *Access to Health Care for People from Black and Ethnic Minorities* (eds Hopkins, A. and Bahl, V.), Royal College of Physicians, London, pp. 1–9.

Baxter, C. (1997) *Race Equality in Health Care and Education*, Baillière Tindall, London.

Beevers, D.G. and Beevers, M. (1993) Hypertension: impact upon black and ethnic minority people. In: *Access to Health Care for People from Black and Ethnic Minorities* (eds Hopkins, A. and Bahl, V.), Royal College of Physicians, London.

British Red Cross (1988) *Red Cross Multilingual Phrase Book*, British Red Cross, London.

Burden, A. (1993) Diabetes: impact on black and ethnic minority people. In: *Access to Health Care for People from Black and Ethnic Minorities* (eds Hopkins, A. and Bahl, V.), Royal College of Physicians, London.

Burke, A.W. (1989) Psychiatric practice and ethnic minorities. In: *Ethnic Factors in Health and Disease* (eds Cruikshank, J.K. and Beevers, D.G.), Wright, London.

Carlisle, D. (1998) Myths of minority care. *Community Care*, 5th March, 10–11.

Daily Telegraph (2001) Asylum claims at lowest level for two years. 26th May, p. 11.

Department of Health [DoH] (1998) *The National Survey of NHS Patients. General Practice*, HMSO, London.

Hammond, M.S., O'Keefe, S.T. and Barer, D.H. (2000) Development and validation of a brief observer rated screening scale for depression in elderly medical patients. *Age and Ageing*, **29**, 511–515.

Henley, A. and Schott, J. (1999) Communication. In: *Culture, Religion and Patient Care in a Multi-Ethnic Society*, Age Concern England, London.

Jitapunkel, S., Lailert, C., Wokakul, P., Srikiakhachorn, A. and Ebrahim, S. (1996) Chula mental test: a screening test developed for elderly people in less developed countries. *International Journal of Geriatric Psychiatry*, **11**, 715–720.

Jones, D. and Gill, P.S. (1998) Refugees and primary care: tackling the inequalities. *British Medical Journal*, **317**, 1444–1461.

Kain, K., Catto, A., Young, J., Bamford, J., Barrington, J. and Grant, P. (2001) Insulin resistance and elevated levels of tissue plasminogen in first degree relatives of South Asian patients with cerebrovascular disease. *Stroke*, **32**, 1069–1073.

Karmi, G. (1993) Management structures for recognising and meeting the health needs of black and ethnic minority patients. In: *Access to Health Care for People from Black and Ethnic Minorities* (eds Hopkins, A. and Bahl, V.), Royal College of Physicians, London.

Karseras, P. (1991) Minorities and access to health care. Part 1: confronting myths. *Care of the Elderly*, 3(9), 429–431.

Lawrence, R.E. and Littler, W.A. (1985) Acute myocardial infarction in Asians and Whites in Birmingham. *British Medical Journal*, **290**, 1472.

Leavitt, R.L. (1999) *Cross-cultural Rehabilitation: An international perspective*, W.B. Saunders, London.

Norman, A. (1985) *Triple Jeopardy: Growing old in a second homeland*, Centre for Policy on Ageing, London.

Phelan, M. and Parkman, S. (1995) How to work with an interpreter. *British Medical Journal*, **311**, 555–557.

Raleigh, V.S. (1997) Diabetes and hypertension in Britain's ethnic minorities: implications for the future of renal services. *British Medical Journal*, **314**, 209–213.

Rawaf, S. and Bahl, V. (1998) *Assessing Health Needs of People from Minority Ethnic Groups*. Royal College of Physicians, London.

Schweitzer, P. (1991) A place to stay: Growing old away from home. In: *Multi-cultural Health Care and Rehabilitation of Older People* (ed. Squires, A.). Age Concern, England and Edward Arnold, London.

Social Trends 30 (2000) *Labour Force Survey*, Office of National Statistics, London p. 25.

Westermeyer, J. (1990) Working with an interpreter in psychiatric assessment. *Journal of. Nervous and Mental Diseases*, **178**, 745–749.

Wild, S. and McKeigue, P.M. (1997) Cross sectional analysis of mortality by country of birth in England and Wales, 1970–1992. *British Medical Journal*, **314**, 705–710.

Will, A. (1993) *Race and Health in Contemporary Britain*, Open University Press, Buckingham.

Young, J. and George, J. (1991) History of migration to the United Kingdom. In: *Multi-cultural Health Care and Rehabilitation of Older People* (ed. Squires, A.), Age Concern England and Edward Arnold, London.

RESOURCES AND FURTHER READING

Alibhai-Brown, Y. (1998) *Caring for Ethnic Minority Elderlys*, Age Concern England, London.

DoH (2001) *The National Service Framework for Older People*, HMSO, London.

Health Education Authority (1994) *Health Related Resources for Black and Minority Groups*, Health Education Authority, London.

Henley, A. and Schott, J. (1999) *Culture, Religion and Patient Care in a Multi-Ethnic Society*, Age Concern England, London.

Hopkins, A. and Bahl, V. (1993) *Access to Health Care for People from Black and Ethnic Minorities*, Royal College of Physicians, London.

Jagee, M. and Saroj, L. (1999) *Religions and Cultures. Guide to Beliefs and Customs for Health Care Staff and Social Services*, Edinburgh and Lothians Racial Equality Council, Edinburgh.

Qureshi, B. (1989) *Transcultural Medicine: Dealing with patients from different cultures*, Kluwer Academic Press, London.

Squires, A. (ed.) (1991) *Multi-cultural Health Care and Rehabilitation of Older People*, Age Concern England and Edward Arnold, London.

Part Two

THE THEORY OF REHABILITATION

4 REHABILITATION CONCEPTS

Rowena D. Plant

AIMS OF THE CHAPTER

The term rehabilitation is subject to the interpretation of the user risking unintended, and often unappreciated, differences in strategic aims across the ever-expanding stakeholder interests. The problem is magnified outside of traditional hospital care with the involvement of other agencies, the lead often being the patient, rather than professional domination. This chapter considers the reasons for differing interpretation and the likely consequences, noting the dilemma of individual freedom versus public safety. It concludes that rehabilitation is a function of services right across the health and social spectrum rather than a discreet service in its own right. Acknowledgement of the differing needs and expectations of participants and acceptance of unanticipated outcomes is a start to implementation of the ultimate goal of personalised rehabilitation. Such an approach, centred on self-management and autonomy asks very real questions of current internal audit of pathways and external assessment of performance against pre-determined standards of care.

DEFINITIONS

Rehabilitation is a complex concept and many definitions exist. Each definition reflects, to some extent, the experience and position of the definer. It is important to be able to articulate both generic and specific definitions and descriptions. Such definitions enable meaningful communication of practice and evaluation both across and within the rehabilitation spectrum. The King's Fund (King's Fund, 1998) determined an emerging consensus as follows:

1 The primary objective of rehabilitation involves restoration (to the maximum degree possible) either of function (physical or mental) or of role (within the family, social network or workforce).
2 Rehabilitation will usually require a mixture of clinical, therapeutic and social interventions that also address issues relevant to a person's physical and social environment.
3 Effective rehabilitation needs to be responsive to users' needs and wishes, purposeful, involve a number of agencies and disciplines and be available when required.
4 An emphasis on restoration enables rehabilitation to be distinguished from primary prevention and maintenance.

It is important to place a caveat on the emphasis on restoration. Those involved in the treatment of older people with complex physical and mental problems will recognise that the concept of restoration can be of limited value. Many of the presenting and underlying conditions within this client group are of a deteriorating and frequently long-standing nature. In these cases rehabilitation has a dual role, restoration, at an impairment level, in the first instance followed by physical, psychological and social adjustment, at a participation level (Ward, 1992). It may be useful in these situations to use an impact driven rehabilitation concept: to minimise the impact of the primary disorder and to maximise (physical, psychological and social) functional activities.

The second edition of the International Classification of Impairment, Disability and Handicap (ICIDH-2) (World Health Organisation, 1999) usefully enables us to place generic and specific definitions of rehabilitation within a model that goes some way to transcending the difficulties of purely 'medical' or 'social' models of disability (McLellan, 1997). Rehabilitation professionals use a mix of models in their practice that include more, or less, of each as appropriate to the situation. It is therefore not surprising to find so many different professionals involved in the rehabilitation process. Similarly, it is entirely reasonable to expect that within the 'skill-mix' of each individual professional, there are both trans-disciplinary and uni-disciplinary skills. The King's Fund (Sinclair and Dickinson, 1998) point to the fact that effective rehabilitation may be achieved by the coordination of complex interventions addressing multiple risk factors, involving multiple professional disciplines and multiple phases of rehabilitation. The interdisciplinary approach is held to be the key to successful and meaningful rehabilitation.

A further useful definition of rehabilitation has resulted from a project designed to develop multi-professional education and training. Rehabilitation is defined as:

> *An enabling process in which societies, communities, agencies and professionals meet the social, psychological, physical and economic needs of the disabled person through knowledge, skill, respect, understanding and agreement. The rehabilitative process includes an assessment of where the individual, community and carer(s) are, where they wish to be, and the contributions each must make to achieve ambitions and meet needs.*
>
> (Baker et al., 1997)

In essence this definition recognises the complexity of rehabilitation, the partnership required by a variety of individuals and professionals, and the willingness of all involved to determine realistic and measurable outcomes. Figure 4.1 begins to pull these concepts together.

Although apparently comprehensive, this definition might be further expanded to consider that ambitions may be unrealistic and that not all needs can be met either through availability of skill or resource. Further, rehabilitation based on an initial assessment and without ongoing monitoring of progress and adjustment of objectives, remains a static process rather than a continuously adjusted activity.

POWER

Central to the above definition by Baker and colleagues (1997) is that the needs or wishes of individuals and the people nearest to them, whether friends, family or employees of the service, are taken into account. Rehabilitation is increasingly a community focused activity and, if benefits are to be maximised, should be enhanced by current changes in the way both health and social services are organised (Ayres *et al.*, 1998). Health Action Zones, Health Improvement Plans and Clinical Governance (see also Chapter 1) are all initiatives that seek to focus on the service user at the centre of both provision and evaluation. The development of Primary Care Trusts places the point of service delivery in the community rather than the hospital (see also Chapter 11). Such developments have the opportunity to facilitate more effective rehabilitation as they begin to blur the barriers between primary, acute, secondary and tertiary care. These barriers have, until now, largely mitigated against effective rehabilitation, which, by its very nature, at individual client, clinical treatment and service delivery levels, is only as successful as it is able to transfer meaningfully into different situations and contexts (see also Chapter 2). It is perhaps helpful to conceptualise rehabilitation as being a function of services right across the health and social spectrum rather than a discrete service in its own right. This juxtaposition is indeed both its challenge and its opportunity. If users and carers are one of the key components in the rehabilitation process, then how they are able to define, articulate and evaluate their wants, desires and needs, which may differ from those of the rest of the team and from each other, is an important pre-determinant of change (see also Chapter 5). For any change to be successful then the degree to which those who seek to benefit are also power holders in the process is pivotal (Crainer, 1998).

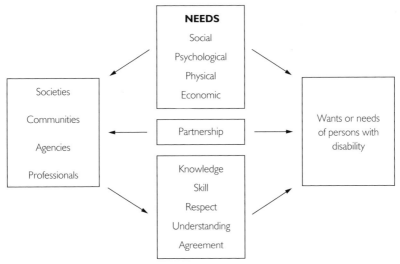

Figure 4.1 The enabling process of rehabilitation

'By empowering others, a leader does not decrease his power, instead he may increase it – especially if the whole organisation performs better' (Griffith, 1997).

This quote is taken from the domain of business management. If we apply it to rehabilitation then can the concept still hold true? If the leader equates with the professional, and the organisation equates with the client (and carer) and the social and/or health service, then we can begin to see that empowering others is health giving not only for the recipient but for the enabler and the organisation in which they work as well. The individual and his/her carers will be central to the rehabilitation programme and will expect to be able, and enabled, to be heard. This shift in emphasis is perhaps subtle but its implications are profound.

Such changes will influence the decisions that are being made about rehabilitation plans and who takes those decisions. Understanding how we frame our beliefs and how we determine and operate power is important, not in the least because we have traditionally worked with disenfranchised individuals in disempowered settings.

ETHICS

Any health-care intervention is held to be a moral endeavour (Seedhouse, 1988) and, as such, rehabilitation is no exception. The ethical or moral perspective of rehabilitation should be built on the four guiding principles of health-care ethics (Gillon, 1985; see Figure 4.2):

- respect for persons and autonomy
- beneficence (doing good)
- non-maleficence (avoidance of harm)
- justice.

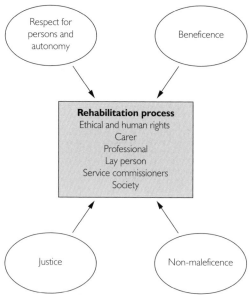

Figure 4.2 Ethical principles that underpin the rehabilitation process

Using these four principles enables examination of the (coherent) moral framework within which rehabilitation seeks to practise. Moral and ethical issues are to be found at personal, team and institutional levels and are contextualised by the social, cultural and religious practices and conventions of society. Furthermore, professionals are bound by the rules and statutes of British and European Law and governing bodies' rules of professional conduct.

When researching practice there are clear obligations to be met, enshrined in three principles (Forster, 1996):

- the validity of the research
- the welfare of the research subject, and
- the dignity of the research subject.

These principles seek to ensure that the research question is important and can be answered, to understand what participating in the research will involve and whether any risks are necessary and acceptable, and finally whether informed consent will be sought and confidentiality respected. Normally, local (or multi-centre) ethics committees adjudge the extent to which proposed research fulfils these principles in health care. However, the process of considering what makes an action (any action) morally acceptable is a question fundamental to clinical practice as well. Such considerations involve the consideration of rights and duties and the contexts in which they are understood.

Three different ways of looking at this fundamental question have usefully been summarised for research ethics committees (Department of Health [DoH], 1997) as:

1 a goal based approach
2 a duty based approach
3 a rights based approach.

In summary, a goal based thinker will argue that the action is good if its goals or outcomes are good. A duty based thinker asks if the action accords with moral principles (e.g. telling the truth), if it does not, then even if the outcome is good, the action is unethical. A rights based thinker will seek to protect the given rights in a society and is concerned that the action does not violate those rights (e.g. confidentiality and consent). Furthermore, the cultures and faiths of our society are also important in shaping and understanding how the concept of rehabilitation may be viewed by different sectors. For example, in Chapter 3, false beliefs about stroke from some minority groups were described, which include that recovery occurs at the same speed as the illness occurred; rest is needed until recovery occurs; recovery is the result of tablets; and that exercise is bad for the affected side.

The common principle concerning rehabilitation is that both the product and process must benefit the older person. The product will be the state of affairs where the individual enjoys an optimal degree of well-being viewed from their own perspective. How 'well-being' and 'optimal' are defined remains open to question. The process of rehabilitation is the actions and outcomes that occur to promote the achievement of goals. How goals are set and achieved, when communication between the individual and others is difficult, remains to be determined (see also Chapter 8). Furthermore, this process takes place within a context, with a number of actors on the stage – user and carer, professional and lay person, local and national service commissioners, and increasingly the wider public to whom ultimate accountability is owed (Figure 4.2). All these stakeholders should and will be involved to some degree in the process. It is easy therefore to begin to imagine the complexity of values that contribute to the rehabilitation process and the possibilities for misadventure that may occur (see also Chapter 5).

Respect for persons and autonomy

The first of the four ethical principles is concerned with being respected and valued as a person, and is essential to human well-being. The definitions of rehabilitation considered that each person is viewed holistically for effective process and outcome. But, what is a person? Suppose 'persons' are defined as 'rational beings with active minds that can make conscious, free choices' and agree that the rational will is a person's most precious possession. Does lack of any of these features fail to qualify an individual as a person and, more importantly, to be treated as one? Do elders lose their definition as a 'person' in certain situations or in certain people's views? Ultimately an individual's view of a 'person' depends on the values they hold. These values may mean that older people more easily become treated as 'non-persons' or alternatively are held in high esteem. In either case we either minimise or maximise the value of the older person's rational will. If we minimise, then we purposefully take away the very essence of their being as a human 'person'. This removal is amoral and could be considered as a criminal act. In this most insidious of ways elder abuse can be most profound, not through actual bodily harm but through neglect of respect and value of the person.

Informed consent is an issue that is becoming central to best practice and forms a major challenge in the development of professional standards and guidelines. It is generally accepted, under Clinical Governance (see also Chapter 1) that such standards are vital to safe and effective practice. An example of a working standard that has emerged is: 'staff will work to ensure that all patients/clients competent to give consent are appropriately informed on their treatment interventions'. Staff working with patients detained under the Mental Health Act 1983 are required to follow the current code of practice (Newcastle City Health NHS Trust, 2000). Could bypassing consent regarding rehabilitation decisions then count as a form of elder abuse (Moon *et al.*, 1996)? Interpretation under the Human Rights Act 2000, which, for example, reinforces the prohibition of inhumane treatment, will rely on definition, explanation and informed consent to activities that could appear less than humane to an observer.

The key question for rehabilitation professionals is: 'To what extent is the personal well-being of the older person, in reality, driving the decision-making process?' Whether this is physical or mental well-being must also be considered – the two may conflict.

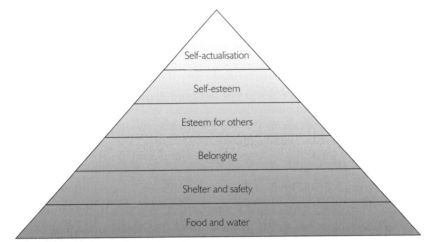

Figure 4.3 Maslow's hierarchy of needs

The next question for us to consider is who decides on what counts as contributing to someone's well-being? Since the impact of rehabilitation is to be found in the lived experience of individuals we need to know what its effect is on a person's well-being. If rehabilitation is to involve more than a mere geographical change, then the quality of life to be enjoyed by the person becomes a crucial factor. One way of defining well-being is to see it as 'the having of achievable personal goals'. Without these, 'persons' are mere puppets. So, rehabilitation outcomes can only be linked to well-being if it is also a goal for the person concerned.

Maslow's hierarchy of needs (Figure 4.3) implies that 'all else being equal, a person is better off and more able to pursue higher goals if basic needs are satisfied first' (Maslow, 1943). These might vary considerably from person to person according to a number of factors such as lifestyle, physique and culture. How far do we minimise the self-actualising, or higher needs of the older person, such as to be seen as still living an independent life, to be responsible for another even if the 'other' is a cat or canary, or, to leave hard earned property to one's family? An older person's basic needs might include the company of pets, the use of tobacco and consumption of alcohol. Professional staff may not consider these as needs at all, rather wants or desires. Equally an older person may not place value on a tidy home, or the necessity of daily bathing, or even the company of others. Such values, when at variance with our own, can make us uncomfortable, yet we would acknowledge that being able to have a degree of choice is also a basic psychological need.

The more self-directed or autonomous people are, the more they will want to determine their own priorities. As rehabilitation is about enabling effective self-management we should not be surprised (or judgemental) when our efforts are successful in enabling self-determination in ways, or domains, that are not our own. Indeed, this could be one of the most meaningful, and challenging, measures of rehabilitation success. Respect for people is ultimately founded on valuing all equally and acknowledging that one person's values are not necessarily those of another. This concept will be further challenged by peer review unless the rationale for unexpected outcomes achieved, measured as successful by the patient, are clearly documented. All of us form our values in social contacts, initially within a family and subsequently through education, social and working life. No two individuals can have identical life experiences, but within a given society values are shared. Within rehabilitation there is an assumed set of professional values, which together with carer values can dominate those of the client. Pain relief is a good example. One would expect the relief of pain to be of primary importance to an individual's sense of well-being. However, Sigmund Freud, as an old man, refused all medication except aspirin, saying 'I prefer to think in torment rather than not to be able to think clearly'. Autonomy as an elder, rather than pain relief, was his primary goal.

The extent to which the individual can play a real part in decision-making about proposals for or against rehabilitation will depend on the degree of autonomy they are able to exercise. This means, in ordinary language, how far a person can be self-directed and to what extent can a free and informed choice be made. It also raises questions as to the degree to which individuals should be, or can be, accountable for their own actions and decisions. The advent of care pathway methodology (Walsh, 1998) holds possibilities for ensuring that elders are consulted and informed about treatment choices and rehabilitation options (see also Chapter 8). Importantly, if used well, they should allow for 'opt-in' as well as 'opt-out' scenarios. The challenge for rehabilitation is fully participative development of trans-disciplinary and flexible 'rehabilitation pathways' that enable the older person to be a full partner in the development and usage of personalised routes. There are, and will remain, older people who no longer seem to wish to be involved in any decision-making – this in itself is a decision. It is always worth remembering, however, that the decisions we see as important are not necessarily shared by the client and vice versa.

An older relative of the author, currently living in a nursing establishment, no longer sees clothing choice as an important decision. A career as a tailoress would probably inform the rehabilitation and care process otherwise. For her, however, decisions regarding food are now central to her sense of self and the ones she feels best able to make. Of course, older people may, perhaps over time, have become conditioned to have decision making taken out of their hands. However, it is important to reflect that even in this they are still exercising a choice, being respected and having a degree of autonomy. Autonomy, like freedom, is a relative concept; no one can be fully free or fully autonomous. The aim of rehabilitation professionals should always be to preserve and promote autonomy as much as is possible. The way in which this can be done is by always attempting to provide a 'window of choice'. Even where autonomy is minimal, small choices can still be made that respect the dignity and integrity of the person. Any person can still show by their actions that they shape their own life to some extent.

Beneficence

The second of our four principles is about doing good. All stakeholders will wish to be perceived as doing good and acting morally. However, 'good' is a relative term. From an ethical standpoint rehabilitation should be presented in terms of benefit to the older person (that is personal benefit, not defined by others in a paternalistic way). The use of the word benefit raises a number of salient questions regarding the evidence base of our practice. As yet we are not in a position, methodologically, that enables satisfactory evaluation of rehabilitation (process and product) reflecting both complex input and personalised outcome. Nevertheless, rehabilitation practice is based on the assumption of benefit, and to withdraw or deny such treatment would be unethical (Plant, 1996). The distinction between 'needs' and 'wants' can usefully be made, as in everyday language these two words are often used synonymously (see also Chapter 5). Individuals are all authorities regarding their own wants or desires; indeed many desires remain entirely unknown to the rest of the world. However, needs are not like this and can be unknown even to the individual themselves. It is in this area where the rehabilitation professional's knowledge and communication skills are so important. For example, an older person envisaging return to their previous environment can be quite unaware of the new and different needs they may have once they leave the comparative safety of the residential or hospital environment. Such different needs may lead to potential conflict, both within the individual themselves and between them and the professional. The desire to return to 'normal' can sit uneasily with the new needs that person may have. And as such the person is in fact not returning to 'normal' but to some other state previously not experienced by themselves, but probably observed in others by members of the team. The way such experience is described will be a key factor in agreeing goals. The perception of what provides benefit will vary according to the perceiver.

Rehabilitation professionals already recognise, operating outside of a simplistic cure paradigm, that 'normal' is not a useful end-point of intervention. However, the challenge is even greater to prepare the older person for a new normality and to do so in such a way as to enable their needs to determine the framework of that normality. It is also worth considering the vexed question of risk and risk taking. Allowing the older person to determine their own strategies regarding the risks they are willing to take (and these go well beyond our limited concepts regarding safety), enabling autonomy, can often appear to be in direct conflict with our imperative to do good. Such an imperative is enshrined in the conduct of health policies, service delivery models and treatment modalities. Compounded by an increasing fear of litigation there is a very real danger that the agenda of the powerful stakeholders and drivers will dominate. In so doing we limit our willingness to take risks and therefore our clients' ability to do likewise (Heyman, 1998).

To benefit from rehabilitation an older person needs to be able to take risks, to experiment and to discover their new needs and wants. The challenge to health and social care practitioners is to provide an overall beneficial frame-work within which this guided and supported process can take place. Pragmatically, the views of the older person and those of professionals towards rehabilitation as a goal, need to gradually converge. Then a truly stereoscopic picture of how resources and policies can complement the prognosis, and balance the needs, wants and motivations of the older person can be made. For effective rehabilitation the two sets of aims should become more or less congruent.

Non-maleficence

The third principle concerns the duty of the avoidance of harm and is not a straightforward opposite of doing good. This principle, like beneficence, is dependent on the degree to which the person is valued. Like negative freedoms it is owed to all people to avoid harming them. We can use the example of risk again here to illustrate this principle, using it in its more constrained meaning regarding personal safety. A useful definition of risk comes from an American lawyer, Charles Fried, who determines a 'risk budget, whereby people decide (however simplistically) the sorts of ends they wish to achieve and the sorts of risks – including risks of death – which they are prepared to take in pursuit of those ends' (Gillon, 1985).

Is rehabilitation and return to a home environment a new or a considerably modified risk? How much modification is of an essential nature and how much is to conform to norms and standards not necessarily owned by the returning older person? Making an environment safer might also make it less familiar. The rehabilitation professional may not want to take risks, partly because the well-being of the patient will be uppermost in his or her mind, but also there is the problem of possible accusations of negligence that might bring the individual, institution or profession into disrepute. The older person may well be taking a risk in having the goal of returning home to a perhaps more hazardous lifestyle than he or she would have in residential accommodation. If it is a calculated risk and is rationally taken it would be illegal and harmful to deny personal autonomy on the grounds of purely personal physical safety. The extent to which professionals have to avoid harm to the patient and others, especially if, in doing this, consent is overridden, will no doubt be debated as the Human Rights Act 2000 is tested.

Informed consent must involve the understanding, agreement, acceptance and actual assent of the client (Purtilo, 1984). In addition it must be made voluntarily, not be coerced, the individual must be sufficiently competent and sufficiently autonomous. This means they must have adequate information; based on evidence not emotion; covering both short-term and long-term consequences; expressed in accessible language on the basis of which they can deliberate, having had adequate time for reflection. Figure 4.4 illustrates the three cornerstones of informed consent.

There are of course challenges in words such as 'sufficiently' and 'adequate', just how much time or information is sufficient or adequate will depend on the individual situation and innovative approaches will be needed where communication is affected by mental or sensory impairment. Furthermore, just how competent or autonomous must such an individual be? Nevertheless, informed consent, action by an autonomous person based on adequate information, remains a cornerstone of ethical rehabilitation practice. Interventions, or doing things to other autonomous persons without their consent, withholding relevant information, distorting the truth due to them, however minor, are all threats to autonomy and respect for the person and cause harm. The fundamental principle underlying consent is the right of self-determination and this principle should never be disregarded.

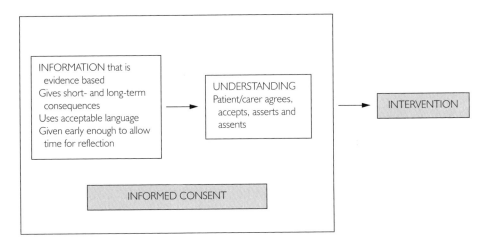

Figure 4.4 Information, understanding and literature: the three cornerstones of informed consent in rehabilitation practice

Professionals will sometimes argue that the information is too complex for the person to understand. This stance is often taken by power holders and always betrays an underlying paternalistic and arrogant attitude. Presenting information in an understandable, informative and interactive way should be a baseline skill for any health professional. Such skill is paramount when the issue at hand is the environment, in which that person will live and enjoy an acceptable quality of life. A wise philosopher noted: 'It is not putting yourself into another's shoes that is morally relevant, it is understanding what it is like for that other person to be in their own shoes that is morally important'.

Deliberate withholding of information relevant to decision-making is a form of deceit. A number of charters within the public (and increasingly the private) sectors seek to provide the relevant information that will enable consumers and users to make informed choices. But does silence, refusal to discuss, the expressed wish not to know or be involved, imply consent? In the past this has often been construed as 'tacit consent', but, strictly, this is not consent at all.

John Stuart Mill (Mill, 1843) argued for the following principle, 'the only purpose for which power can rightfully be exercised over any member of a civilised community against his will is to prevent harm to others'. Mill thought that a person's own good might be a motive for reasoning with them or attempting to persuade them about a course of action. However, the line between this and moral coercion is rather fine. A person's own good is obviously concerned with their welfare and happiness, and as such principles of legitimate intervention, rules which distinguish acceptable from unacceptable ways of affecting other people's freedom, are perhaps more useful to rehabilitation than those of non-interference.

Justice

The final of our four principles is concerned with the equal rights of persons to enjoy the goods of society and to be protected equally by the law of the land. Forcing an older person to leave his or her home because they cannot demonstrate the ability to function independently is direct physical interference, and justification of this needs to be very soundly based on risk assessment data. As considered above, any intervention occurring without consent can be construed as an assault upon the person and the position of older persons can mean that they may be more easily harmed through a misuse of such power. It is not a defence of indoctrination to say that people want their minds to be made up for them. Some individuals may genuinely want the responsibility of decision-making taken from them. To be sure that this is the case, full assessment of mental competence will be needed, and the skills of an advocate made available. While health-care staff are facilitating rehabilitation, relatives may be unwilling for an older person to be rehabilitated because of an increased financial, physical or social risk, and may be tempted to indoctrinate the older person with persuasive arguments and by carefully selected information. For example, they may make them believe they are more dependent than they might otherwise be by highlighting areas of weakness and dependency.

The NHS Plan (DoH, 2000) emphasises the role of the patient advocate. It is the business of advocacy to facilitate the views and rights of the user and it is the business of government in a good society to ensure there are checks on how such power is exercised. It is a cornerstone of European policy to improve the quality of life of older people in the European Union by promoting measures that increase independence and self-determination, even when very frail (European Comunity, 1999). The older person often lacks power for economic reasons and the 1990 Reforms (DoH, 1989) sought to give older people the right to choose between different care service providers by giving them back power, by means of the power to purchase.

Coercion and deception cause a person to become an instrument of someone else's will, which is against natural justice. Of course, a person wishing their liberty to be restricted in certain ways also exercises their own autonomy; if the reasons for doing this are rationally and freely considered. The dilemma for statutory and voluntary carers is clarifying what is actually in the individual's best interests, and does this in any way conflict with the equity, freedom and safety of others? If an older person is not able to argue articulately and forcefully for him or herself, and there is a possibility of injustice, then an advocate is needed who has no vested interest in the decision-making. The aim of advocacy is to empower the individual, not to persuade them to bend to the will of others.

Together with the implicit and covert nature of belief systems that operate, unwittingly, within health and social care professionals themselves, the circumstances in which they are likely to be impartial advocates are few and far between. Whether people ought to be persuaded of a particular course of action and what counts as a genuine claim to provide true information in the best interests of individuals and society at large is the business of ethics. Arguing from authority is a common type of fallacy; the truth or falsity of a given statement does not rest solely on the authority of the person who makes it. It is not the prestige of an authority (which includes all rehabilitation professionals) that makes a statement true or false, but rather the citing of evidence either to confirm or refute the statement. Moral questions therefore cannot be settled by appeals to authority and this is especially relevant in rehabilitation. There is no stronger case that can be put for always having access to an advocate, who is independent of the relevant authority, whether that authority is statutory, voluntary or professional. The function of the advocate is to transfer power back to the client and assist in pleading the cause of the person who is not sufficiently autonomous to do this for themselves. The essential criteria for advocacy have been summarised by the five Cs (Table 4.1) of Compassion, Competence, Confidence, Conscience and Commitment (Roach, 1987). Advocacy is justified and required where there is reduced autonomy, for those who are confused, those who feel powerless and anyone who cannot effectively act for themselves.

Table 4.1   The five essential criteria for advocacy

- Compassion
- Competence
- Competence
- Competence
- Commitment

(Roach, 1987)

ETHICAL THEORIES

Ethical theories relevant to rehabilitation include those of those of Mill (Mill, 1843) and Kant (Paton, 1948). Mill espoused a consequentialist theory best known as utilitarianism in which actions are right or wrong, according to the consequences of those proposed actions. The best consequences are those that provide the greatest amount of good. Mill further insisted that all should be treated equally and that no one man's pursuit of the 'good' should cause harm to another. The utilitarian argument is for maximising 'pleasure' (the good), while avoiding pain. Utility is the factor that is the measure of satisfaction in life. However, is a life without pain necessarily a life with full quality? Conversely, does a life, in which all wants and needs are met, allow an individual to be valued as a person? One problem is that preferences change, we may plan for a more independent lifestyle, but when the move is imminent we may resist such an option, from fear perhaps. Does informed choice rest inevitably on making decisions about what we already know about? Many long for congenial company without having experienced it, but we would not say this was an uninformed choice. Utilitarianism argues for the greatest good to the greatest number but that this should avoid significant harm to others. Suppose the older person really does just want to be left alone to die? Can we and should we respect this choice if we have no good reason to doubt his or her rationality. It is a question of trade-offs of the 'goods' of life. Griffin (1986) compares the ingredients of a particular quality of life to ingredients in cooking – 'we can measure the quantities of wine, beef and onions separately but we can only measure their value to the dish by considering them in various combinations'. The value will also be unique to the individual.

By contrast, Kant (Paton, 1948) illustrates a duty-based approach to ethics. This approach holds that consequences of actions should not be the prime consideration; instead moral reasoning should be governed by duty. Kant believed in the freedom of the will of rational beings that would recognise a self-imposed rational law. In colloquial terms this would be 'do as you would be done by'. It is more easily applied as a theory within the relationship between client and professional, whereas utilitarianism is more easily applied to public and service policies. Above all, Kant's thinking recognises respect for persons as a driving force in ethics, and he valued a combination of freedom and responsibility. Autonomous man, insofar as he is autonomous, is not subject to the will of another. From this basis we have a moral duty to keep promises and honour contracts, and this leads us to believe we have a moral right to expect this from others. Is it therefore acceptable to assure an older person that they will be rehabilitated, as it cannot be any single person's duty to carry this out? Since any promise or contract imposing a duty on another cannot be valid unless that other person has been involved, such promises should never be made. The process of ethical rehabilitation is therefore based on interdisciplinary assessment, which includes the views of the user and carer, goal setting which meets user and carer needs, intervention in which the user and carer are active participants, and review which includes evidence of achievements and opportunities for progress. These are further considered in Chapter 8.

SUMMARY

Whichever ethical theory we espouse there will be no rubric, or set of right/wrong answers about when to rehabilitate, or when it might be justified, or what rehabilitation itself might actually mean for the person in question. What is needed is a very careful grounding of both the process and product of rehabilitation in a commonly held definition and concept. In communicating and actioning such rehabilitation we will, covertly or overtly, examine and use concepts such as person-hood, well-being, autonomy, rights and freedoms, duty of care and responsibilities, needs and wants, justice and fairness, informed choice, and quality of life. Such concepts are contextualised by experiences of team members, users and other interested parties – all potentially different. Rehabilitation is in a unique position in its potential to impact upon the very essence of being human. In the rehabilitation of the older person we have the very real potential to add life to years so long as the differing experiences and consequent care planning processes we all engage in are shared and understood.

REFERENCES

Ayres, P., Wright, J. *et al.* (1998) Achieving clinical effectiveness: the new world of clinical governance. *Clinician in Management*, 7, 106–111.

Baker, M., Fardell, J. *et al.* (1997) *Disability and Rehabilitation: Survey of education needs of health and social service professionals*, Disability and Rehabilitation Open Learning Project, London.

Crainer, S. (1998) *Key Management Ideas*, Pitman Publishing, London.

Department of Health [DoH] (1989) *Caring for People*, HMSO, London.

DoH (1997) *Briefing Pack for Research Ethics Committee Members*, Department of Health, London.

DoH (2000) *The NHS Plan*, The Stationery Office, London.

European Comunity (1999) *Towards a Europe for all Ages*, Commission of the European Communities, Brussels.

Forster, C. (ed.) (1996) *Manual for Research Ethics Committees*, King's College, University of London, London.

Gillon, R. (1985) *Philosophical and Medical Ethics*, Wiley, Chichester.

Griffin, J. (1986) *Well Being*, Clarendon Press, Oxford.

Griffith, V. (1997) It's a people thing, *Financial Times*, London.

Heyman, B. (ed.) (1998) *The Management of Risk in Health Care: A critical approach*, Edward Arnold, London.

King's Fund (1998) *Trends in Rehabilitation Policy: A review of the literature*, King's Fund and the Audit Commission, London.

Maslow, A. (1943) A theory of human motivation. *Psychological Review*, **40**, 370–389.

McLellan, D. (1997) Introduction to rehabilitation. In: *The Rehabilitation Studies Handbook* (eds Wilson, B. and McLellan, D.), Cambridge University Press, Cambridge.

Mill, J. (1843) John Stuart Mill 1806–1873, Utilitarianism. In: *Utilitarianism and Other Essays*, Penguin Classics, London (1987).

Moon, J., Pethybridge, J. *et al.* (1996) Gaining patient consent to supported discharge following stroke-patient empowerment. *European Journal of Neurology*, 3(Suppl. 2), 90.

Newcastle City Health NHS Trust (2000) *Professional Standards and Guidelines*, P. A. Forum, Newcastle City Health NHS Trust, Newcastle upon Tyne.

Paton, H.J. (1948) *'The Moral Law' – Translation of Kant's 'Groundwork of the Metaphysic of Morals'*, Hutchinson, London.

Plant, R. (1996) Towards meaningful research in rehabilitation. *British Journal of Therapy and Rehabilitation*, 3(5), 245–246.

Purtilo, R.B. (1984) Applying the principles of informed consent to patient care. *Physical Therapy*, **64**(6), 934–937.

Roach, S. (1987) *Caring as a Responsibility: A response to value as the important-in-itself*, 2nd International Congress on Nursing Law and Ethics, Tel Aviv.

Seedhouse, D. (1988) *Health: The Foundation for Achievement*, Wiley, Chichester.

Sinclair, A. and Dickinson, E. (1998) *Effective Practice in Rehabilitation: The evidence of systematic reviews*, King's Fund Publishing and the Audit Commission, London.

Walsh, M. (1998) *Models and Critical Pathways in Clinical Nursing: Conceptual frameworks and care planning*, Harcourt Brace, London.

Ward, C. (1992) Rehabilitation in Parkinson's Disease. *Reviews in Clinical Gerontology*, **2**, 254–268.

World Health Organization (1999) *ICIDH-2: International classification of functioning and disability*. Beta-2 draft. Full version. World Health Organisation, Geneva.

5 MEETING THE CHANGING NEEDS OF STAKEHOLDERS

Amanda J. Squires

AIMS OF THE CHAPTER

Historically, health care has been a contract between the provider and the user. Internal and external influences have created worldwide change towards market style health-care provision. This introduces a third stakeholder, the commissioner or funder. These three groups have their own needs as individuals and as stakeholders. In addition, users will have needs specific to their cohort and care group. While there is recognition that we now have an ageing population, the social significance of this demographic change is not widely understood (Vincent, 1999). This chapter attempts to unravel the concept of stakeholder satisfaction as it applies to rehabilitation of older people. Key stakeholders are defined as users, providers and funders, each having basic, expressed and anticipated needs that they measure against their perception of the service provided. While, predominantly, funders pursue a business model, providers pursue a scientific model. Elderly users have to date pursued a social model, many remembering the pre-NHS days and eternally 'grateful' for what they receive. Newer cohorts are, and will be increasingly, different. They will be more informed and willing to challenge just at a time when their partnership in the provision of care is increasingly needed (Chapter 1). The chapter concludes by suggesting that how these individuals are identified and their contribution used will provide a productive opportunity for the proactive stakeholder – and a serious threat to the reactive stakeholder.

CREATION OF THE NHS

The formation of the British National Health Service in 1948 has been well documented, and indicates a post-war population deferent to powerful autonomous medical expertise (Strong and Robinson, 1990). A stable, paternalistic relationship developed with almost universal acceptance and gained support across political parties.

Changing expectations, epidemiology, technology, demography and economics are driving health service review worldwide (Ranade, 1994). Those particularly pertinent to the UK include: limited tolerance for higher taxation by workers; rising expectations by welfare recipients; unprecedented medical advancement; a widespread belief in the right of citizens to the best available health care; availability of technology for improved biological survival and functional independence; and an ageing population with chronic disability. Rising expectations have been shown to be the main influence, exceeding even the more publicised impact of ageing (Abel-Smith, 1994).

NHS REFORM

A relatively small miscalculation in the NHS budget produced a massive financial crisis in 1988. Thousands of beds were closed before a particularly harsh winter, significantly ending 40 years of the sacrosanct, all-party support for the service. The Confidential Review of the NHS resulted in reform towards a more responsive culture through a managed or quasi-market, limited to internal competition (Department of Health, 1989). Responsiveness was mainly directed at identifying and meeting the largely assumed needs of users by competition between providers. The needs of other stakeholders (providers and commissioners) were largely overlooked.

The 1998 reform aimed to make the NHS 'Modern and Dependable' (NHS Executive, 1997), replacing paternalism and competition with partnership. Funding, referring and some responsibility for provision going to Primary Care Trusts, the key medical and nursing members of which would carry a caseload and listen to patient preferences on a daily basis. They would influence placement of business accordingly. Health Authority commissioners have been too far removed from this valuable qualitative intelligence, relying, to the potential detriment of the service, almost solely on quantitative evidence, unrepresentative anecdotes and complaints. The potential for change as a result of this reform has been largely underestimated.

The NHS Plan (Department of Health [DoH], 2000) (see also Chapter 1) includes further investment and reform to provide a health service fit for the twenty-first century. Stakeholder interests are widened to include Care Trusts to commission health and social care in a single organisation, a concordat with private providers for NHS patients, and a drive to overcome unnecessary boundaries between professions and agencies. This was reinforced in 2001 (DoH, 2001), where a reduced number of Health Authorities will be co-located with regional government offices with the appointment of a Regional Director of Health *and* Social Care.

NEEDS OF STAKEHOLDERS

For a partnership to be successful, the needs of the now three stakeholder groups (user, provider and commissioner) must be identified, understood and met. Kano *et al.* (1984) categorise needs to be satisfied as basic, expressed and unanticipated to explain the responses that they categorise respectively as expected, wanted and exciting.

Basic needs

Basic needs are generally unnoticed by individuals, as are the assumed responses that may be technical and defined by experts.

Expressed needs

Expressed needs are described by the individual; they must be heard and understood to elicit the wanted response, which should also include the response to integral basic needs. These wanted responses are foremost in the individual's mind, are generally functional and symbolic, and will have strongly contributed to the 'choice' decision to engage in the activity.

Unanticipated needs

Unanticipated needs are shown in responses over and above those wanted and expected. These may be exciting to pursue and can elicit an excited response from individuals – so long as the integral basic and expressed needs are met.

Only expressed needs have the potential consistently to achieve mutual satisfaction, underlining the importance of encouraging articulation of needs by stakeholders. The risk of falling into the pit of dissatisfaction when basic needs remain unmet is forever present, irrespective of the higher level of need met. When unanticipated needs are met *in addition* to those expected and wanted, customer satisfaction is maximised.

THE CONCEPT OF SATISFACTION

The ratio between expectation and perception of the experience results in a level of satisfaction for the individual making the judgement. The differentiation between experience and perception of the experience is important; the *perception* is what counts. The customer therefore is *always right* as they compare *their* perception of the experience with *their* expectation (Pike and Barnes, 1996), any dissatisfaction being caused by inappropriate expectation (either through commission or omission of information in an appropriate medium or inappropriate provision – both being provider and funder responsibilities).

All individuals have generic needs (irrespective of the product or service), of convenience, control, cost and effectiveness, and additionally for services, of responsiveness. Such individuals also have service-specific needs. For example, in health care, participants will have generic service needs and specialised health-care needs, in addition to those for their user, provider or commissioner position and some may be antithetical, for example control, which all will nevertheless pursue. These generic, service specific and stakeholder needs will be further subdivided into basic, expressed and unanticipated, further complicating the picture. This complexity of the concept of quality in health care is reflected in the sparse literature, resulting in poorly understood causes of dissatisfaction and risks inappropriate resolution.

Maxwell (1984) conceptualised six dimensions of health care to which all stakeholders can probably subscribe. These generic health-care needs are:

- **Accessible** – overcoming boundaries of geography, money, time, age, language, etc.
- **Relevant** – the match between the communities' patterns of disease or handicap, and the service given
- **Effective** – optimising the prognosis for the individual patient
- **Equitable** – fair allocation between patients or communities
- **Acceptable** – what the consumer thinks about the manner of care
- **Efficient** – the lowest unit cost per unit of output.

These have traditionally been *basic* needs but the individual components are fast becoming *expressed* by different groups, in different combinations for unique circumstances.

NEEDS OF USERS

Although only a small percentage of the population use the health service at any one time, availability is of interest to all – the public in general, users and their carers and referrers.

The public

In general, the British public are poorly informed about health care; their beliefs have been influenced by experience, hearsay and the mass media. The history of the British health service from charitable to welfare provision, through a strong medical model and within a culture of deference to authority, encouraged by providers, has largely contributed to this situation (Harrison and Pollitt, 1995) (see also Chapter 1).

The public generally see health care as an art (Neuberger, 1993); they are experts in assessing human and social qualities (Haines and Iliffe, 1993), and have undertaken many of the routine caring, domestic, home-making and organisational tasks that they will assess others performing with an experienced and critical eye; they are also the least satisfied with cleanliness (Hardy and West, 1994). The state of the non-staff toilet is frequently viewed as an indicator of management performance, and now to be a specific target for improvement (DoH, 2000).

A literature search has shown that the public appear to have *basic* needs that can be categorised as follows and that become *expressed* when a response is wanted as personal needs become threatened.

- **Availability** – presence of medical care resources; accept that resources are limited, affecting decision-making (Hopkins *et al.*, 1994) for others.
- **Environment** – comparison with standards and amenities experienced in other (private) services such as banks, bakeries, restaurants and hotels (Vuori and Roger, 1989; Ellis and Whittington, 1993; Brindle, 1994), particularly convenience, control and choice (Herzlinger, 1997).
- **Finances** – investment in health care – but vote to pay less tax (Allsop, 1993); effective, rather than necessarily *cost*-effective, treatments.
- **Scope** – might or might not be expected to include those who pursue activities that push the boundaries of life beyond reasonable limits (Rivett, 1998) without enhanced contribution.
- **Preservation** – of services and particularly premises that they or their family subscribed to build, for example, the rural cottage or war memorial hospital (Banyard, 1997), which the community feel should be retained irrespective of inefficiencies.

The unexpected but exciting needs include:

- **Technical advancement** – irrespective of quality of life.

Patients

Short-term patients, both elective and emergency, represent the majority of health-care episodes, although not the greatest costs. Such transient use weakens interest and influence; it is the area most likely to be compared with the private sector; and incorporates mainly reluctant users – avoidance of ill health being the norm. Long-term patients represent the greater comparative cost resulting from the content and especially duration of their episodes; they and their carers are the most knowledgeable about their condition and the service, but their consumerist power is weakened by physical dependence and smaller numbers. The comparative needs of these groups clearly differ.

The interpersonal component

Ware and Davies (1983) particularly emphasise the importance of the 'inter-personal' component of acceptable service delivery, the need for which increases in ill health. The subject usually features strongly in any patient survey on human services. The interpersonal component includes the way in which providers interact personally with patients, particularly their:

- **attitude** (Donabedian, 1980; Enthoven, 1988)
- **information** on treatment and risks (Hopkins and Maxwell, 1990), options (Lawrence, 1992), choice (Seedhouse, 1995) and consent (Rigge, 1997)
- adequate **time** with provider (Lawrence, 1992)
- individualised **attention** (Calnan and Cant, 1993)
- **involvement** as partner (Patients' Association, 1995) on discharge (Hopkins and Maxwell, 1990; Lawrence 1992; Hopkins *et al.*, 1994) and other decisions (Hopkins and Maxwell, 1990)
- **consistency** of message (Calman, 1987).

Every interpersonal contact has the potential for concern or satisfaction; each also influences subsequent contacts by revising the expectation baseline. The policy to increase community-based care is having particular consequences for the interpersonal skills of staff, who will increasingly work within the *patient's* domain and expectations (see also Chapters 3, 4 and 10).

It appears from the sparse literature that UK health-care patients increasingly value and expect services that offer high, non-technical attributes, that is, a *social* model of health care. In the absence of more meaningful measures of success, patients apply proxy social and tangible measures, such as short waiting times and more quantity (Hopkins *et al.*, 1994), the last developing in tandem with commercialism, but without the accompanying investment.

Cohort and care groups

Within generic and specialised health-care needs, there are those of particular cohorts (people having a personal characteristic in common) and care groups (people with a health need in common). Entry into a cohort is usually insidious, for example, by age.

For the cohort of older people Cornwell (1989) found that coordination of multi-agency/multi-service health care, consistency of message and empathy were sought. Partridge *et al.* (1991) found that the same group also sought someone who listened and took account of individual perceptions and family dynamics, confidence in the treatment, individualised delivery, continuity of the carer and making the patient feel at ease. Luker and Waters (1993) found that explanation, undisrupted routine, slow pace and individualised care were sought. Most of these are *expected,* perhaps due to the characteristics of the cohort described. The needs of other cohorts may differ and might also be more clearly *expressed.* For example, a recent King's Fund survey found that older people value continuity of care and are prepared to wait to see the same GP, while younger people wanted immediate access to the NHS and were happy to see any health professional (Malbon *et al.*, 1999).

Herzlinger (1997) draws attention to knowledgeable, energetic, financially secure, health-promoting health activists. Such individuals are undertaking or commissioning database searches on their health topic of interest. Their aim is to confront providers on a more equal, and in some cases superior, knowledge basis. This can feel threatening to staff, although it has the potential for mutual benefit through partnership. Recent BBC research has identified that 4 million older people in the UK now own a PC, of whom 80 per cent find it easy to use and 25 per cent spend more time in front of a PC than a TV (Gann, 2000).

Entry of individuals into a care group will, in general, have been overt resulting from medical and/or functional needs (see also Chapter 2); their expectations are therefore more likely to be focused, expressed and gaining support from peers. An example of the needs of a care group are patients who seek podiatry. This group have an expectation of life-long treatment, including nail cutting (Jay, 1987), by competent staff with good social skills (Hares *et al.*, 1992); with the health gain objective of comfort in wearing shoes (Kemp and Winkler, 1983), reducing foot pain (Jay, 1987) and improving mobility (Cartwright and Henderson, 1986).

Members of cohorts and of care groups may be combined into a powerful force that have achieved national and charitable status, are financially secure, may have political and media support, and can run sophisticated campaigns to get their needs recognised. For example, older people who are podiatry care group members through support from the charity, Age Concern England, succeeded in getting government endorsement of social nail cutting (NHS Executive, 1994).

Carers

Unpaid carers are an increasing part of the unit of care both for the ageing population and for people of all ages with disabilities (see also Chapter 12). Recent legislation (Carers Recognition and Services Act 1996) gave carers the right to be consulted and assessed for their own need as a potential carer. Some have anticipated their role (caring for ageing parents, fostering disabled children), but some have not (caring for a partner or child with acquired disabities). Surveys have consistently shown that carers are predominantly women over 50 who are married, with some caring for more than one dependant. Changing employment circumstances are likely to affect the gender of those available to care; this has its own consequences, including enthusiasm for, and acceptability of, provision of personal care in some situations. Changing social expectations, particularly in a welfare system, are likely to also change willingness to *provide* care. A change in style of provision, for example, grades of insurance premium or enhanced benefit, may encourage it.

Carers are becoming increasingly assertive in their service demands, which many find easier to make on behalf of a third party in a welfare system. If this expressed need is added to that of the local or national group representing those for whom they care (for example, people with stroke), the pressure for a response can be substantial.

Carers' basic, and increasingly expressed, needs include:

- information and advice (Lewis, 1993)
- comprehensive response through systematic patient-centred care packages (Lewis, 1993).

Carers' expressed needs are:

- recognition and response to the resulting personal, physical, psychological and social consequences of caring, wanting respite, information, physical help, money and continuity of contact (Anderson, 1987).

Referrers

As health care has become more formalised, specialised and complex, referral systems exist to enable access to appropriate skills. Registered practitioners of most disciplines are now legally autonomous and referral may occur freely between them. For efficiency and effectiveness, the scope of practice, referral criteria, agreed goals and progress reports from those to whom patients are referred are the minimum standard that should be expected. Although responsibility and accountability are integral to autonomy, referrers will increasingly wish to be assured of the competence of those to whom they refer their patients and whom they may employ; this will be particularly important where known providers have been replaced as a result of competitive tendering.

These qualities that referrers expect of their providers are encompassed within the Maxwell six dimensions above, and will be more likely to be *expressed*.

NEEDS OF PROVIDERS

Providers of health care are usually regarded as professionals who are paid to do so. The definition should also include those paid and trained individuals with no professional qualifications who provide most of the routine formal health care under the supervision of professionals, but whose needs have been little investigated.

The basic needs of professional providers are:

- **altruism** – best interests of patient (Ellis, 1991)
- **patient survival** – against the odds (Ellis, 1991)
- **technical skill** – sophisticated practice (Stocking, 1992; Ellis, 1991)
- **individual health gain** – improvement in clinical condition as a result of intervention.

Their expressed needs are:

- **autonomy** – freedom to act on initiative (Ellis, 1991)
- **unconstrained** – by policy and resources (Pollitt, 1990).

Their unexpected, exciting needs are:

- **advancement** of provision and career through specialisation and recognition.

These needs particularly parallel the career path of clinicians where, on qualification, basic needs are inherent; through ambition, more political needs are overtly expressed; with the goal of advancement through specialisation ahead. This in itself can be problematic, when unrepresentative but exciting conditions are pursued for personal advancement resulting in public demand.

NEEDS OF COMMISSIONERS

Users in a managed market rely on the commissioner to ensure quality, both non-clinical and clinical. Such commissioners may or may not have a clinical background. Where they are themselves clinicians, they may have little or no accredited expertise in the field under review or will have only a rusty knowledge of the service. They will have been appointed on the basis of other skills, for example, knowledge of health policy, analytical skills, management experience and, particularly, the ability to make objective decisions based on the often poor evidence provided.

In a quality-managed quasi market, the commissioner is responsible for ensuring that the values and expectations of the three parties are identified, understood and acted upon. Resolution will be needed between potential conflict of values. For example, the commissioner remit of cost-effectiveness will sit particularly uncomfortably with the user value of functional effectiveness, irrespective of cost, and the provider value of lack of constraint.

Commissioners are more likely to pursue uncontroversial markers within safety, effectiveness and efficiency (Debrah, 1994) – a business model. Where commissioners have extended their vision to more qualitative measures, they will require the expert help of users and providers to synthesise dynamic and contextual expectations into prioritised, meaningful, acceptable, achievable and measurable quality standards. As has been noted, values and expectations are dynamic and contextual, and their acquisition should be appropriate and continuously fed into the process for service improvement.

Basic needs of commissioners are:

- **clinical and non-clinical quality** – provision within statutory requirements.

Expressed needs are:

- **objective decisions** – based on indisputable fact
- **equity** – of provision on the basis of evidence and morality
- **resource constraint** – to meet central objectives
- **cost-effectiveness** – to maximise value of the resource.

Unanticipated and exciting needs are:

- **population health gain** – aggregated response to basic and expressed needs.

CAPTURING EXPECTATIONS

To simplify the capture of the expectations of stakeholders in any area of health and social care, the Stakeholder Quality Expectation Model is proposed. This provides a framework for any service. The example below (Table 5.1) summarises stakeholders' expectations of chiropody for older people and incorporates evidence described above.

Table 5.1 Stakeholder Quality Expectation Model – chiropody for older people

Generic stakeholder needs	
General needs	Convenience, control, cost-effectiveness
Service needs	Responsiveness
Health-care needs	Accessibility, relevance, effectiveness, equitability, acceptablility, efficiency
User needs: User as patient needs User as referrer needs	Availability, scope Interpersonal Competence
Carer needs	Information, advice, comprehensibility, recognition
Provider needs	Altruism, survival, skill, individual health gain, advancement
Commissioner needs	Total quality, objectivity, equity, resource constraint, cost-effectiveness, population health gain
Service-specific needs	
Cohort, e.g. older people	coordination, consistency, empathy, responsiveness, assurance, explanation, continuity
Care group, e.g. chiropody	Life-long, nail cutting, shoe comfort, reduction of pain, improvement of mobility

PATIENT-CENTRED CARE

Patient-centred care is the objective of modern responsive health care. It can be seen from the discussion above that the basic, expressed and unanticipated exciting needs of patients may differ in interest and level of need from those of other stakeholders potentially compromising this objective. Numerous points of mismatch lead to potential dissatisfaction by the participants, but opportunities also exist for matching and satisfaction.

User satisfaction

The aspects of care have been described by Donabedian (1980) as falling into structure (the organisation), process (the treatment) and outcome (change in health status attributable to the structure and process). Patient satisfaction is largely sought on process, with a growing interest on their view of outcome.

Those most likely to report satisfaction are:

* older people, women and those who are married (Beaumont, 1992)
* lower socio-economic groups (Calman, 1987)
* minority groups (ethnic, social and physical) (Craig, 1990).

These characteristics equate with the least influential and those most in need and dependent on the service.

User dissatisfaction

Although 'voice' is virtually the only option for the dissatisfied in public health-care, complaints reflect only the tip of the iceberg of dissatisfaction. For example, 40 per cent of NHS patients have wanted to complain at some time, with only 4 per cent taking action (Newman and Pyne, 1995), but probably all the dissatisfied relay their story to at least ten other people. The reasons why so many who are dissatisfied fail to complain may be perceived powerlessness, barriers, personal reasons and low expectations.

The dissatisfied are disproportionately influential and those most likely to complain are:

* **higher socio-economic groups** with higher expectations (Calman, 1987) and capacity
* **carers** (Allen, 1992) who will fight more for a third party than for self
* **younger users** who are less tolerant (Craig, 1990)
* **those who were refused** what they felt was their right to expect (Scott, 1994)
* **those requiring complex interventions** (Hall *et al.*, 1990).

Most complaints are about specific issues a lay person can confidently relate to such as:

* **interpersonal skills**
* **misunderstanding**
* **patient/provider disputes, policy issues and interface discontinuity** in the 'chain' of health care amounting to around 75 per cent of complaints (McKenna, 1995).

SATISFACTION OF PATIENTS, PROVIDERS AND COMMISSIONERS

The general factors resulting from the perspectives of stakeholders identified in this review are that predominantly:

* **Users are pursuing a social model** – as a result of reluctant and deferent use; cohort experience; poor information; media influence; importance of attitude;

and proxy measurement of non-technical aspects. There is an assumption of infallibility of the body/clinical care, the provider being blamed for failure.

- **Providers are pursuing a scientific model** as a result of protection of professional values; and assumption of user values. Lack of evidence to support a scientific approach results in failure being blamed on the idiosyncratic user.
- **Commissioners are pursuing a business model** as a result of public service equity values; lack of clinical experience; and the drive for business success factors. The lack of evidence to support clinical practice leaves the commissioner reliant on provider autonomy.

These positions provide the ammunition for both healthy collaboration and unhealthy conflict (see also Chapter 7). The former will ensure that the changing interests of the groups are represented, with participatory education and specification reducing the interface gaps over time.

Figure 5.1 portrays these relationships and indicates that, when stakeholders' needs are congruent, mutual satisfaction with the service could be said to exist. Congruence will depend on equal partnership, reciprocal education, common assessment of need, shared information, mutual understanding, agreed values and clear specifications. To avoid complacency and a static culture when expectations are known to be forever changing, ongoing review of standards will facilitate the ultimate goal of a service pursuing continuous quality improvement (CQI).

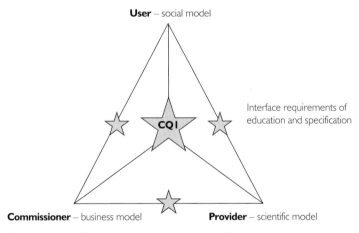

Figure 5.1 Stakeholder satisfaction through continuous quality improvement

DEVELOPMENT OF A MODEL FOR ACHIEVING STAKEHOLDER SATISFACTION

As part of a research project to develop a model to achieve stakeholder satisfaction (Squires, 2002), it was agreed by a stakeholder group that specifications for the quality improvement process would consist of three parts:

1 'Core' standards developed for all providers as a result of statutory requirements or central guidance such as those emanating from the National Institute for Clinical Excellence (NICE)

2 'Care Group' standards drawn from national best practice for all providers of that service to the authority such as those emanating from National Service Frameworks (NSF); this would also include national accreditation schemes
3 'Service Specific' standards developed from the unique quality improvement needs of individual providers to meet local stakeholder requirements.

It is anticipated that the new initiatives from the National Institute for Clinical Excellence (NICE) (Clinical Standards Board in Scotland) and the National Service Frameworks (NSFs) will address many of the issues in Core and Care Group standards (see Chapter 1). Locally, the three sets of resulting standards would be documented, implemented, monitored, the results added to other quality intelligence received during the period and the process repeated within the contracting cycle with the aim of achieving continuous quality improvement.

Service Specific standards were identified by the stakeholder group as key to quality improvement in unique local situations. As expectations are likely to differ at each stage of the care process, each stage will need to be considered separately; Ovretveit (1994) has provided a visual cue – the patient's path – to cover the stages in an episode of care from selection and assessment, through treatment and review to discharge. This generic model can be adapted for diverse specific situations, for example, community nursing, stroke units and outpatient physiotherapy.

The Quality Pathway Matrix

A Patient Pathway Quality Matrix has been developed (Squires, 2000) so that the three stakeholders can jointly and overtly identify areas of concern along the local pathway of care and against the six dimensions of quality health services (Maxwell, 1984) described in Figure 5.2.

The hypothetical patient can be tracked through the system, each step being audited against stakeholders' perceptions and evidence of achievement on the relevant quality dimension (a triangle acting as a reminder). The lack of agreement within and between disciplines on criteria and interventions makes the patient's journey along this 'chain' of health care difficult, increasing inequitable variation, decreasing satisfaction, confusing service scope, compromising meaningful audit and raising more questions. Rehabilitation of older people relies on complex multi-agency relationships and interactions, the complete chain of care probably only being known by the patient and/or carer.

After experimentation with the pilot matrix, a column for 'development' was added to ensure that planned service changes were similarly addressed, so that quality becomes an integral part of planning from inception.

Structure, process or outcome?

There are assumed links between the structure, process and outcome (SPO) components of any issue. For example, adequate preconditions are more likely to produce an acceptable process and outcome (Vuori and Roger, 1989), because at least the structures of staffing and organisation are present; and that adequate process produces an acceptable outcome (Donabedian, 1988). Although these

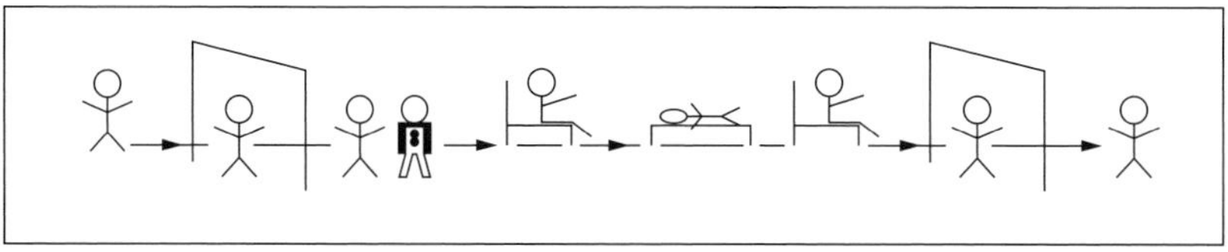

	Selection S/P/O ∇	Entry S/P/O ∇	1st contact S/P/O ∇	Assessment S/P/O ∇	Intervention S/P/O ∇	Review S/P/O ∇	Closure S/P/O ∇	Follow-up S/P/O ∇	Development S/P/O ∇
Effective									
Acceptable									
Efficient									
Accessible									
Equitable									
Relevant									

S – Structure
P – Process
O – Outcome

Figure 5.2 Quality Pathway Matrix

have yet to be proven, common sense makes them seem likely to be conducive to a higher quality of service. Identification of whether the identified issue of concern was structure, process or outcome enables setting of clear standards and criteria, and 'SPO' in the model was used as a cue for such identification.

Setting standards

Starting with the highest priority, the issues can be prioritised by the group and developed into standards or goals following recognised best practice of meeting SMART and RUMBA criteria (specific, measurable, achievable, relevant, theoretically based, understandable and behavioural).

The resulting standards, including wording and the pace of implementation, should be agreed by commissioner, provider and patient representative. The next stage is for the commissioner and provider to agree the pace of implementation of the contracted standard, using the project cycle of Plan, Do, Check and Act (Table 5.2).

Table 5.2 Project implementation cycle

P = Plan:	Completed indicates a plan is in hand
D = Do:	Completed implies the plan is executed
C = Check:	Completed implies the plan is monitored
A = Act:	Completed implies the results are incorporated into a timetabled action plan with review

Expected (E) performance is agreed within the contract, and the provider required to report on *actual* (A) achievement each quarter (Q). This has proved a highly efficient and effective process in that reporting is brief but informative. A concise summary each quarter to provide the context, and exception reports added as appropriate or requested.

Two examples of the resulting standard in a podiatry service for older people are provided in Table 5.3.

Based on the manual system, software has been developed to enable the quality progress reports to be input by the provider with conversion to a graphic report, and sent by e-mail to the commissioner, further reducing the need for paper, the bane of most quality systems. Figure 5.3 shows the screen view of provider progress on a specific standard.

Table 5.3 Examples of service specific standards in a chiropody service

Standard 1:	an analysis of the cause of inappropriate referrals will be undertaken by the provider and an appropriate action plan implemented.
Target:	All inappropriate referrals.
Measure and report:	Quarterly progress report on implementation of system. Full review in annual report.

Plan	Do	Check	Act
E Q1	Q2	Q3	Q4
A Q1	Q2	Q3	Q4

Exception report attached
yes/no
Additional comments
1st quarter: Planning the project
2nd quarter: Project being implemented
3rd quarter: Review of inappropriate referrals
4th quarter: New policy in place Report submitted

Standard 2:	The provider will review a sample of clients receiving just foot care, identify common factors, especially contact with formal carers and suggest an action plan.
Target:	Sample of clients receiving just foot care.
Measure and report:	Evidence of a system to analyse and quarterly progress report on implementation and action plan. Full review in annual report.

Plan	Do	Check	Act
E Q1	Q2	Q3	Q4
A Q1	Q2	Q3	Q4

Exception report attached
yes/no
Additional comments
1st quarter: Planning the project
2nd quarter: Sampling undertaken
3rd quarter: Common criteria identified
4th quarter: Working with HA on nail-cutting project

The commissioning aim, which the right or standard supports, has a target measure. The agreed pacing of the quality cycle is depicted as expected input, and can be compared with that achieved depicted as actual input. The expected output compliance and actual output compliance achieved are compared.

In the example, the standard and its aim are documented. It was jointly anticipated that there would be 90 per cent compliance each quarter. During the year the provider would have a process for quality improvement in hand, the anticipated progress on each standard being negotiated as part of the contract. In this example, a plan will be completed in the first quarter, implemented in the second, monitored in the third, with action on findings in the fourth. What actually occurred was progress as agreed in the first quarter, no progress in the second providing an indicator for possible investigation, implementation in the third quarter and checking in the fourth. Action on the results was not achieved within the period and 90 per cent compliance was only reached in the fourth quarter, being 60 per cent in the first quarter, 70 per cent in the second and 80 per cent in the third. Any lack of adherence might trigger a focused investigation. For standards documented for non-NHS services funded by the Health Authority, such as private or independent provision or joint funding for social care, the process works in the same way.

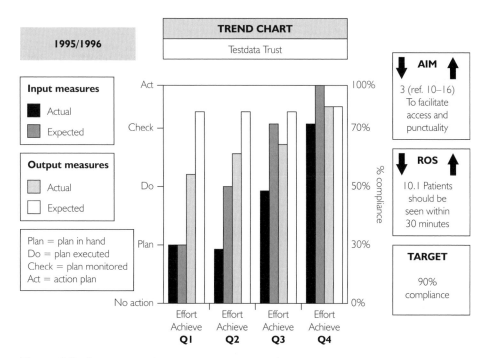

Figure 5.3 Screen view of progress on quality standard

Key to Figure 5.3

ROS:	Right or Standard	**Actual status:**	plan/do/check/act achieved
AIM:	aim of the Right or Standard	**Expected output:**	numerical target expected
Target:	numerical target for compliance	**Actual output:**	numerical target achieved
Expected status	plan/do/check/act negotiated position	**Q1.95, Q2.95, Q3.95, Q4.95:**	quarters in 1995

SUMMARY

The identification of needs of the stakeholders in health care is essential if a partnership approach is to be successful. These needs are different both in content, context and intensity. Services for older people have to date been largely exempt from expressed and rising public expectations. This has been due to the cohort effect of the user group, many remembering the pre-NHS days and eternally 'grateful' for what they receive. Newer cohorts are, and will be increasingly, different.

The potential size of this group of newly/early retired users, who have much to give, little to lose, available resources and a lifetime of contacts and experience is an influence *very seriously* underestimated by the service. Having lost the opportunity for efficient proactive partnership, the service will ultimately respond in a costly reactive way. How these individuals are identified and their contribution used will provide a productive opportunity for the proactive – and a serious threat to the reactive. The inclusion of service users within key parts of the current NHS reforms provides an opportunity for a proactive partnership.

REFERENCES

Abel-Smith, B. (1994) How to contain healthcare costs: an international dilemma. Lecture, 15 November, London School of Economics, London.

Allen, I. (1992) Older people: their choice and participation. In: *Towards a Social Policy on Ageing: A consultation report* (ed. Lively, B.), The Research for Ageing Trust/Academic Department of Medicine for the Elderly, Chelsea–Westminster Hospital, London.

Allsop, J. (1993) The voice of the user in healthcare. In: *In the Best of Health* (eds Beck, E., Lonsdale, S., Newman, S. and Patterson, D.), Chapman & Hall, London.

Anderson, R. (1987) The unremitting burden on carers. *British Medical Journal*, **294**(6564), 73.

Banyard, R. (1997) Out in the field. *Health Service Journal*, **107**(5538), 30–31.

Beaumont, D. (1992) Consumer relations. *Care of the Elderly*, **4**(10), 456–457.

Brindle, D. (1994) Less is often more. *The Guardian*, 22 June, 12.

Calman, M. (1987) *Health and Illness: The lay perspective*, Tavistock, London.

Calnan, M. and Cant, S. (1993) You pays your money. *Health Service Journal*, **103**(5353), 31.

Cartwright, A. and Henderson, G. (1986) *More Trouble with Feet*, HMSO, London.

Cornwell, J. (1989) *The Consumer View: Elderly people and community health services*, King's Fund, London.

Craig, A. (1990) Buying health care for the community: The role of health authorities as purchasers. Royal Institute of Public Health and Hygiene Symposium, London, 25 July.

Debrah, Y.A. (1994) Evolution and implementation of a quality improvement programme: a case study of two organisations. *Total Quality Management*, **5**(3), 11–25.

Department of Health [DoH] (1989) *Working for Patients*, HMSO, London.

DoH (2000) *The NHS Plan,* The Stationery Office, London.

DoH (2001) *Stiking the Balance of Power in the NHS,* The Stationery Office, London.

Donabedian, A. (1980) *Explorations in Quality Assessment and Monitoring,* Health Administration Press, Michigan, IL.

Donabedien, A. (1988) The quality of care. How can it be assessed? *Journal of the American Medical Association,* **260**(12), 1743–1748.

Ellis, R. (1991) Competence in the caring professions. In: *Professional Competence and Quality Assurance in the Caring Profession* (ed. Ellis, R.), Chapman & Hall, London.

Ellis, R. and Whittington, D. (1993) *Quality Assurance in Health Care: A handbook,* Edward Arnold, London.

Enthoven, A.C. (1988) *Theory and Practice of Managed Competition in Health Care Finance,* NHC Publishers, North Holland.

Gann, B. (2000) Patient participation in an electronic age. Presentation to *Involving and Empowering People.* 21 September, Harrogate Management Centre Ltd, London.

Haines, A. and Iliffe, S. (1993) Primary health care. In: *In the Best of Health?* (eds Beck, E., Lonsdale, S., Newman, S. and Patterson, D.), Chapman & Hall, London.

Hall, J.A., Feldstein, M., Fretwell, M.D., Rowe, J.W. and Epstein, A.M. (1990) Older patients' health status and satisfaction with medical care in an HMO population. *Medical Care,* **28**(3), 261–270.

Hardy, G. and West, M. (1994) Happy talk. *Health Service Journal,* **104**(5410), 24–26.

Hares, T., Spencer, J., Gallagher, M., Bradshaw, C. and Webb, I. (1992) Diabetes care: who are the experts? *Quality in Health Care,* **1**, 219–224.

Harrison, S. and Pollitt, C. (1995) *Controlling Health Professionals,* Open University Press, Buckingham.

Herzlinger, R. (1997) *Market Driven Healthcare,* Addison Wesley, New York.

Hopkins, A. and Maxwell, R. (1990) Contracts and quality of care. *British Medical Journal,* **300**, 919–922.

Hopkins, A., Gabbay, J. and Neuberger, J. (1994) Role of users in health care in achieving a quality service. *Quality in Health Care,* **3**, 203–209.

Jay, M.W. (1987) Quality – in whose eyes? *The Chiropodist,* **42**(8), 319–327.

Kano, N., Seraku, N. and Takahashi, F. (1984) Attractive quality must be equitable. *Quality* **14**(2), 39–44 (in Japanese), cited in Bergman and Klefsjo (1994).

Kemp, J. and Winkler, J.T. (1983) *Problems Afoot: Need and efficiency in footcare,* Disabled Living Foundation, London.

Lawrence, R.N. (1992) Assessing the true cost of minimally invasive surgery. *Care of the Elderly,* January, 14.

Lewis, J. (1993) Community care: policy imperatives, joint planning and enabling authorities. *Journal of Interprofessional Care,* **7**(1), 7–14.

Luker, K. and Waters, K. (1993) The six o'clock shock. *Health Service Journal,* **103**(5349), 20–22.

Malbon, G., Jenkins, C. and Gillam, S. (1999) *What do Londoners Think of Their General Practice,* King's Fund, London.

Maxwell, R.J. (1984) Quality assessment in healthcare. *British Medical Journal,* **288**(1), 470–471.

McKenna, H.P. (1995) A multiprofessional approach to audit. *Nursing Standard,* **8**(42), 20–21.

Neuberger, J. (1993) What's on the outcomes agenda? *Outcome Briefing,* **2**, 23–24.

Newman, K. and Pyne, T. (1995) Contracting for quality: a study of purchaser practices. *Journal of the Association for Quality in Healthcare*, **3**(1), 16–24.

NHS Executive (1994) *Feet First*, NHS Executive, London.

NHS Executive (1997) *The New NHS: Modern and dependable*, NHS Executive, London.

Ovretveit, J. (1994) Roads to recovery. *Health Service Journal*, **104**(5407), 32–33.

Partridge, C.J., Johnstone, M. and Morris, L. (1991) *Disability and Health Services: Perceptions, beliefs and experiences of elderly people*, King's College Centre for Physiotherapy Research, London.

Patients' Association (1995) *Patient's Voice*, Summer, 68, 1.

Pike, J. and Barnes, R. (1996) *TQM in Action*, Chapman & Hall, London.

Pollitt, C. (1990) Doing business in the temple? Managers and quality assurance in the public services. *Public Administration*, **68**, 435–452.

Ranade, W. (1994) *A Future for the NHS: Healthcare in the 90's*, Longman, London.

Rigge, M. (1997) Keeping the NHS customer satisfied. *Health Service Journal*, **107**(5577), 24–27.

Rivett, G. (1998) *From Cradle to Grave – Fifty years of the NHS*, The King's Fund, London.

Scott, E. (1994) Don't keep patients in the dark. *Management in General Practice*, **12**, 50.

Seedhouse, D. (1995) The logic of health reform. In: *Reforming Health Care* (ed. Seedhouse, D.), Wiley, Chichester.

Squires, A.J. (2002) Stakeholder quality in healthcare: synthesising expectations for mutual satisfaction. PhD Thesis, City University, London.

Stocking, B. (1992) Promoting change in clinical care. *Quality in Health Care*, **1**, 56–60.

Strong, P. and Robinson, J. (1990) *The NHS Under New Management*, Open University Press, Milton Keynes.

Vincent, J.A. (1999) *Politics, Power and Old Age*, Open University Press, Buckingham.

Vuori, H. and Roger, F. (1989) Issues in quality assurance – the European scene. *Quality Assurance in Health Care*, **1**(2/3), 125–135.

Ware, J.E. and Davies, A.R. (1983) Behavioural consequences of consumer dissatisfaction with medical care. *Evaluation and Programme Planning*, **6**, 291–297.

6 THE NATIONAL SERVICE FRAMEWORK FOR OLDER PEOPLE: TIMELY AND CHALLENGING

Amanda J. Squires

AIMS OF THE CHAPTER

As part of the UK government's drive to improve quality and reduce variation in the NHS (Department of Health [DoH], 1998a), a series of National Service Frameworks (NSFs) have begun to set the standards for local service delivery in the NHS in England and Wales. Parallel arrangements are being developed for Scotland and Northern Ireland. Frank Dobson, Secretary for State for Health in 1999, launched the initiative as a whole by declaring:

> *National Service Frameworks are not statements of pious hope. In the future they will improve services all over the country and make sure the NHS delivers top quality services for everybody, no matter where they live. They will also spell out the practical arrangements which will be put in place to prevent and treat the various conditions they cover. Standards will be set and they will be met.*

NSFs will also provide a means whereby related policies are linked, reinforced and targeted towards a single direction (Swage, 2000). This centralising force responds to a range of criticisms about variations in quality and levels of provision.

An external reference group will be formed to bring together the key stakeholders of providers, users, commissioners, partner agencies and other advocates. This consensus approach is designed to steer each Framework advising the Department of Health on the whole system of care in the following areas:

- improving the quality of care and health outcomes using the best available evidence of clinical and cost-effectiveness
- reducing undesirable variations in health care
- setting out the expectations of NHS care to the public and providers.

Each NSF includes:

- a definition of the scope of the Framework
- the evidence base underpinning intervention including assessment of need; current performance; evidence of clinical and cost-effectiveness; and identification of significant gaps and pressures in the service
- national standards and timescales for delivery
- an assessment of key interventions and associated costs
- commissioned work to support implementation, including the NHS research and development programme; critical appraisal of good practice; benchmarks; and outcome indicators
- supporting programmes including workforce planning; education and training; personal and organisational development; and development of information management and technology

• a performance management framework for commissioners to monitor progress.

These arenas are not new but based on the public health agenda (DoH, 1998b) (see also Chapter 1). They stand in contrast to the Patient's Charter, which set out a series of expectations, that arguably were difficult to meet (see also Chapter 5).

Following publication, local committees will be formed to oversee implementation through local clinical governance frameworks, inter-agency working and inclusive participation. Some flexibility to meet local needs is anticipated, although national consistency is a prominent theme. Local monitoring will be through the performance management framework, with ultimate monitoring through the Commission for Health Improvement as part of its remit to specifically review progress on NSFs, as well as through routine clinical governance reviews. Gaps in the current evidence base will be used to inform the research and development agenda. NSFs have already been produced for Mental Health and Coronary Heart Disease. The third to be published is that specifically for Older People, although some components such as stroke and falls also have application to younger age groups.

THE NSF FOR OLDER PEOPLE

After much work by all groups represented in this book and campaigning organisations for older people, but with delay explained only by the complexity of the subject, the NSF for Older People was published without ceremony in March 2001 (DoH, 2001a). It describes itself as a ten-year programme addressing the needs of older people by linking services to support independence and promote good health. The time span is important, not only to enable phased implementation by providers, but also to recognise that the needs and particularly expectations of successive cohorts of older people and their carers, attitudes of society, the roles of providers, medical developments, assistive technology and information technology will change over this period (see also Chapter 5). Such a time span also means that progress can be hard to judge, as rising expectations will necessarily exceed solutions designed for previous needs.

Although a lot of effective work is known to exist within services for older people, the many reported variations in service provision and quality have caused public and professional concern. The NSF aims to develop higher quality services for older people, specialised services for key conditions, and a culture change that will ensure that all older people and their carers are always treated with respect, dignity and fairness. A key strategy for successful implementation will be the active engagement of primary, secondary and tertiary care.

The NSF specifically addresses those conditions that are particularly significant for older people and that have not been covered in other NSFs: stroke, falls and mental health problems associated with older age. Older people will also benefit from the earlier NSFs on Mental Health and Coronary Heart Disease, as well as those forthcoming on Diabetes, Chronic Neurological and Renal Diseases. Conditions such as stroke and falls and even dementia addressed in the Older People NSF are not limited to older people, and the standards and service models will apply for all who need them, regardless of their age. The deadlines for implementation are tight, with the entire Framework to be delivered by April 2005. The new arrangements are to be funded by investment included in the NHS Plan (DoH, 2000).

Professional bodies and user groups have broadly welcomed the framework, with shared concerns that such high standards, low resources and aggressive, tight deadlines will result in an unreasonable mismatch between vision and reality; and the fear that younger people might perceive improving access to treatment for older people as discriminatory, and fuel a dangerous backlash.

Despite such caveats, those who have for so long fought largely rearguard actions to improve health and social services, organisation and attitudes for the benefit of older people (see Chapter 1) now have the opportunity to do so in partnership both across agencies and with increasingly knowledgeable, assertive and organised user groups (see Chapters 5 and 12). The reason for such delay in publication and haste in implementation can only be surmised as realisation that the plan is not fully deliverable, not least because of the lack of knowledge, resource and skills; growing concern at what expectations might be unleashed; and the potential support of 18 per cent of the adult population eligible to vote in any election, who, being the most likely to vote, actually make up 25 per cent of adult voters; as well as the complexity of the subject.

In Scotland, *Comunity Care: A Joint Future* (Scottish Executive, 2000) intends that older people will have more 'joined up community services' that will similarly make a difference, together with a tight timetable for rebalancing the care of older people. The emphasis in Scotland is very much on partnership working between health, social work and housing to ensure that older people are enabled to remain at home in their community. The challenge for health professionals will be in sharing skills across traditional service boundaries, developing multi-skilled, generic support workers and putting the older persons' needs at the centre of the care. The Chief Medical Officer for Scotland has formed an expert group that will review the care of older people in acute and primary health care services in Scotland and the Clinical Standards Board for Scotland (CSBS, 2001) will launch standards for health care of older people in the autumn of 2001.

The NSF provides a blueprint for change, focuses on improvement and reduction in inequalities, reinstates and progresses specialist care, facilitates investment and provides a clear agenda for implementation and progress (Wilson, 2001). The absence of specificity; lack of knowledge, skills and resources; and in some cases the inability to influence a much wider agenda will make implementation as well as achievement of the standards challenging (Johnson, 2001). There will need to be mutual local realisation about what is achievable within competing agendas. In comparison, the NSF for Cancer services is specific and deliverable, the underpinning science is good, treatment is well researched and the targets can, and are already, being achieved. The advantage that the NSF for Older

People has over others is that all those responsible for implementation can anticipate being recipients, which may add energy to the development of services that will find wide acceptability.

Key features

Older people are the main users of health and social care. The NSF provides a strategy to draw together new and existing requirements for services to be fair, high quality and integrated to support independence, promote good health, provide specialist services where necessary and treat older people with respect and dignity. Not only is the number of older people increasing, but so are their expectations, particularly those just entering old age who have had different life experiences (see Chapters 1 and 5). For this group, promotion of a healthy active life will be the goal. For those, usually older, groups beginning to experience health and social needs, the goals will be early identification of problems and provision of effective and timely responses. For those who have become frail in old age, the goals will be to anticipate the interaction of needs and ensure integration of response.

The NSF also considers the changing components of the older population, particularly the increasing number of older people from ethnic minorities (see Chapter 3); those with sensory disability (see Chapters 17 and 20); learning disability (see Chapter 9); those in prison (see Chapter 10); and carers of older people (see also Chapter 12).

The NSF also accepts that older people may receive services from a range of agencies within a range of environments. The NSF applies to services provided by health, social services and the independent sector, delivered at home, in residential care, nursing home, hospital or intermediate care facility.

Not surprisingly, the NSF was broadly welcomed by the professions who have nevertheless responded with consistent themes:

- concerns about the capacity of the current workforce to deliver the NSF along with other initiatives
- disquiet that workforce planning arrangements to meet this and other initiatives are all reliant on overstretched health and social care staff
- anxiety that education and training at all levels, together with curricula that incorporate the key messages and themes, are insufficient to support implementation.

The NSF in detail

Four main themes constitute the NSF, supported by eight standards:

Theme 1: Respecting the individual

Standard 1: Rooting out age discrimination
NHS services will be provided, regardless of age, on the basis of clinical need alone. Social care services will not use age in their eligibility criteria or policies, to restrict access to available services.

Standard 2: Person-centred care
NHS and social care services treat older people as individuals and enable them to make choices about their own care. This is achieved through the single assessment process, integrated commissioning arrangements and integrated provision of services, including community equipment and continence services.

Theme 2: Intermediate care

Standard 3: Intermediate care
Older people will have access to a new range of intermediate care services at home or in designated care settings, to promote their independence by providing enhanced services from the NHS and councils to prevent unnecessary hospital admissions and effective rehabilitation services to enable early discharge from hospital and prevent premature or unnecessary admission to long-term residential care.

Theme 3: Providing evidence based specialist care

Standard 4: General hospital services
Older people's care in hospital is delivered through appropriate specialist care and by hospital staff who have the right set of skills to meet their needs.

Standard 5: Stroke
The NHS will take action to prevent strokes, working in partnership with other agencies where appropriate. People who are thought to have had a stroke have access to diagnostic services, are treated appropriately by a specialist stroke service, and subsequently, with their carers, participate in a multidisciplinary programme of secondary prevention and rehabilitation.

Standard 6: Falls
The NHS, working in partnership with councils, takes action to prevent falls and reduce resultant fractures or other injuries in their populations of older people. Older people who have fallen receive effective treatment and rehabilitation, and with their carers, receive advice on prevention through a specialist falls service.

Standard 7: Mental health and older people
Older people who have mental health problems have access to integrated mental health services, provided by the NHS and councils to ensure effective diagnosis, treatment and support, for them and for their carers.

Theme 4: Promoting an active, healthy life

Standard 8: The promotion of health and active life in old age
The health and well-being of older people is promoted through a coordinated programme of action led by the NHS with support from councils.

Implementing the NSF

Implementation will be led by the newly appointed National Director for Older People, Professor Ian Philp, who has met with professional bodies to discuss how they can support implementation. There will be regional leads to monitor the progress on the action points. Local implementation of the NSF will require consultation with older people and their carers; a shared vision and partnership working appropriate to the diverse needs of the local population; leadership; inclusive planning; and communication. Local arrangements were to be in place by 30 June 2001 (communications strategy by May 2001) include designated leads, plans and identification of gaps.

Five programmes will support implementation:

1 **Finance** – additional financial resources for services for older people, intermediate care and promotion of independence
2 **Workforce** – timely availability, recruitment, development and retention of the right number and skill of staff as well as new ways of working
3 **Research and development** – through targeted research funding, particularly reduction of disability and promotion of independence; needs of carers and minority groups; innovation
4 **Practice development** – through focused use of existing services, such as the Cochrane Collaboration, NHS Centre for Review and Dissemination, NICE and Social Care Institute for Excellence
5 **Information** – a strategy to provide local information and to support care such as electronic and coordinated standards and records.

Monitoring implementation

Local performance measures already include some relevant components, such as joint investment plans (JIPs), NHS Service and Financial Frameworks (SaFFs) and Performance Assessment Frameworks (PAFs). These will be complemented by regular user and carer surveys; existing reviews and inspections (through Social Services Inspectorate (SSI), Audit Commission, Commission for Health Improvement (CHI), Best Value and National Care Standards Commission); and a combined and focused approach to services for older people by SSI, CHI and the Audit Commission.

The Modernisation Board supported by the Taskforce for Older People will provide a national overview of progress.

PRACTICAL CONSIDERATIONS

There is much to applaud within the NSF. It states formally many principles that are already included within this book and that have long been acknowledged as 'best practice'. Hopefully, inclusion within this strategy will ensure that these principles become accepted as the 'norm' everywhere and not just in isolated centres of excellence. The contributors to this book have made reference to the NSF in their chapters, and bring together here their integrated comments on the practical issues that will face local interdisciplinary/agency teams now charged with implementing the strategy. These comments are under the eight standards, implementation support and requirements, and monitoring.

Standards

> *Standard 1: Rooting out age discrimination*
> NHS services will be provided, regardless of age, on the basis of clinical need alone. Social care services will not use age in their eligibility criteria or policies, to restrict access to available services.

It is perhaps a sad reflection on our society and culture that this needs stating at all. Age-related judgements in access, organisation and delivery of health care have and will continue to be made; the important feature is that they should be evidence based. Older people with health problems from black and minority ethnic groups can be particularly disadvantaged and are likely to suffer more discrimination in accessing services (see Chapter 3). Greater involvement of older people at all levels in both health and social services will do much to educate, as well as ensure relevant policies are not discriminatory but still allow individuals' views about their care to be expressed.

The background to such attitudes by society, providers and indeed older people themselves, needs to be understood and the attitudes consistently challenged in education programmes. There will also need to be further research into effectiveness of care at various ages, with better understanding regarding the links between biological and chronological ageing, so that clinical need will be the driving force (see Chapter 2). Those falling within agreed, objective criteria will need to be encouraged to access services; those falling outside will expect a full and reasoned explanation and alternative care and/or advice to meet what they perceive as an unmet need (see Chapter 5).

Meeting this standard will be challenging for primary care organisations, which will have to set up information systems that can monitor variations in access to and use of services by older people.

The availability of staff from the full range of specialist services to meet different demands will also have to be addressed. For example, anti-ageist values and person-centred care have been central to many social workers' practice but often thwarted by lack of resources and organisational problems. Person-centred care may result in opportunities for staff to work in a range of environments, in which conditions of employment may have to be negotiated and the risk to service fragmentation considered (Chartered Society of Physiotherapy [CSP], 2001). Much progress has been made in changing attitudes and perceptions at both undergraduate and postgraduate level towards working with older people. Much remains to be achieved. For example, there is evidence (Finn, 1986; Morris and Minichello, 1992) that very few physiotherapists express a desire to work in the speciality, citing lack of professional status as one of the reasons for this. Developments in intermediate care and rehabilitation services, together with implementation of the NSF, will afford the opportunity to create nurse and therapist clinical specialist and consultant posts in older people's services offering the clinical leadership required to move services forward and to shape education at both undergraduate and post graduate level.

Social care services will no longer be able to use age in their eligibility criteria to restrict access to services and the additional funding made available for community equipment (see Chapter 16) will potentially enhance the lives of many older people who wish to remain independent within their own homes. The resource issue will need to be addressed by the growing mismatch between expectation and reality.

There will therefore need to be consideration of representation, education, research, comprehensive availability, career opportunity and the relevant resources for this standard to be addressed, and acknowledgement that ageism is part of a much wider system of social structure.

Standard 2: Person-centred care
NHS and social care services treat older people as individuals and enable them to make choices about their own care. This is achieved through the single assessment process, integrated commissioning arrangements and integrated provision of services, including community equipment and continence services.

The purpose of rehabilitation is to facilitate the return of individuals to their chosen lifestyle, and by definition should be person-centred. There remain numerous opportunities for providers to develop better skills in eliciting what perceptions individual older people and their carers have of their abilities and opportunities. They will need to match these more effectively with the availability of skills and resources, in particular communication skills to explain any gap that exists between perception and reality. The added opportunity to develop services that meet perceived needs more appropriately is a prime task for commissioners, particularly to meet the needs of the growing numbers of older people from minority groups entering old age.

While education for all staff at all stages in their careers can support this standard, users need to be informed and empowered to take part confidently in decisions about their care. Many still hold the traditional view that the 'professional' knows best, but this will doubtless change as future generations of older people will be more used to a consumer-orientated culture (see also Chapter 5). All professionals will need to negotiate with and respond appropriately to and learn from the complaints, criticisms, concerns and compliments of articulate users.

A single assessment process to ascertain needs is also very welcome, and numerous examples of partial progress exist. The level of assessment will need to be clarified: will it be generic screening or a series of specialist assessments? It has been well established that older people who have complex co-morbidities associated with older age are best assessed and treated by specialists (see Chapter 2). It is commendable that nurses are to be involved with assessment of nursing needs. Other disciplines likewise should be involved in assessments that either require their specialist assessment skills or advice on provision of their services. In circumstances where this is not feasible, relevant disciplines will need to ensure that colleagues are well briefed and trained on transferable assessment skills (see Chapter 8).The outcome will also need to be clarified: will it be based on need or service availability, and who will have responsibility for delivering what (CSP, 2001)? It is essential that it is a means to an end not just a process to be achieved.

Assessors will need to be highly skilled, and this task should become the centre of activity. Whether a single individual can accomplish this is unlikely, although some assumptions of ability will continue to be made. The example of continence assessment is a prime example (see Chapter 21), where the issue may be the most crucial need to the individual, but few if any in a conventional core team will have the expertise for a thorough approach. The most important skill for the care professional involved in assessment will be the ability to appreciate their personal limitations and knowledge of the local networks and avenues available to obtain specialist support.

Assessment determines use of resources and outcome and requires finely honed skills of all participants. For this to be comprehensive and effective across all disciplines and agencies it will require mutual education, mutual trust and respect – true interdisciplinary working (see also Chapter 7), as well as the technology to support communication across agencies and disciplines, inside and beyond the core team. The development of an effective national tool for assessment will be a further challenge, together with the training of all staff in the skills to implement it. Without a national, valid and reliable assessment tool acceptable to all participants, the ambition of reduction in variation cannot be achieved.

The drive to integrated commissioning and provision through the accelerated development of Primary Care Trusts, formation of Strategic Health Authorities, and particularly the co-location and unified management of health and social care (see Chapter 1) should at last bring together the two key statutory agencies, as well as the independent sector in commissioning and providing health and social care for older people. The ultimate opportunity of Care Trusts, formed, subject to legislation, through a formal partnership between local government and an NHS Trust, could enable an integrated budget for commissioning and provision, ensuring clarity of direction and promoting unification of all services that facilitate health and its care for older people and others. Its staff, however, will need to become more used to sharing decisions and different perceptions of need and risk.

Locally, PCTs will need to develop robust systems that can identify and meet the needs of local people, develop an effective single assessment process, ensure that provision is similarly integrated and that services to meet the identified needs both currently and in the future in an appropriate timescale are available. Efficiencies can be gained where time has been spent in duplication of roles, or repairing the damage caused to those who have fallen through the net.

At an operational level, some disciplines represented in this book have traditionally been employed within one agency, while a few have worked across both statutory agencies, for example social work, occupational therapy, dietetics and podiatry, and some have experience of the independent sector, for example, physiotherapy and nursing. The majority of pharmacists are employed within the private sector and their current contract with the NHS is such that they only get reimbursed for items dispensed – not for advice or any other contribution. Although many will actively wish to be involved with the NSF, it will currently be on a voluntary basis, although negotiations are in hand to change the system. There will be a need for all disciplines now to understand alternative organisational cultures and statutory requirements in order for such integration to be successful.

The increased funding and proposed integration of community equipment services (DoH, 2001b) will enable many older people to retain their independence and to remain at home, as well as save staff time accessing equipment across organisational and funding boundaries (see also Chapter 16). There will need to be clarification regarding the financial criteria for access to such services, which currently differ between health and social services. Integration of continence services based on good practice, policies, procedures, guidelines and targets is considered further in Chapter 21.

Standard 3: Intermediate care
Older people will have access to a new range of intermediate care services at home or in designated care settings, to promote their independence by providing enhanced services from the NHS and councils to prevent unnecessary hospital admissions and effective rehabilitation services to enable early discharge from hospital and prevent premature or unnecessary admission to long-term residential care.

Slow-stream rehabilitation patients have been moved into the independent sector since the 1980s, where care has been largely custodial. The provision of 'intermediate care', of which rehabilitation is a key component, in partnership with local social services departments, will be a challenge to this sector, which will need a comprehensive programme of skill development and support from NHS colleagues where the skills largely remain. It will also be another major challenge for PCTs, which will become the conductor of a different interdisciplinary orchestra (see Chapter 11).

Many successful local schemes have been developed over the past few years. The key to this next phase of intermediate care development is integrated and shared care, including primary and secondary health care, social care and involving the statutory and independent sectors as equal partners. Ensuring access to acute services and intermediate care at the time they are needed will be crucial. The fact that the duration is stated as six weeks (with the opportunity for review) may compromise those with long-term rehabilitation needs who could avoid admission to long-term care (CSP, 2001). In some senses, provision of the increased numbers of beds is the easy part, while building up such increased provision with appropriate staff, which is used most effectively within a culture of realistic cure rather than just care, will be the challenge. Specialist staff will need to consider how they develop their role along either a generic or specialist route; and as 'treater' of older people or 'teacher' of their other carers, or a mixture of both (CSP, 2001).

Intermediate care services should include the full range of disciplines outlined in this book, with support from care assistants and administrative staff, and involvement of users and carers. The methodology for determining physiotherapy staffing for a range of services for older people in a range of settings has been described in Chapter 10 and is transferable to other disciplines. Similar demands for the involvement of allied health professions in a number of other initiatives, for example, preservation of good health, prevention of ill health, acute rehabilitation, and support and maintenance of those discharged from institutional care, should result in more robust and visionary workforce planning. Innovative ways of managing available resources including models of working, skill mix and skill share, and effective utilisation of support staff, together with appropriate training, supervision and development, need to be developed.

There will also need to be greater recognition of systems based approaches, which recognise that appropriate and timely entry to and exit from intermediate care is just as important as the provision of intermediate care itself. It will be essential that care pathways extend into intermediate care, requiring both involvement and training across health and social care.

Standard 4: General hospital services
Older people's care in hospital is delivered through appropriate specialist care and by hospital staff who have the right set of skills to meet their needs.

It is disappointing that a National Service Framework that sets out to promote best practice has a standard addressing specialist skills in hospital care, without a parallel standard for similar skills in primary care. The current emphasis on developing primary care and the promotion of whole system care makes this even more compelling. There is also a lack of information on the whole issue of interdisciplinary specialist care, skills needed and access criteria. A few individual disciplines have promoted their own visions, but until these are mutually acceptable, effective and comprehensive, specialist care will remain an enigma. This book has tried to bridge this important gap.

There is no doubt that specialist services promote the best practice in care for older people (see Chapter 2), exemplified by the interdisciplinary team (See Chapter 7). The potential for these teams to reach further into the pathway of care followed by an older person, in Accident & Emergency departments, other specialities and primary care, should be emphasised and explored. Likewise, traditional services in secondary care might be equally effective when adapted for a primary care setting, for example nurse triage and discharge management. All staff whose work includes older people will need the necessary skills to address their needs, in whatever settings they appear. This will require greater emphasis in pre-registration curricula, and the impact on recruitment will require consideration (CSP, 2001). In addition to nurses, other disciplines require professional leadership skills to develop their service and staff, so that all can equally contribute to the development of the whole.

The management of medication is another service, which transcends primary and secondary care. The NSF aims are to ensure older people 'gain maximum benefit from medication to maintain or increase quality and duration of life' and that they 'do not suffer unnecessarily from illness caused by excessive, inappropriate or inadequate consumption of medicines'.

It provides detail about ways to achieve this but basically centres on the following:

• prescribing advice and support
• active monitoring of drug therapy
• review of repeat prescribing
• medication review
• education and training.

These present many opportunities for pharmacists from all areas of the profession who are regarded as 'core members of specialist teams for older people' with 'an emerging role as experts in drug management'. The NSF requires that pharmacists carry out an annual medication review for those over 75 on regular medication (six-monthly for those taking more than four medicines, which constitute a high proportion); provide more help to older people in using their medicines (e.g. assess ability to open bottles or understand direction); and work with PCTs to improve the quality of cost-effectiveness of prescribing for older people (i.e. that they are obtaining maximum benefit from the treatment options available). This will require a much greater number of pharmacists employed/contracted by PCTs. Two main challenges emerge from this:

1 **Training** – to ensure that there is appropriate training for some of these new pharmacy roles and that it is uniform across the country; and
2 **Recruitment** – there is already a huge national recruitment problem in pharmacy due to extending the degree course and increasing demand.

> *Standard 5: Stroke*
> The NHS will take action to prevent strokes, working in partnership with other agencies where appropriate. People who are thought to have had a stroke have access to diagnostic services, are treated appropriately by a specialist stroke service, and subsequently, with their carers, participate in a multidisciplinary programme of secondary prevention and rehabilitation.

This condition will be a prime test for the success of single assessment systems, and there has been considerable research into specialist interdisciplinary/agency stroke services, the key being local leadership, irrespective of discipline. This chapter sets some very challenging targets and all sectors will need to agree protocols for the following groups:

- those at risk of having strokes
- those with transient ischaemic attacks
- those who have had a stroke.

In addition PCTs will also need to set up disease registers and information systems that will allow them to audit whether or not the protocols are being implemented. Much of this is already in place but further emphasis will provide a lever for further service development, particularly a continuum of care, as appropriate, from the stage of prevention; the stroke episode through admission, assessment, acute rehabilitation, intermediate care and long-term support; and prevention of further episodes. This process, from the viewpoint of all the different disciplines in the book, has been described through the case study of 'Susan Hunter' in Chapters 8, 9 and 11–21. The evidence based impact of a number of disciplines in the successful rehabilitation of people with stroke points to the need for considerable expansion of the specialist workforce in this area, just at a time when the same disciplines are being sought for their expertise elsewhere.

> *Standard 6: Falls*
> The NHS, working in partnership with councils, takes action to prevent falls and reduce resultant fractures or other injuries in their populations of older people. Older people who have fallen receive effective treatment and rehabilitation, and with their carers, receive advice on prevention through a specialist falls service.

This standard offers a further opportunity to test the advantages of single assessment systems, and again there has been considerable research into specialist interdisciplinary/agency strategies for falls, the key again being local leadership, irrespective of discipline. There will be a need to address issues of primary, secondary and tertiary prevention of falls, as well as agreeing protocols for the interdisciplinary/agency assessment and management of people who have fallen.

- **Primary prevention** will need to focus on provision of physical activity programmes that maintain strength, balance and coordination, and on physical, social and psychological risk reduction within the home.
- **Secondary prevention** will need to focus on the development of systems that can identify those at most risk, such as people with Parkinson's Disease, osteoporosis or those who are taking certain prescribed medicines. These groups may then benefit from targeted interventions, which reduce their risk.
- **Tertiary prevention** will have to be focused on reducing the risk of further falls in those who have already fallen. This will need to include appropriate medical interventions, exercise programmes to increase strength and coordination, and attention to the social causes of falls. The development and implementation of joint guidelines by physiotherapists and occupational therapists (AGILE/ACPC/OCTEP, 1998; CSP/College of Occupational Therapists [COT], 2000) College of Occupational Therapists [COT] have gone a considerable way to addressing this need (see Chapter 15).

Standard 7: Mental health and older people
Older people who have mental health problems have access to integrated mental health services, provided by the NHS and councils to ensure effective diagnosis, treatment and support, for them and for their carers.

Services for older people with mental health problems have made significant strides over recent years to become integrated across agencies. Social workers have recognised that their services, and those of many members of the multidisciplinary team, are often brought in too late for real preventive work to be done, or to be able to work with people around their own choices and priorities. The emphasis on early diagnosis and support for people in this standard is welcomed, and can only make an impact on a still largely marginalised area of care for older people. Whether the knowledge base, resources and skills are available for implementation will determine the outcome.

A major task for PCTs will now be to establish, implement and monitor protocols to diagnose, treat and care for people with depression or dementia. It is likely that practices will need support from community psychiatric nurses, clinical psychologists and occupational therapists if they are successfully to deliver this standard. The physical problems of old age are often superimposed on mental health problems, and sharing of skills across both specialities can have mutual advantage.

The NSF also focuses on the needs of older people with learning disabilities, as this group increasingly survive into old age. Much less is known in services for older people about how to meet such combined needs, but shared learning between colleagues and between disciplines on this subject will indicate the opportunities available.

While this book was in its final stages of preparation a further government policy document, the White Paper, *Valuing People* (DoH, 2001c) has drawn attention to the requirement to respond to the needs of older carers, particularly elderly parents who care for their learning disabled adult son or daughter at home. This group of older people who may be both service users and carers simultaneously in respect of their own health needs and those of their adult offspring, require the sensitive attention of practitioners who combine skills from traditionally separate arenas.

Standard 8: The promotion of health and active life in old age
The health and well-being of older people is promoted through a coordinated programme of action led by the NHS with support from councils.

This standard includes some very specific, as well as some broader targets. PCTs and their component practices will need to be able to report annual improvements in flu immunisation, smoking cessation and blood pressure management. More broadly they will need to engage with local authority and voluntary sector partners in order to promote the development of exercise, welfare benefits uptake, home energy efficiency schemes and healthy eating programmes. There are concerns about the lack of staff, underdeveloped knowledge base for implementation and lack of outcome measures available with which to monitor achievement.

There is an obvious link between this and Standard 6 in relation to strategies aimed at promoting physical activity that will reduce levels of dependency and frailty – and there are numerous opportunities to work across agencies and with multiple disciplines to achieve this standard.

Activities that can promote healthy active life for older people include the following:

- Access to mainstream health promotion and disease prevention programmes of specific benefit to older people, tailored where necessary to reflect cultural diversity. These include programmes for increasing physical activity, improved diet and nutrition, immunisation and management programmes for influenza.
- Wider initiatives involving a multi-sectorial approach to promoting health, independence and well-being in old age: exercise services, healthy eating, Keep Warm Keep Well campaign, and Home Energy Efficiency Scheme.
- Occupational and leisure opportunities for older people, despite disability or distance from mainstream activities can be facilitated by occupational therapists (see Chapter 16).

Other resources that will support successful implementation of this standard include a focus on carers (Chapter 12), podiatry (Chapter 18), psychology (Chapter 9), dietetics (Chapter 20A), dentistry (Chapter 20B), optical (Chapter 20E) and hearing services (Chapter 20F). Adult education in later life, and life-long learning as a whole, should also play a major part.

Implementation support and requirements

Local implementation of the NSF will require consultation with older people and their carers; a shared vision and partnership working appropriate to the diverse needs of the local population; leadership; inclusive planning; and communication.

Local arrangements include designated leads to address plans and gaps. Five programmes will support implementation:

- Finance – additonal financial resources for services for older people, intermediate care and promotion of independence
- Workforce – timely availability, recruitment, development and retention of the right number and skill of staff as well as new ways of working
- Research and development – through targeted research funding particularly reduction of disability and promotion of independence; needs of carers and minority groups; innovation
- Practice development – through focussed use of existing services such as the Cochrane Collaboration, NHS Centre for Review and Dissemination, NICE and Social Care Institute for Excellence
- Information – a strategy to provide local information and to support care such as electronic and co-ordinated standards and records.

The NSF for Older People has assigned a range of major tasks and responsibilities to PCTs. There are some concerns about the ability of PCTs to discharge these responsibilities at the same time as they are setting themselves up as new organisations, taking on many of the responsibilities of Health Authorities and being expected to meet the requirements of other NSFs. Some of the milestones, such as the single assessment and the development and monitoring of protocols for stroke and falls will only be achieved by increasing the level of skills, competencies and capacity within the PCT. If they are going to be successful PCTs will need to take the following steps:

1 Mapping of existing resources and skill mix within the PCT and within voluntary and statutory service partners. This will need to cover all relevant professional groups.
2 Training, recruitment and capacity building to meet any identified gaps both in terms of the range of professional groups and range of specialist skills.
3 Development of realistic protocols in which primary care professionals have a sense of shared ownership and commitment.
4 Development of effective IT systems, which can share, with agreed safeguards, information across practices, health and other social care providers.
5 Development of effective monitoring and audit systems, which can close the quality loop by providing feedback to practices about their performance.
6 Development of workplace, inter-agency and inter-professional training, which is targeted at performance deficiencies and ensures that all those within the locality are working collaboratively to meet agreed targets and milestones.

7 Development of robust systems for involving, listening to, and acting upon the views of older people and their carers.

For service providers, opportunities abound for innovation and establishing evidence of effectiveness of intervention. For too long, much of the latter has remained unproven, but must now be evidence based and age specific. For the nursing and therapy professions, the standards offer opportunities for advanced and consultant practitioner posts. While finance is a major element, the need to change the culture and mindset of those involved in service provision, across agencies and disciplines, is probably the biggest challenge. Integration will add further challenges for compatible and mutually accessible but protected information systems and shared assessments, plans, progress and other records.

- Local performance measures already include some relevant components.
- A national overview of progress will be provided by the Modernisation Board supported by the Taskforce for Older People.
- Much is already in place that will absorb monitoring of this initiative, and the detail should be developed in tandem with implementation of the standards so that all involved are clear regarding the criteria to be used. Whatever the political measures used, the key to effectiveness will be whether older people, their carers and care providers feel that services are equitable, person-centred, comprehensive and integrated.

SUMMARY

After much deliberation on the organisation of services for older people the NSF is welcome in the focus it provides. The emphasis on opportunities for all disciplines for specialisation, integration and innovation await the enthusiasts. There will never be a better time to accept the challenge, or a worse time to reject it as the number of older people in the population continues to rise, and their expectations grow along with their political power.

There may be few surprises, but achieving the delivery of these standards, rather than debating them, will be the real challenge. This will require inter-agency collaboration to establish actual need, evidence on which to base interdisciplinary practice, and monitoring of impact from the perspective of the older person or their carer, where relevant.

Such seemingly simple principles will in themselves require education and training, capacity and resources, and above all copious goodwill to transcend well-established boundaries. The challenge will be for disciplines and agencies to work together, across traditional boundaries, to grasp these opportunities in order to benefit older people throughout the continuum of health and social care services.

ACKNOWLEDGEMENTS

Anne Fenech, Pre- and Post-Registration Officer, College of Occupational Therapists

Gwyn Owen, Professional Adviser, Chartered Society of Physiotherapy

Gwilym Wyn Roberts, Group Head, Education and Practice, College of Occupational Therapists

Contributor colleagues: Fiona Bevan, Chris Drinkwater, Margaret Hastings, Suzanne Hogg, Jill Manthorpe, Jill Mantle, Kiran Shukla, Olwen Finlay, Jennifer Wenborne

REFERENCES

AGILE/ACPC/OCTEP (1998) *Guideline for the Collaborative Rehabilitative Management of Elderly People Who Have Fallen*, Chartered Society of Physiotherapy, London.

Chartered Society of Physiotherapy/College of Occupational Therapists (CSP/COT) (2000) *The National Collaborative Audit for the Rehabilitative Management of Elderly People who have Fallen – Final Report*, CSP/COT, London.

CSP (2001) *Policy Briefing Paper: National Service Framework for Older People*, Chartered Society of Physiotherapy, London.

Clinical Standards Board for Scotland (CSBS) (2001) *Older People in Acute Care*, Clinical Standards Board for Scotland, Edinburgh.

Department of Health [DoH] (1998a) *A First Class Service: Quality in the new NHS*, HMSO, London.

DoH (1998b) *Our Healthier Nation: A contract for health*, HMSO, London.

DoH (2000) *The NHS Plan*, The Stationery Office, London.

DoH (2001a) *The National Service Framework for Older People*, The Stationery Office, London. http://www.doh.gov.uk/nsf/olderpeople.htm

DoH (2001b) *Guide to Integrating Community Equipment Services*, Department of Health, London.

DoH (2001c) *Valuing People: A new strategy for learning disability for the 21st century*, Department of Health, London.

Finn, A.M. (1986) Attitudes of physiotherapists towards geriatric care. *Physiotherapy*, **72**(3), 129–131.

Johnson, M. (2001) The NSF for older people – what are the issues to be addressed? Presentation at CAPITA Conference, London, 23 May 2001, Capita Business Services, London.

Morris, M. and Minichello, V. (1992) Why choose to work in geriatrics? Factors which affect physiotherapists' decision to work with older people. *Australian Physiotherapy*, **38**(1), 121–128.

Scottish Executive (2000) *Community Care: A joint future – report of the Joint Future Group*, Scottish Executive, Health and Community Care Department, Edinburgh.

Swage, T. (2000) *Clinical Governance in Healthcare Practice*, Butterworth-Heinemann, Oxford.

Wilson, K. (2001) Implementing the NSF for older people. Presentation at CAPITA Conference, London, 23 May 2001, Capita Business Services, London.

7 TEAM WORKING IN REHABILITATION

Margaret B. Hastings

AIMS OF THE CHAPTER

The delivery of health care for older people requires a variety of specialist knowledge and skills together with general care. No one individual can deliver the complexity of interventions alone, and skills and knowledge will be shared among the group of individuals involved with the older person. Groups of staff from different agencies need to be developed and enabled to work together as a team. This chapter considers the social and interpersonal skills needed by each member of the team to ensure effective rehabilitation of the older person. Many health professionals graduate with little knowledge and understanding of the core skills and competencies of their colleagues as joint learning at undergraduate level is not yet shared in the UK. Apart from learning about other team members, the team also needs to acknowledge the process of team development and the influence new members to the team may have on the effective working of the team.

INTRODUCTION

The process of rehabilitation has been described as 'continuous and multifactorial . . . which is dependent on multiple inputs' (Squires, 1994), and a 'mixture of clinical, therapeutic and social interventions' (King's Fund, 1998). The way in which these inputs are linked, through those concerned with the patient's management and support working closely together and sharing knowledge and skills, is essential for rehabilitation to be effective, efficient and acceptable to the patient. Chapter 4 outlines how the agreed goals of rehabilitation are subject to a range of influences affecting both the process and outcome. Team working is about groups of people taking responsibility for their own combined actions.

WHAT IS A TEAM?

Concepts of teams and team working vary widely within health, social services and the business sector. Within health and social care there may be teams that include users and/or carers or advocates where appropriate, for example in goal setting and discharge planning; or non-clinical teams of professionals dealing with internal service issues. This chapter considers the principles of team working, irrespective of the membership.

Definitions of a team vary from a group of people working together, to a specific number of people who share their expertise, organising themselves purposefully to accomplish shared goals.

Caird *et al.* (1994) describe the characteristics of a team as:

- having two or more members
- members contribute their skills within inter-dependent roles towards shared goals
- team identity is distinct from individual members' identities
- there are established methods of communicating within the group and with other teams
- the structure is explicit, task and goal oriented, organised and purposeful
- the effectiveness of the team is reviewed periodically.

Rehabilitation requires a range of competencies and expertise not available from any one individual member of the team. Staff from different agencies, e.g. health, social, voluntary and private services, need to work together with the user. The team's tasks and goals cannot be achieved by individuals alone due to time and resource constraints, and no individual can possess all the relevant competencies, capabilities, breadth of ideas and experience. The supportive nature of working in a team coping with unique complex issues, should not be underestimated. Team members will provide different levels of input at any one time, dependent on need. The strongest teams are those where input is truly reciprocal and not measured against a balance sheet – equity of input rather than equality.

Lewis (1992) identifies four faces to a team, which indicate the breadth of skills required:

1 adapting to the environment and utilising organisational resources effectively in order to satisfy the requirements of the team sponsor

2 relating effectively with people outside the team in order to meet the needs of the consumer, whether internal or external to the organisation

3 using systems and procedures appropriately to carry out goal-oriented tasks

4 working in a way that makes people feel part of the team.

The value of team work

The skills required for effective team working can be learned and developed to ensure that the sum of the parts of the team is greater than the whole. Above all team work involves trust, knowledge and effective communication skills. Team working is most valuable when members have to work together with a common purpose to achieve a consistent quality of service within the resources available. A well-managed team will work effectively and efficiently, ensuring that resources (mainly costly professional time) are used appropriately. There will be transfer and sharing of skills to ensure patients' needs are met and provider and service user time is not wasted.

In the continually changing health and social care sector, effective and flexible team working will be essential in sharing the workload to meet deadlines and in providing support to team members. Much psycho-social and physical support will be provided by effective team working. Especially in sharing the stresses individuals face when working in vulnerable situations such as in isolation; with emotive problems, e.g. working with people with dementia; and in high risk areas, e.g. community rehabilitation in an area of social deprivation and high addiction rate.

Groups or teams?

The variety of the tasks within rehabilitation require different problems to be addressed by either groups (number of people sharing an interest) or teams (number of people working together). Team work is more appropriate where there is a need for people to work together towards a common purpose. The development of relationships is the key to success. Groups, perhaps formed from a larger team, will work best for short-term specific tasks. Team working will be more costly in resource terms, with members requiring time to meet together to plan, negotiate and share a common purpose. It can take longer to make decisions, with increased discussion and problem analysis from a well-structured team (Gorman, 1998). For some tasks within rehabilitation, e.g. the design of an interdisciplinary record, it may be more effective to use a group for initial decision-making before wider consultation with the team. The following chart (Table 7.1) suggests the factors that affect the choice of working in groups or teams and is drawn from the Open University (1994):

Table 7.1   Factors affecting the choice of working in groups or teams

When to use groups	When to build teams
• Simple tasks or 'puzzles'	• Highly complex tasks or problems
• Co-operation sufficient	• Consensus essential
• Minimum discretion	• High level of choice and uncertainty
• Fast decision needed	• High commitment needed
• Few competencies required	• Broad range of competencies required
• Members' interests inherently conflicting	• Members' individual objectives can motivate
• Organisation credits individuals for operational and vision outputs	• Organisation rewards teams for strategy building
• Innovative responses sought	• Balanced views sought

(Open University, 1994)

Multi- or interdisciplinary?

Multidisciplinary implies many different groups of professionals. Interdisciplinary infers professionals working together. Gorman (1998) suggests that the inter-disciplinary label indicates that all members and disciplines of the team recognise the abilities, skills and critical contributions of each of the others. Rehabilitation of older people has long been the natural home of team working in the health service, albeit not always inclusive of the patient. In striving to provide quality services, staff should now be actively pursuing interdisciplinary working with comprehensive membership and good coordination.

Team formation

There are many instances in health and social services where groups of people have historically arrived together to form a team without the necessary organisational structure. They may evolve into chaos, where conflict, differing values (see also Chapters 4 and 5) and inter-personal difficulties reflect poorly on the team work philosophy, or by pure luck, find common ground and solve the problem. A dysfunctional team can be one that is muddling along and not fulfilling its potential in problem-solving. It is essential that consideration is given to the formation and management of all the teams working in rehabilitation of older people. The proposed Leadership Centre to develop management and clinical leadership in the NHS Plan (Department of Health, 2000) could do much to progress this ambition.

Health and social care practitioners are likely to be members of several different teams:

- **intra-disciplinary** – own discipline with peer support
- **interdisciplinary** – patient-focused care team
- **project team** – specific development or management function.

The individual expectations of, and contributions to, each team will vary but all teams will require a variety of roles to be performed within the team and to develop through the stages of team building. All teams require a defined organisational structure, which provides an environment that will survive the inevitable changes in membership and demands (Ovretveit, 1994). Within health and social care, team work skills need to be learned, and all new members of a 'team' need timely development to enable them confidently and effectively to fulfil their team role from the start.

TEAM TYPES

The organisational structure of teams varies widely due to the resource available and the need to be addressed. Ovretveit (1994) identified eight different team types:

- client team and care manager provider team
- network association teams
- formal
  (i) fully managed multidisciplinary team (see Figure 7.1, e.g. community learning disability team with different disciplines managed by a budget manager)

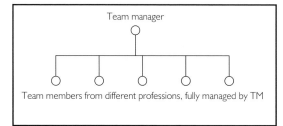

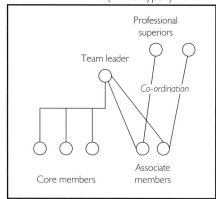

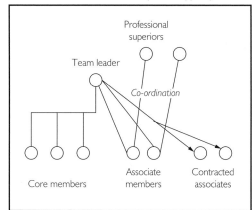

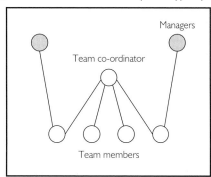

Figure 7.1 Fully managed MDT (formal type i)

Figure 7.2 Managed core + coordinated associate team (formal type ii)

Figure 7.3 Managed core + coordinated associate + contracted associate team (formal type iv)

Figure 7.4 Leader coordinated (formal type v)

(ii) managed core and coordinated associate team (see Figure 7.2, e.g. ward nursing team with different disciplines attached to ward but managed by own discipline)

(iii) managed core and contracted associate team

(iv) managed and coordinated core and contracted associate team (see Figure 7.3, e.g. as above but with disciplines under contract from other organisations)

(v) leader coordinated team (see Figure 7.4, e.g. Locality Community Team)

(vi) leader contracted team.

Mapping the different patterns helps to summarise the complexities of team working within health and social care.

TEAM ROLES

No one team member can possibly be expected to have all the necessary competencies to perform key skills. Each member must identify their own strengths and weaknesses, and know the roles they are most competent at providing. Belbin (1993) has identified eight roles for team members. Those required in each team will depend on the task to be performed. The eight team types are as follows:

- **The implementer** – disciplined, reliable, conservative and efficient. Turns ideas into practical actions. *Weaknesses:* somewhat inflexible; slow to respond to new possibilities.
- **The coordinator** – mature, confident, a good chairperson. Clarifies goals, promotes decision-making, delegates well. *Weaknesses:* can be seen as manipulative; delegates personal work.
- **The shaper** – challenging, dynamic, thrives on pressure. Has the drive and courage to overcome obstacles. *Weaknesses:* can provoke others; hurts people's feelings.
- **The plant** – creative, imaginative, unorthodox. Solves difficult problems. *Weaknesses:* ignores details; too preoccupied to communicate effectively.
- **The resource investigator** – extrovert, enthusiastic, communicative. Explores opportunities. Develops contacts. *Weaknesses:* over-optimistic; loses interest once initial enthusiasm has passed.
- **The monitor evaluator** – sober, strategic and discerning. Sees all options. Judges accurately. *Weaknesses:* lacks drive and ability to inspire others; overtly critical.
- **The team worker** – co-operative, mild, perceptive and diplomatic. Listens, builds, averts friction, calms the waters. *Weaknesses:* indecisive in crunch situations; can be easily influenced.
- **The completer-finisher** – painstaking, conscientious, anxious. Searches out errors and omissions. Delivers on time. *Weaknesses:* inclined to worry unduly; reluctant to delegate; can be a nit-picker.

Everybody will use several roles to a varying degree and conflict can arise when holders of similar roles are perceived to be competitive. Group roles can be learned by observation and practice, and behaviour can be constrained and modified. Belbin recommends individuals to perfect the team roles already held; work at those which are weaker to hold in reserve; and forget those which feel unnatural.

All members of an interdisciplinary rehabilitation team will also have a specialist role in their own area of clinical expertise. Within a well-developed and balanced team there will be a willingness to share non-specialist skills among team members with trust allowing collaborative practice within the statutory and professional framework. Demarcation disputes over professional boundaries are less likely to arise and there will be more flexibility of roles at times of increased pressure to enable the performance of the task. The model shown in Chapter 1 (Figure 1.2) demonstrates the strengths and opportunities of such best practice.

STAGES OF TEAM DEVELOPMENT

Bion (1961) and Tuckman (1965) have modelled four stages of team development, and each in turn has four dimensions that need attention: group behaviour, group tasks/issues, interpersonal skills and leadership issues (Table 7.2). Gorman (1998) adds mourning, the social process of disengagement on completion of the task. Team working skills should be a fundamental component of basic training for all disciplines, particularly where continuous policy change affects consistent team membership, with teams needing to form and work together in increasingly shorter time spans.

Table 7.2 The life cycle of teams

Tasks/issues	Leadership	Stages	Interpersonal	Behavioural patterns
Membership definition Similarities/differences Orientation and introductions	Dependence	FORMING	Inclusion	Move to similarities Anger and frustration Superficial, polite, ambiguous, confused
Decision-making process Power/influence	Counter-dependence	STORMING	Control	Establishing operating rules Attempts made to create order Attacks on leadership Emotional response to task demands
Functional relationships	Inter-dependence	NORMING	Affection	Cohesion Negotiation
Productivity		PERFORMING		Growth/insight Collaboration
Evaluation Completion of task	Reflective	MOURNING	Disengagement	Recognition of achievements

Forming stage

At this stage the team is in its infancy and members need to come together before any output can be achieved.

- **Group behaviour** – likely to be superficial with polite ambiguity and confusion. Compatibility among team members and linking of people with similar needs will be evident.
- **Group tasks/issues** – establish basic criteria for membership. Orientation and introductions within the team and the role of the team defined.
- **Interpersonal issues** – establishment of safe patterns of interaction and evaluation of the inclusion criteria.
- **Leadership** – crucial role at this stage to focus on team members' needs of getting to know one another and clarifying the goals, roles, responsibilities and procedures that are relevant to the team's role.

Storming

This can be likened to adolescence and is a vital stage of development to deal with power and decision-making. Unless this stage is recognised and the unpleasantness tolerated the team will not move on to the productive stages.

- **Group behaviour** – establishment of operating rules and creation of order. There will be attacks on the leadership that will be emotionally charged and in response to the demands of the task.
- **Group tasks/issues** – power/influence issues need to be identified together with the agreed decision-making process within the team.
- **Interpersonal skills** – members work through their own control needs to regain their individuality, power and influence, and thus achieve a sense of direction and purpose they are comfortable with.
- **Leadership issues** – need to help resolve the issues by listening, providing feedback and encouraging working towards shared goals. Conflict needs to be recognised and managed to clear the air and help the team to become more cohesive.

Norming

The team becomes a cohesive unit and begins to negotiate roles and processes for achieving its task.

- **Group behaviour** – cohesion and negotiation.
- **Group tasks/issues** – functional relationships built. Readiness to tackle tasks.
- **Interpersonal skills** – affection, sharing of insight, recognition of individual skills.
- **Leadership issues** – ensuring cohesiveness and individual member's interdependence on team's purpose and values.

Performing

This stage consists of the achievement of tasks within the team in an effective and efficient manner.

- **Group behaviour** – growth and insight lead to meaningful functional relationships and collaboration in performing the task.
- **Group tasks/issues** – group identity, recognition of factors that contribute to or hinder success. Productive.
- **Interpersonal skills** – trust and collaborative working.
- **Leadership issues** – evaluation of team work, recognition of team effort rather than individual efforts to avoid disruption, competitiveness and hostility.

Teams will need to recycle back through various stages as the team changes, with new members, new leadership and differing roles. From the author's experience of many different team types, it is common to find that where problems are developing within the team, one stage has not been properly addressed and the process needs to be revisited to allow the performing stage to be achieved.

Mourning

All teams will eventually complete their task and need to be transformed. This may be by redefinition by establishing a new purpose or structure, or disengagement/termination so that its members can accept the different challenges ahead. Successful teams will try and stay together to retain the strong bonds within the team, and although the team must be allowed to disengage, social bonds may remain and prove fruitful future contacts.

Continuity has been an accepted value in public services, and staff in such environments may find disengagement particularly difficult. Gorman (1998) has termed this stage 'mourning', which is characterised by two important activities – evaluation and recognition of the team's achievements. Evaluation should consider how effective the team has been and what lessons have been learned. Recognition of the collective achievements and the development of individual team members will help to finalise the process.

OBJECTIVES AND TEAM GOALS

For effective team building, the role of the team should first be identified together with the competencies required to achieve the goals. This will lead to the composition of the team specification, which will identify the team roles needed, together with the likely membership size, life span, objectives and review plans. Any team should only exist for as long as the need is evident. Staff should be appointed to the team who have the necessary skills or who are willing and able to develop these competencies. When team members change it is an ideal opportunity to review the objectives and competencies required before appointing new members. This is the theory, but few job descriptions yet identify team roles and interdisciplinary working as required competencies in the rehabilitation field. Where teams are intra-disciplinary, consideration may need to be given to the natural characteristics of that discipline to ascertain whether the range of skills is likely to be present, or whether such a team will be weighted towards certain roles.

All team members must know what the team goals and objectives are. They should be discussed and formally recorded, and review dates set. It is important to make sure that all new team members have the objectives and goals explained to them from the start to integrate the new member into the team and ensure their effective working. Where objectives are unclear, opportunity for dominance between disciplines exists. For example, Reed (1993) has identified subtle power playing, particularly between nursing and physiotherapy. Two settings were reviewed: acute/rehabilitation where there was collaborative working; and long-term care where collaborative working did not exist, and 'referral', mirroring the medical model, was used by nurses to obtain the required results. Reed (1993) puts this variation down to the different philosophies at play. In acute/rehabilitation, the medical model of cure provides a united goal with physiotherapy staff primarily dedicated to the unit. In long-term care the medical and social models are inter-twined, with nurses caring and therapists attempting to 'cure' with their time spread over a range of other activities. The goal of cure was seen as disruptive in the nurses' domain and sabotage was employed by them to achieve their own goal. Although this research compared two distinct settings, misunderstanding of the goal for a particular patient in any setting could conceivably lead to a similar situation (see Chapter 8).

Purpose of teams

The purpose of a team should be specific, e.g. 'To provide a high quality rehabilitation service to the patients in the rehabilitation unit'. The defined purpose of the team will allow the necessary processes to achieve this purpose to be agreed. The required process for any service delivery will have inputs and outcomes (see Figure 7.5), and the advantages of a team-based approach to defining and reviewing such issues will meet commissioners' interest in contracting through processes or pathways of care.

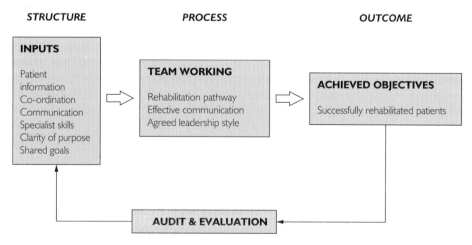

Figure 7.5 Team working in rehabilitation

Pathways are being developed as part of the response to calls for evidence based, equitable and outcome oriented care. A care pathway determines locally agreed interdisciplinary practice, based on guidelines and evidence where available, for a specific patient/client group. It forms all or part of the clinical record, documents the care given, and facilitates the evaluation of outcomes for continuous quality improvement (Swage, 2000). These are necessary in specialities such as rehabilitation of older people, where interdisciplinary input is paramount in providing care to patients with many problems resulting from multiple pathology. Where inter-professional pathways are developed participatively, team work and collaboration will be enhanced.

Pathways incorporating guidelines, standards and audit tools can include:

- referral procedures
- assessment by whom/when/where
- timing of investigations
- treatment plans
- care plans
- drugs
- mobility/functional activity measures
- diet
- discharge planning process
- additional information.

Outcomes

In health and social care the outcome is the impact of that care on the user, including the costs of providing that care. 'Outcome is more difficult to define than structure and process standards and is arguably the most important of the three' (Koch, 1991).

Outcomes should be understandable to the patient. If the care package is for rehabilitation of an older person, then the outcome may be achievement of agreed functional goals to maintain optimal quality of life in the chosen environment. Any differing views between patient and team, and even within the team, as to what constitutes a goal 'to maintain optimal quality of life' requires open discussion. Explanation of the various options and consequences, and mature acceptance of a patient led plan that may not fit established pathways and standards, should lead to a positive outcome (see also Chapter 4). Inexperienced clinicians may fall into the trap of assuming outcomes always to be a forward progression in functional ability, but maintenance of a functional level or adequate pain control in a deteriorating condition are equally acceptable outcomes, and should be recorded as such (see also Chapters 5 and 8). A model for identification of structure, process and outcome issues for improvement along the patient pathway is described in Chapter 5 (see Figure 5.2).

A problem that will arise in successful interdisciplinary practice will be the immature requirement to measure the outcome attributable to an individual discipline for audit purposes. Teams will need to have adequate measures of patient-centred outcome and resist pressure to dissect the contributions unless required to do so for performance measurement or other exercises.

Skill identification

In setting up a new interdisciplinary team the objectives and goals of the team will have been considered and the list of skills required in carrying out its function should have been identified. For successful team working, members will have to contribute their skills and expertise to the team's goals. Not all members will be natural team players, although they may have the necessary client based skills. In a career in rehabilitation, especially with older people, these interpersonal skills are essential and can be acquired where there is a genuine desire to learn. All teams will have a mixture of task and people functions, which requires a variety of skills. Skills found to have a positive effect on team working are:

- good interpersonal relationships with understanding of each other's values and management style
- the ability to discuss issues openly without arousing undue sensitivity or tension
- a high level of trust in each other
- to be approachable and able to accept objective feedback and criticism
- sufficient discipline and cohesion to implement agreed decisions
- the capacity to discuss and understand both long-term and short-term issues. (Alderson, 1992).

Meetings

In rehabilitation of older people two types of team meetings will be required:

- **Case specific** – where all team members contribute to the discussion on the progress of the patient/service user, identifying goals and their achievement and planning discharge from the service. This will need to consider the users' problems from a psycho-social model, not solely a medical model, and include the view of the user and their carer.
- **Team performance** – where the structure, objectives, goals, policies and strategies can be discussed and the team performance evaluated. Team perceptions of achievements will need to be tested with external customers, such as referrers, who may have a different, more objective, view.

To be a valuable use of time, everybody participating in the team meeting should know the purpose of the meeting and what contribution they are expected to make. New technology can facilitate meetings by e-mail, telephone or video conferencing. Agreed formats for patient meetings should be followed and an agenda circulated for all other meetings. An agreed method of recording decisions and actions to be taken, by whom and by when must be made and adhered to. This record and action on results should be auditable.

Conflict

Teams that are in total harmony and avoid conflict will not work effectively, as such teams will be working in a closed system and encouraging group think, rather than lateral and innovative thinking. Interdisciplinary teams can bring together different perspectives and skills in a coordinated manner to provide for the needs of the individual user. Conflict and differences are to be expected and need to be handled positively for the good of the user and the creativity of the team. Areas of possible conflict identified within teams are role ambiguity, role conflict and role overload due to expectations of different disciplines (Embling, 1995). Where role and hierarchy cultures (Handy, 1985) are dominant within an organisation, then conflict will be prevalent. Supportive and achieving cultures will encourage service user rather than role focus and reward effective teams (Harrison, 1987). Sharing roles and trusting other team members to appropriately represent other disciplines shows maturity and support within a team. Reciprocity of such representation will strengthen relationships. Sharing and representing may be particularly difficult for recently qualified professionals still learning their own role and concerned about 'who does what' issues. Even in mature teams, a representative can only report what they have been briefed on, and will need to have the confidence to admit the need to seek out further information and report back if the answer to a problem is not known.

Decision-making processes must be identified and agreed within the team. Ovretviet (1994) identifies four types of decision that reflect on health-care team members and their level of management accountability:

1 Profession-specific decisions about patients – confidence needed in professional role.
2 Care management decisions about one patient – knowledge and experience of local situation and/or alternative actions.
3 Policy and management decisions about how all patients will be served and about how care coordination will be done – ability to carry out any changes required.
4 Planning decisions – what level of authority is required to implement the change process. Do all members of the team have the same level of authority?

The size of teams will also affect the level of conflict. The larger the team the more chances of interpersonal conflict and the less chance of consensus in decision-making as a result of the increased number of interactions. Teams should be no larger than 12 members. Larger teams will perform better by restructuring into smaller groups to achieve the team goals. The ideal team is one that is as small as possible, but which encompasses all the expertise required to meet the team goals.

Management of teams

Teams will founder when they lose their sense of purpose and objective, which should have been clearly documented and agreed at the start (Gorman, 1998). Perhaps the time has come to disengage, realise that objectives have never been clearly set or that they need to be revised in line with surrounding change. All teams must take time to explore their vision and sense of purpose, and analyse the tasks they have to complete within the timescale. The team leader will have to allow capacity for this and ensure that all team members feel supported enough to be able to share their views. Within rehabilitation of older people the task may be to enable the user to reach the optimal functional level to return or remain at home. With the decreased length of inpatient stay that objective may change, and the required functional level at discharge from hospital may be lower, with increasing demands on rehabilitation services in the community to enable further function to be reached. It is likely that the skill mix of community based teams will change as more unqualified support workers help to provide the care. Such workers bring different values and skills (see Chapter 4) and different roles will be expected of them as team members. It is unwise to translocate a hospital based team into the community without providing the opportunity to develop the required competencies (see Chapter 10).

The level of staff required to join the team will also vary between agencies and on the issues, e.g. policy making, budget control. This can lead to problems where certain team members are unable to make a decision without referring to a higher authority and can be very frustrating to more autonomous members. There may also be tensions between different organisational cultures, e.g. valuing choice in social care/social work (see Chapter 19) and providing suggestions of appropriate behaviour in health care. Is the patient allowed to stay in bed all day from personal choice or should he/she be encouraged to get up and sit in the chair to prevent pressure sores and flexion contractures, and facilitate mobility? (For more on this, see also Chapter 4.) For a user-focused approach choice is essential, but it must be informed choice based on evidence not emotion (see Chapter 4). How a team will cope with rejection of informed best practice by increasingly assertive service users will be an issue for the future. The different conceptual models held by users, providers and commissioners have the potential for both unhealthy conflict and healthy collaboration (see Chapter 5). The balance of views within the team, from a social, scientific and business perspective, should lead to collaborative practice.

Review

The traditional acute care based model of rehabilitation of older people is changing towards intermediate care/community provision. Team members are being encouraged to benchmark their services against others and note what they can do to ensure that their service best meets the patients' needs and wishes. Increasingly multi-agency working will provide care in a variety of environments. Challenges to traditional patterns will lead to disruption of teams and new teams will have to be reformed with different agendas and management. Change is inevitable and a good practitioner in rehabilitation of older people will be an adept team player. Membership of interdisciplinary rehabilitation teams is continually changing due to variations in contracts, personnel, management structures and needs of the care group. Even where there has been little change among participants of the team, it is necessary to review the membership to ensure that it has not become stagnant and closed. For these reasons, regular reviews of the team need to be carried out. Areas to be considered are:

- team objectives
- team goals and timescales
- team values
- skills required to perform the task
- staff development
- leadership role
- team effectiveness.

TEAM WORK IN PRACTICE

Joining an established team can cause anxiety, but consideration and development of appropriate competencies can make the process more effective and enjoyable. An objective analysis of the situation can be enlightening.

Professional competencies

Are members sure what their professional role in this area is? Are there specific competencies they need to have, such as assessment skills or neurological rehabilitation skills? Do they know which validated tools to use? What specific skills is each contributing, which no other team member can provide? Which skills overlap with other team members that can be shared? Are there tasks that can be delegated? Are there any skills that need to be developed? Are participants aware of the current research in the field? Are individuals able to objectively justify their decisions assertively, without using aggression?

Strengths and weaknesses

What are individuals' preferred team roles? Which ones need to be cultivated? Which ones will be ignored, and which ones will never be achieved? Do such decisions leave role gaps to be filled? Have participants increased their knowledge about the objectives and goals of the team? Are individuals prepared to share their weaknesses with other team members? Is the culture of the team supportive enough for each to share these weaknesses? Is confidentiality established?

Interpersonal skills

Effective communication among all members of the team is essential for successful team working (see Chapter 17). Time must be taken to ensure that communication systems are appropriate, utilised and functioning. There will be the written or electronic communication of case record-keeping and the verbal (and non-verbal) communication of personnel interactions.

How is the information contained within the team recorded? Does the team have ownership of the interdisciplinary record and access to it when necessary? Does the user/carer member of the team know the procedures for access to such documentation? Does the record meet current professional standards of record-keeping or do supplementary records need to be kept? How easy are the records to audit? Can the relevant information be found when needed? Many teams have been surprised that, following audit, record-keeping is highlighted as a major weakness. There should be a record of interdisciplinary problems and goals to be achieved with review dates.

Communication can be a powerful tool. Not all communication is verbal, and gesture and other extra information may be lost in telephone or electronic communication. What happens when one team member 'talks down' to a new team member? How do you react to criticism? A knowledge of Transactional Analysis (Berne, 1966) can be very useful in understanding the positions held or assumed between communicators, helping to prevent a breakdown in communication.

The skills of communication that all team members need to have or develop are:

- presenting ideas, information and opinions clearly
- listening to others
- giving feedback
- advising and supporting
- participating in discussion and decision-making.

Hidden agendas and conflict are common barriers to communication within the team (Reed, 1993). Within a trusting and supportive culture these can be countered. Conflict will always happen within progressive teams and should be utilised to promote a variety of solutions to the complex problems the team has to manage. Members will always bring different skills, experience, knowledge and values to the task. Where this is recognised and understood, respect and trust will develop, and the team will develop procedures to face and resolve conflict.

Every team member will have some form of power within the team. Conflict from power struggles may arise and it is important that the leader is aware of any underlying issues. Power is an essential component of organisations, enabling the astute to use appropriate avenues to achieve objectives. Swage (2000) recognises a number of sources of power in organisations determined by:

- **authority** – recognition by others of the individual's role within the organisation
- **expertise** – technical knowledge and skills, with power directly related to its exclusivity and usefulness to the organisation
- **resources** – usually including physical, financial or information with power directly related to the resources most valued by the organisation
- **personal attributes** – such as interpersonal skills and ability to influence, and emphasised by personal charisma
- **gate keeping** – usually through control of access to people, information and resources, and can be effectively wielded at low levels within the hierarchy.

The power of dependence is also added to the list by Swage:

- **dependence** – the giving or withholding of willing co-operation.

Apart from expert power, positive use of dependence power will be the most important to ensure effective team working (Paton, 1985). Position power of the leader and/or team members will also reflect the complex interpersonal relationships within a team. Power struggles within the team will challenge the leader to facilitate effective and cohesive activity.

Leadership

The leadership style of the team is aimed at getting the task done and encouraging team-building. The expert power of the doctor is valued by the health-care organisation due to its exclusivity, usefulness and political links. Such power does not necessarily equate with good leadership, although the doctor has traditionally assumed the team leadership role.

Increasingly key workers are being identified from within the team to lead implementation of the care package, especially in arranging discharge from hospital. At different stages throughout the patients' health-care journey this leadership role will be passed to the most appropriate person. The example of leadership will depend on the natural style of the potential leaders:

- whether they tend to an authoritarian or participative approach
- the nature of the team – what types of roles the team members tend to adopt
- power – more responsibility leads to greater authority
- the structure of the task – less structure allows a more participative leadership style
- continuity of membership.

The leader will need to be aware of the informal communication network, the power strata and the preferred roles and learning styles of the team members. Building a cohesive team has to strike a balance between 'preventing conformity' and 'group think'. Ways in which cohesion can be promoted are:

- giving open and supportive feedback, avoiding backbiting and malicious gossip
- confronting interpersonal problems
- tolerating differences of opinion and criticism that is constructive
- allowing disaffected members to withdraw
- being aware that individual objectives may be distinct from team objectives
- avoiding blaming particular team members for particular problems.

Learning

The emphasis on continuing professional development should ensure that professionals evaluate their own learning needs. Increasingly such education will include team building and leadership. For successful team work and organisational development it is essential that teams learn and develop through the processes they carry out. Again there are stages in the ability of teams to learn. Initially members will follow their *individual* learning styles, framing and reframing the problem within their own values and understanding of the world. This is followed by *shared* learning, where members will consider joint hypotheses from different perspectives and starting to cross boundaries to gather information and views. *Joint* learning will see the team as a whole sharing meanings, values and beliefs with integrated perspectives.

Summary

Good social and interpersonal skills are needed by each member of an inter-disciplinary team to ensure effective rehabilitation of the older person. An understanding of the roles, development, purpose and leadership of teams will facilitate success and enjoyment for team members. An effective team will be committed, encouraged, nurtured and be in a good state of organisational health.

References

Alderson, S. (1992) *Reframing Management Competence: Shifting the focus away from the individual and onto the top management team*, Paper presented at Reframing Management Competence, Bolton, November.

Belbin, R.M. (1993) *Team Roles at Work*, Butterworth-Heinemann, Oxford.

Berne, E. (1966) *Games People Play: The psychology of human relationships*, Andre Deutsch (Penguin), London.

Bion, W.R. (1961) *Experience in Groups and Other Papers*, Tavistock Publications, London.

Caird, S., Mabey, C., Adams, R. and O'Sullivan, T. (1994) *Working in Teams: Managing personal and team effectiveness*, Open University Press, Buckingham.

Department of Health (2000) *The NHS Plan*, HMSO, London.

Embling, S. (1995) Exploring multidisciplinary teamwork. *British Journal of Therapy and Rehabilitation*, 2(3), 142–145.

Gorman, P. (1998) *Managing Multidisciplinary Teams in the NHS*, Kogan Page, London.

Handy, C. (1985) *Understanding Organisations*, Penguin, Harmondsworth.

Harrison, R. (1987) Organisation culture and quality of service: a strategy for releasing love in the workplace. In: *What is Making a Difference in Organisations?* (ed. Cunningham, I.), Association for Management Education and Development, Polytechnic of Central London, London.

King's Fund (1998) *Trends in Rehabilitation Policy: A review of the literature*, King's Fund and the Audit Commission, London.

Koch, H. (1991) *Total Quality Management*, Longman, London.

Lewis, R. (1992) *Team Building Skills*, Kogan Page, London.

Open University (1994) *Working in Teams: Open University from managing personal and team effectiveness*, Management Education Scheme by Open Learning, NHS Training Directorate, Open University Press, Buckingham.

Ovretveit, J. (1994) *Coordinating Community Care – Multidisciplinary teams and care management*, Open University Press, Buckingham.

Paton, R. (1985) 'Conflict', *Managing in Organisations*, Units 9–10 of T244, Open University Press, Buckingham.

Reed, J. (1993) The relationship between semi-professions in acute and long term care of elderly patients. *Journal of Clinical Nursing*, 2, 81–87.

Squires, A.J. (1994) Key issues for purchasers and providers in hospital, day hospital and community rehabilitation services for older people. In: *A Unique Window of Change, NHS Health Advisory Service, Annual Report 1992–93*, HMSO, London.

Swage, T. (2000) *Clinical Governance in Healthcare Practice*, Butterworth-Heinemann, Oxford.

Tuckman, B.W. (1965) Development sequences in small groups. *Psychological Bulletin*, **63**, 384–399.

8 THE PROCESS AND OUTCOME OF REHABILITATION

Margaret B. Hastings

AIMS OF THE CHAPTER

This chapter considers the building blocks of the rehabilitation process (Assessment, Goal setting, Interventions) and how their effective delivery will result in the positive outcome for the older person. It also considers the roles of different team members in the assessment process and finishes with the introduction of the case study that is used throughout the rest of the book by each professional to consider their specific role in the rehabilitation of a stroke patient. Stroke rehabilitation is used as an example, as the interventions required for a successful outcome requires effective team working between many specialists and carers. The previous chapter has considered the basic structure of rehabilitation – the interdisciplinary team of people who:

- work together towards common goals with each patient
- involve and educate the patient and family
- have relevant knowledge and skills
- can resolve most of the common problems faced by their patients.

This chapter considers the process of rehabilitation and its key components of:

- assessment
- goal setting
- interventions
- outcome.

THE REHABILITATION PROCESS

Rehabilitation is a cyclical process incorporating assessment, goal setting, interventions, reassessment and review, all directed at a measurable outcome. Where an evidence based clinical pathway exists for an uncomplicated and specific condition, the process is simplified. Fractured neck of femur is a useful example. The challenge of medicine in old age is the multiple pathological and social conditions that each patient presents, requiring a tailor-made approach by each practitioner, combined into a coordinated interdisciplinary package to maximise impact (see Chapter 7).

The personalised rehabilitation process in elderly care will include interdisciplinary assessment using standardised assessment measures where possible; problem identification using disease specific measures where relevant; goal setting using goal attainment scales where available; and clinical interventions based on evidence based practice where reported (see Figure 8.1).

Within the holistic approach of interdisciplinary team working with older people there will be a plethora of assessment tools and outcome measures used. Assessment tools and outcome measures are not interchangeable. Assessment tools will focus on aspects of impairment or pathological dysfunction. Outcome measures need to provide data on the progress of patients receiving an intervention and enhance communication between team members and feedback to patients themselves. Health-care providers need aggregated outcome indicators for specific conditions to audit the success of interventions. Health-care comissioners need aggregated outcome indicators for specific conditions to benchmark and compare different providers. All should be reliable, valid, responsive, specific and sensitive (Bowling, 1997). Standardisation is not always inclusive of cultural and ethnic groups, which requires consideration. Given the wealth of tools available, there is usually no need to devise a local tool so long as that selected is appropriate and used as validated. The benefits of benchmarking a service against others by using standardised measures will enhance the clinical effectiveness knowledge base in rehabilitation of older people. The risk is that personalised outcomes to meet the unique requirements of individuals may not fit a 'standardised' performance measurement model.

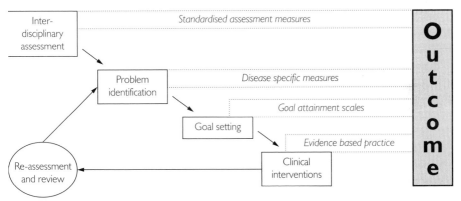

Figure 8.1 The rehabilitation process

Assessment

Older people rightly complain about the number of assessments they complete for different agencies and professionals (Sutherland, 1999; Scottish Executive, 2000a, b). Assessing the need for social and health care in old age should be facilitated by a single screening tool. This will identify what services are required and which other professionals need to provide a more specialist professional analysis of the identified problems. (see *www.doh.gov.uk/scq/sap/*)

Assessment within the speciality of medicine of old age encompasses not only clinical diagnosis but also the evaluation of mental and physical function and the social circumstances of older people (Royal College of Physicians/British Geriatrics Society [RCP/BGS], 1992) Assessment is a continuous process by which the acquisition of relevant, quantified and other data will result in the formulation of treatment plans relating to goals that have been actively set with the patient. In 1989 the World Health Organisation recommended the following domains for assessment of older people:

Activities of Daily Living (ADL)
- physical activities of ADL, i.e. maintaining basic self-care
- mobility
- instrumental activities of ADL, i.e. being a functioning member of society and coping with domestic tasks.

Mental health functioning
- cognitive
- presence of psychiatric symptoms.

Psycho-social functioning
- emotional well-being in a social and cultural context.

Physical health functioning
- self-perceived health status
- physical symptoms and diagnosed conditions
- health service utilisation
- activity levels and measures of incapacity.

Social resources
- accessibility of family, friends and a familiar/professional, voluntary helper
- availability of these resources where needed.

Economic resources
- income as compared to an external standard

Environmental resources
- adequate and affordable housing
- siting of housing in relation to transport, shopping and public services.

These dimensions can be reflected within the World Health Organisation's International Classification of Impairment, Disability and Handicap – 2 (World Health Organisation, 1999):

> IMPAIRMENT – *loss or abnormality of body structure or of physiological or psychological function.*
> DISABILITY (ACTIVITY) – *something a person does, ranging from very basic, elementary or simple to complex.*
> HANDICAP (PARTICIPATION) – *the nature and extent of a person's involvement in life situations in relationship to impairments, activities and contextual factors.*

This is graphically shown in Figure 8.2, which identifies a holistic care approach over the three dimensions of impairment, activity and participation.

All members of the interdisciplinary team will have a specialist contribution to make to the holistic assessment process. The measurement of the various domains suggested above will produce a comprehensive picture of the functional ability of the older person. Within a well-functioning team the various components of the assessment will be shared among the team without unnecessary duplication of effort for the patient or the team. How clear members are about their contribution and how it impacts on the values of colleagues will affect overall success (see also Chapter 4).

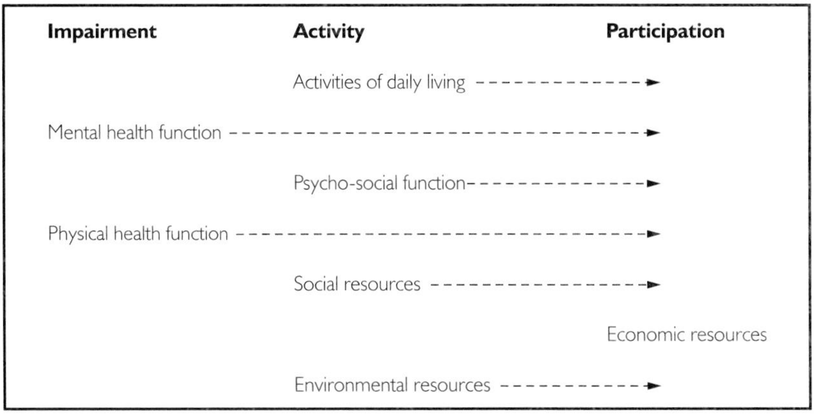

Figure 8.2 Assessment domains and relationship to WHO classification 1999

Older people classically present with multiple pathology; this is due to the lifetime accumulation of degenerative diseases, such as osteoarthritis, osteoporosis, cataract (Chapter 2). Best practice (RCP, 2000) identifies that pre-illness function as well as function levels on assessment and at discharge from health intervention should be documented. Follow up after discharge is equally important as ongoing independence is after all the purpose of all the foregoing activity and results can provide a useful learning tool. It is essential that assessment tools can be used in and across community, acute care and rehabilitation settings.

No single tool will be specific to all the complexities of case mix found within rehabilitation of older people. A report by the RCP and BGS (1992) identified a Cascade Assessment Scheme for the Elderly (Figure 8.3). The 'over 75' screening tests within general practice can be an initial tool, although Swift (see Chapter 2) demonstrates that returns on time spent are low in such blanket approaches, more focused approaches being more cost-effective. The joint working of health and social care on a single screening tool, which is targeted to identify real needs will identify when more detailed and specific tests are necessary. These will provide more detail about problems within the assessment domains and are described below. (See *www.doh.gov.uk/scq/sap/*).

Local teams may wish to standardise the assessment tools that they already use to ensure conformity across a Trust or Health Authority area. For example, Essex Rivers Healthcare has produced a standardised assessment battery for use across its service providers of:

- Elderly Mobility Score (Smith, 1994)
- Berg Balance Score (Berg *et al.*, 1992)
- Rivermead Mobility Index (Collen *et al.*, 1991)
- Modified Barthel ADL (Shah *et al.*, 1989)
- Hodkinson Mental Test (Hodkinson, 1972)
- Geriatric Depression Scale (Sheik and Yesavage, 1986)
- Speech & Language Therapy Outcome Measurement (Conradie, 1997; Enderby, 1997)
- Nutrition Assessment Tool
- Patient Dependency Score.

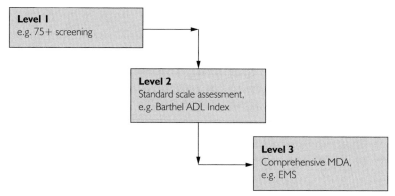

Figure 8.3 Cascade assessment scheme for the elderly
(Adapted from RCP and BGS, 1992)

As older people will experience a range of problems, a combination of assessment methods and tools is often required. Teams may wish to consider the following when selecting an assessment tool:

- the data that needs to be obtained
- the nature of the problem that has precipitated the need for assessment
- factors that previously affected performance
- environment
- sensory abilities
- cultural background
- frame of reference and model of practice used within the service.

The Barthel Index (Mahoney and Barthel, 1965; Table 8.1) is the most commonly used functional indicator. It was one of the first activity of daily living indices, whereby a person is observed performing a functional activity and then scored according to whether or not it can be performed independently.

This index is easy to use and recognised by the majority of medical practitioners and should be considered as a minimum data set for elder rehabilitation. It is a sound basic Activities of Daily Living data set for assessment but does have a ceiling effect and patients with high Barthel scores should be assessed with a more detailed ADL index (Rodgers *et al.*, 1993) (see Chapters 15 and 16).

Table 8.1 Barthel Index of Activities of Daily Living (ADL)

Function	Score	Description
Bowels	0	Incontinent (or needs to be given enema)
	1	Occasional accident (once a week)
	2	Continent
Bladder	0	Incontinent or catheterised and unable to manage
	1	Occasional accident (maximum once per 24 hours)
	2	Continent (for more than 7 days)
Grooming	0	Needs help with personal care
	1	Independent face/hair/teeth (implements provided)
Toilet use	0	Dependent
	1	Needs some help but can do something alone
	2	Independent (on and off, wiping, dressing)
Feeding	0	Unable
	1	Needs help in cutting, spreading butter etc.
	2	Independent (food provided within reach)
Transfer	0	Unable (no sitting balance)
	1	Major help (physical 1 or 2 people) – can sit
	2	Minor help (verbal or physical)
	3	Independent
Mobility	0	Immobile
	1	Wheelchair dependent, including corners, etc.
	2	Walks with help of one person (verbal or physical)
	3	Independent
Dressing	0	Dependent
	1	Needs help but can do about half unaided
	2	Independent (including buttons, zips, laces etc.)
Stairs	0	Unable
	1	Needs help (verbal, physical, carrying aid)
	2	Independent up and down
Bathing	0	Dependent
	1	Independent (Bath: must get in and out unsupervised and wash self. Shower: unaided/unsupervised)

The responsibilities and integration of the interdisciplinary health-care team have been described (see Chapter 1, Figure 1.2). This indicates that the primary nurse holds a key role in team communication.

Nursing

The nursing team are often the first point of contact with the elderly rehabilitation team. Much of the initial demographic and social database will be collated and verified by the nursing team. It is essential to identify potential areas of overlap and designate specific tasks to individual disciplines to avoid duplication. This saves resources and avoids users becoming tired and frustrated. The nursing assessment will usually follow a recognised model, such as Roper, Logan and Tierney (1996). This will provide screening information for other members of the team and start to identify potential problems and difficulties to be addressed. (See Chapter 14 for more detail.)

Medical

Within primary care it is normal for a general practitioner to refer a patient to a secondary care consultant physician, and increasingly to consultants in other disciplines, for a specialist opinion about the patient's problems, to make a diagnosis and provide advice on the medical management of the patient.

The physician will concentrate on:

- disease processes and relevance to current problems
- diagnosis
- drug management
- mental state.

(See Chapter 13 for more detail.)

Physiotherapy

The aim of assessment of physical function is to quantify the inter-relationship between ageing, disease processes and problems relating to function: physiotherapy assessment must therefore incorporate measures both of impairment and activity. The relationship between physical performance and functional ability is well documented (Young and Dinan, 1994; Gill *et al.*, 1996; Spirduso, 1996) and physiotherapists have a key role to play in the assessment of manual handling risk, movement and mobility. (See Chapters 15 and 18 for more detail.)

Occupational therapy

The importance of occupation in the domains of activity and participation ensures that an occupational therapy assessment is also a fundamental component. Routine use of standardised assessments is limited, due to a combination of issues, for example, the very nature of what is being assessed – occupation and doing – is incredibly complex, so constructing standardised assessments is difficult. (See Chapter 16 for more detail.)

The initial screening by these core professions may identify that other professional input is required; this will probably most frequently be podiatry, social work, dietetics and speech and language therapy, but may also include dental, continence, pharmaceutical, hearing and optical advice (see Chapters 17, 18, 19 and 20 for more detail).

Podiatry

Nail and foot pathology may require assessment and prompt intervention to ensure good functional gait and independence is facilitated. Footwear can affect the outcome of tests, for example, the Functional Reach Test, Timed Get Up and Go and 10-metre walk test. For these tests women move fastest in walking shoes, slower barefoot and slowest wearing 'dress' shoes; thus footwear should be documented and remain constant from one test to another (Arnadottir and Mercer, 2000) (see Chapter 18 for more detail).

Social work

The need for social work assessment and intervention will be identified early in the screening process. The nurse will have had early contact with relatives and visitors and will be documenting information about home and social circumstances. The functional and cognitive activities carried out by the occupational therapist will also help to identify any social care needs. All members of the team should be aware of the indicators of elder abuse (see Chapter 19 for more detail).

Dietetics

The need for nutritional support or weight management programmes, as well as dietetic intervention in specific medical conditions, will be identified as part of the initial screening assessment. The dietician can provide advice and management of these problems to the team, having assessed the individual's need and considered their biochemical and nutritional status. The state of the mouth and dental hygiene will be highly important in this area (see Chapter 20 for more detail).

Speech and language therapy

Ensuring communication abilities to maintain participation and self-esteem is an important contribution to participative rehabilitation. Speech and language therapists are also routinely asked to assess problems with dysphagia (see Chapter 17 for more detail).

Problem identification

Problem identification, as part of assessment, precedes goal setting. Problems will be identified as active (i.e. something that concerns the patient and can be worked on) or inactive (an impairment/disability that cannot be resolved or does not affect the patient).

GOAL SETTING

Due to the nature and scale of illness and disability in the older person, the number of emerging problems may overwhelm team members. By focusing on functional problems, together with the person's own perception of the problems, the team should be able to prioritise them with the patient, and carer if relevant. This stage of clinical decision-making is, however, often dependent on the 'intuition' of experienced staff. Textbooks and research may indicate the way ahead for individual conditions, but cannot when they commonly present in unique combinations. This skill of setting a functional goal from a mix of problems is the specialist skill of teams who work successfully with older people.

Decisions are particularly difficult when the appropriate approach is not to inter-vene where rehabilitation is unlikely to be of benefit (Squires and Wardle, 1988) (see also Chapter 4). Such decision should be made objectively, overtly and clearly recorded. In some cases the physical problem will be associated with an environmental or social cause. Such problems will involve the physiotherapist, social worker and occupational therapist working in close conjunction with each other, and increasingly with agencies external to both health and social care (see also Chapters 15, 16 and 19).

Rothstein and Echternach (1986) made the argument for drawing up the problem list *before* physical examination of the patient. They stress the patient's problems are those identified by the patient and 'problem lists generated after physical examination often have departed from dealing with the patient's prob-lems because they have included clinical impressions, diagnostic information or professional jargon.' This provides a valuable caution to team members and encourages a patient centred approach emphasised in the National Service Framework for Older People (see Chapter 6). Starting with the patients' perceived problems, carrying out a thorough assessment and comparing the two should result in a relevant active problem list. This approach could achieve greater user satisfaction where it is a comparison between their expectation and perception of the experience that satisfaction is rated (see Chapter 5). At least the expec-tation that their problem was being noted would be perceived.

Setting goals

As in problem identification, goal setting can be a complex process. Goals should always relate to the older person's informed expectations. Goals are the purpose of the subsequent intervention (Johnson, 1997), and must be realistic, meaningful, achievable and measurable. This will be facilitated by setting both long-term and short-term goals. The former should be directly related to the achievement of the latter. Different team members will have different aims for their own interventions, which should contribute to the ultimate goal. Each team member must be aware of the effect their approach may have on others, and be prepared to compromise for the benefit of the older person – the person who matters. A therapeutic/rehabilitative or a prosthetic approach can be utilised to achieve the same functional goals with individual patients. In the former, the physical impairments/disabilities are treated; in the latter they are not, but appropriate aids and adaptations are provided, and advice is given to allow the same func-tional level to be achieved. A consistent approach from the different team members, crucially including carers, is essential for success, and may require objective debate to agree the approach to be used. Health-care resources will be wasted if a rehabilitative intervention is chosen and the carer at home is only able or willing to follow a prosthetic approach.

The goal setting process has been characterised as an active relationship incorporating opportunities for feedback (see Chapter 9). Patients should take as much responsibility as possible for developing their own goals (Bergquist and Jacket, 1993). The General Mobility Index was developed by physiotherapists to combine assessment of key activities with personalised functional goals and their achievement, and is adaptable for use with whatever key activities the team requires (Squires *et al.*, 1991).

Goal Attainment Scaling was developed in the US for use in Community Mental Health (Kiresuk and Sherman, 1968), and has been developed and evaluated in many different areas of health care. More recently Reid and Chesson (1998) considered its use in stroke care and the setting of physiotherapeutic goals. In this study patients were inclined to define very broad goals that were more difficult to scale and record achievement. Time for negotiation and the setting of more realistic targets was required. It was felt that through goal attainment scaling, clinical practice was enhanced and there was evidence of developing reflective practice. Schut and Stam (1994) identified that Goal Attainment Scaling was an appropriate vehicle for team working and goal setting that may increase the motivation of the rehabilitation team. The TELER system (Le Roux, 1993) is a computerised programme that allows individual goals to be set and the outcomes measured, recorded and evaluated.

For rehabilitation to be successful, team members, including patients and carers, must develop and agree the goals and work towards their achievement. Negotiation skills and patience are essential competencies for all members of the rehabilitation team (see also Chapter 12).

INTERVENTIONS

Having agreed the goals with the patient and carer an intervention plan will be agreed by members of the team with a role to play. Intervention plans will focus on problems and have specified evaluation intervals. In wound care this may be at every treatment; continence management may be reviewed weekly; and functional mobility goals may take several weeks to achieve. It is essential, in any rehabilitation setting, that good communication systems are in operation for 24 hours a day, 365 days per year, hence the role of team communicator being assigned to the nurse. Specialist staff will provide specialist interventions within their professional and legal remit (for example physiotherapy, occupational therapy, podiatry), and all members of the team will carry out the routine practice of different skills and endurance activities. Rehabilitation is the responsibility of all staff working with the patient. Finlay (1994) adapted the Mobility Index (above) as a communication chart for functional mobility within a ward area. With the patient's consent, this can be made available to all staff to make it easy to see how the patient is progressing.

Integrated care pathways

The development of clinical guidelines has recently become a business opportunity – threatening to overwhelm already pressed practitioners. From systematic, evidence based national guidelines (see Chapter 1), adaptation will be needed for local circumstances. Within pathway development it is essential to realise the rights of the individual to self-determination and ensure that care is patient focused not system focused – some patients may not wish to follow the intended route (see Chapter 4).

Integrated care pathways (ICP) (also known as coordinated care pathways, care maps and anticipated recovery pathways) aim to facilitate the introduction into clinical practice of clinical guidelines and systematic continuing audit (Campbell *et al.*, 1998), and is a fundamental component of clinical governance (Chapter 1). Systematic recording within the pathway system facilitates audit of variances. Such audits aim to improve clinical practice through implementation of the recommendations or the changes required, always the most challenging part of the quality cycle.

Care pathways have been used in the US for many years and their growing use in the UK is in recognition of the tool they provide in enabling the implementation of locally agreed interdisciplinary guidelines (Kitchiner and Bundred, 1998). The complexities of multiple pathology encountered within elder rehabilitation will mean that there may be more variances than successful completion of pathways. This factor needs to be appreciated by commissioners measuring supposedly comparative performance.

Within the therapy professions work has been done in trying to develop Therapy Outcome Measures directly related to the goals of the service. Enderby (1998) has focused her work on the ICIDH-2 dimensions of Impairment, Activity and Participation. She argues that for therapists in rehabilitation there is a need to add a fourth concept of Distress/Well-being, as much effort is focused on improving patients' adjustment to disability and developing coping strategies (see also Chapters 16 and 17).

The Therapy Outcome Measure allows staff and patients to describe the relative abilities/difficulties of the patient in the four domains (as above), in order to monitor changes over time. Patients (and carers) are scored on an ordinal scale in the four dimensions. The scales allow clinical judgement to be accurately reflected within the complexities of rehabilitation. Detailed scales have been developed for:

- anxiety
- cardiac rehabilitation
- cerebral palsy
- cognition
- complex and multiple difficulty
- dyspraxia (children)
- head injury
- incontinence
- learning difficulties
- mental health
- multi-factorial conditions
- musculo-skeletal
- neurological disorders
- respiratory care

- schizophrenia
- stroke
- wound care.

Patients are grouped according to case mix – medical diagnosis + functional diagnosis. This work has been well accepted by speech and language therapists, and is developing within occupational therapy, physiotherapy, nursing and podiatry.

OUTCOMES

Outcome refers to the effectiveness of the rehabilitation interventions in achieving the expected goal (Bowling, 1997). The key is that the goal was agreed by all participants. Thus outcome measures are used to assess the relative change within the rehabilitation process. Health outcomes are the results on health of any type of process (Baumberg *et al.*, 1995). They can be affected by housing, social care and employment as well as health services. The Clearing House for Health Outcomes (www.leeds.ac.uk/nuffield/infoservices/UKCH) is based in Leeds and gives advice on specific measures of health outcome in a variety of conditions, for example stroke. Health outcome measurement is required to:

- define and monitor health needs over time
- link the effects on health to the process involved, so that the effects are shown to be outcomes, not just a different state of health
- identify any mediating factors.

The structure of health outcomes considers:

- primary prevention of disease
- secondary prevention of disease
- mortality
- complications/service morbidity
- multi-dimensional health status profiles and indices.

Traditionally, health outcomes have related to what has been required and easily measurable, e.g. death, number of new patients, length of stay. Such measures of input have become used as proxy measures of quality of the intervention process (see also Chapter 2). The emphasis on cost-effectiveness, outcome measurement and evidence based practice since 1990 has developed the methodology of measuring clinical outcomes and allowing qualitative performance indicators to be identified.

The National Centre for Health Outcomes Development published a series of Health Outcome Indicators in 1999 covering Asthma, Breast Cancer, Cataract, Diabetes Mellitus, Fractured Proximal Femur, Myocardial Infarction, Severe Mental Illness, Stroke and Urinary Incontinence – all relevant to the older population. They intend to make recommendations about the 'ideal' indicators for specific conditions and especially about outcomes that may be attributable to interventions or the lack of them. An indicator is an aggregated statistical measure that is derived from a specific population. It provides a benchmark to allow reflective practice. For each condition a menu of indicators has been suggested that will be applicable to different groups of people and for different purposes. They also aim to reflect population-wide, clinical, patient and carer perspectives. It should be noted by elderly rehabilitation specialists that these are aggregated indicators, which cannot be personalised for unique patient specific outcomes.

The indicators have a general structure of:

Title – identifies indicator

Intervention aim – reflects the stages of intervention in the health-care process

Characteristics – classifies the indicator in the four dimensions of specificity; perspective; time frame; outcome relationship

Indicator definition – specifies variable aggregation; sets of denominators; how longitudinal change is to be measured

Rationale – reasons and objectives of the indicator and a range of potential alternatives

Potential uses – local management of practice/local audit/provider based comparisons/population based comparisons/assessment of regional and national trends or progress towards targets

Potential users – national/regional policy makers; provider management; commissioners; clinicians; consumers/public

Possible confounders – identifies the population risk factors likely to influence the indicator that may aid interpretation

Data sources – identifies current systems and systems that may need development

Data quality – limitations of completeness and accuracy

Comments – considers definition, validity, practicality

Further work required – identifies further research and development needed

Conclusions and priority – Working Group's assessment of the priority for implementation

References – appropriate references used in the construction of the indicators.

An example of the complexity of rehabilitation: stroke

To give a practical example of the complexity of the interdisciplinary rehabilitation process and ways of mapping the use of outcome indicators with older people, a case study of a patient with stroke will be described in this chapter, with the authors of Chapters 9 and 11–20 each addressing their contribution to comprehensive care.

Stroke outcome measures have been classified primarily according to the ICIDH-1 (WHO 1999) model of impairment, disability, handicap and are multidimensional. Additionally outcomes related to prognosis, adverse reactions or complication, patient/carer satisfaction and expectations and clinical process were added. In all, 24 indicators have been identified (Fairfield and Long, 1996). Table 8.2 demonstrates the complexity of the available tools to measure the outcome of stroke care.

Table 8.2 Range of stroke outcome measures

Outcome	Classification	Examples
IMPAIRMENT	Arousal	Glasgow Coma Scale
	Motor	Ashworth Scale, Motricity Index, Motor club assessment. Fugl–Mayer assessment
	Cognition	Paced Auditory Serial Addition Test; Behavioural Inattention Test; Frenchay Aphasia Screening Test; Rivermead Perceptual Assessment Battery; Rivermead Behavioural Memory Test; Mini Mental State Examination; Clifton Assessment Procedures for the Elderly; Boston Diagnostic Aphasia Examination; Weschler Adult Intelligence Scale
	Psychological	General Health Questionnaire; Hospital Anxiety and Depressions Scale; Wakefield Self-assessment Depression Inventory
	Severity	A variety of stroke scales
DISABILITY	Physical interaction (mobility and personal care)	ADL activities of daily living – Barthel ADL Index; gait speed; functional ambulation categories; Frenchay Arm Test; Nine-hole Peg Test
	Psychological Interaction	Hodkinson Mental Test; Rivermead Behavioural Memory Test; Frenchay Aphasia Screening Test
	Global disability	Extended ADL, e.g. Nottingham, Rivermead; Frenchay Activities Index; OPCS Disability Scales; functional independence measure
HANDICAP	Orientation, mobility, dependence Self-sufficiency, occupation, social integration	Nottingham Health Profile; Rankin Score; Life Satisfaction Index; Frenchay Activities Index; Nottingham EADL; Edinburgh Rehabilitation Status Scale; Functional Autonomy Measurement; London Handicap Scale; Oxford Handicap Scale; WHO Handicap Scale
MULTI-DIMENSIONAL	Global outcome	Nottingham Health Profile; Quality of Life Well-being Scale; SF-36
	Quality of life	Life Satisfaction Index, Sickness Impact Profile
OTHER	Prognostic outcomes	Incontinence, conscious level; Allen Score
	Negative outcomes	Mortality, complications
	Patient/carer satisfaction, expectations, etc. Process (proxy) outcomes	Pound Questionnaire; Caregiver Strain Index; Cohen, Hoberman Inventory; Kellner's Questionnaire Key Worker, stroke register, re-admissions, discharge destination, number of patients on aspirin

(Rudd et al., 1999)

Of people with a stroke 30 per cent will die and 90 per cent of these deaths will be in the over 65 age group. Government targets involve the halving of mortality rates from stroke by 2010 (Departament of Health [DoH], 1998). With the ageing of the population, how will these targets be achieved and what will be the consequence for morbidity of survivors? What will happen to outcomes of clinical care if quality of life measures and measures of carer strain are recorded? The mortality rate is very easy to measure from death notification requirements. Measures of impairment and disability are common and some are easy to use, but these are not often easily accessible for population data analysis. Handicap is much more complex to measure as it is strongly influenced by psycho-social factors and there is no norm to measure against. Thus, proxy measures of outcome are often used. These are easy to collect and may measure the *process* of care rather than the outcome. Using a Continuous Quality Improvement approach (see Chapter 5) standards set for the process of care that are congruent with stakeholders' needs are likely to result in error-free processes leading to positive outcomes. This relates back to the initial assessment process and its level of complexity and completeness. Resource considerations and patients' wishes will influence decisions. For example, ensuring that all stroke patients have a dysphagia screen within 24 hours of admission is more cost-effective, preventive and patient centred, than measuring the number of patients who aspirate within 72 hours of admission, which requires all patients to have an X-ray at 3 days post-admission.

The plethora of research on the development of bigger and better outcome measures appears to be following the belief that the better the measure the better the outcome. Unless the problem and goal are clearly identified and defined, the outcome can never truly be measured. Wade (1999) states it is 'highly unlikely that the outcome of the service will be influenced greatly by any one profession – this is the nature of team work'. There is still little information about the nature and strength of the factors influencing rehabilitation and Wade recommends that rehabilitation has a greater need for more well-designed studies than for improvements in outcome measures. Locally, teams should agree which measures they will use and then be willing to benchmark their results with colleagues to encourage multi-centre audit and evaluation of clinical practice.

CASE STUDY INTRODUCING SUSAN HUNTER

To give a practical example of the multidisciplinary rehabilitation process, a case study of a patient with stroke will be described, with contributors to Chapters 9 and 11–20 each addressing their contribution to comprehensive care. In accordance with the patient's wishes derived during the initial social assessment by the nurse, Mrs Hunter is called Susan Hunter by the team.

Name:	Susan Hunter
Date of birth:	13.08.19
Social history:	Lives alone in a 2-bedroom ground floor flat. Nursed her husband through terminal illness. He died 3 months ago. She has a daughter who works part time and lives 3 miles away. Her son (a psychiatric nurse) lives with his wife in the next street. Mrs Hunter has 6 grandchildren who all call in and see her. While she was nursing her husband she had carer support, which allowed her to keep up her hobbies of bowling and the local church groups.

Past medical history:	1983 Non-insulin dependent diabetes mellitus
	1988 Osteoarthritis right hip and knee
	1990 Right total hip replacement
	1992 Mild hypothyroidism
	1998 Decreased vision left eye (early cataract)
	1999 Loss of appetite and weight loss – 4 months

Presenting history: Sudden onset of left hemiplegia with left hemianopia, visuospatial disturbance and swallowing difficulties. Fluctuating conscious level for 48 hours and double incontinence. CT Scan showed Total Anterior Circulation Infarct. Gained sitting balance at 6 weeks and could control bowel but remains urinary incontinent. At 3 months is able to get in and out of bed with assistance, to stand with supervision for 10 seconds. Can walk with the help of one person 5 metres. She has increased tone in her left shoulder and elbow and low tone in left ankle and knee. She requires orthotic management of her unstable left ankle. She has been a bit weepy during treatment and is finding that she is regularly getting a lot of pain in her right knee when standing. Her family visit her regularly and try to help her with treatment. They feel that recently she is becoming more detached and not always responding to what they are saying.

Interdisciplinary record-keeping

Patient information needs to be accessible to all members of the interdisciplinary team within the standard confidentiality rules. Why, then, are separate records kept by doctors, nurses, therapists, social workers and so on? Consider the patient's journey from primary care to acute medical care, to rehabilitation, to discharge back home with day hospital to follow and, finally, discharge back to primary care. How many sets of patient records will be started? As Henwood (1994) states, discharge from one area is admission to another area of care. It is important that the information given to patients and carers is documented to ensure consistency of approach and inform all members of the team. (For a fuller discussion on the psychological effects of confused communication see Chapter 9.)

It is intended in the NHS Plan (DoH, 2000) that records should accompany the patient in the form of smart cards. This should include all the medical test results, nursing interventions and therapy assessments, the rationale for the goals set and the achievement of these goals measured as outcome measures, plus discharge support arrangements.

Home care support in primary care should be identified automatically to acute medical care as care transfers, and clarification is needed as to whether this new initiative will be so comprehensive.

In the meantime electronic records may make existing arrangements easier. Staff must agree what is the minimum data they need to have. Electronic links between primary care and acute/intermediate care must be established. Training needs to be given on what the information means and why it is important. If team members understand how they and others can use the information it is more likely to be collected with accuracy and enthusiasm. The development of integrated care plans is one method of ensuring interdisciplinary record-keeping. There may be a need to review professional regulations to ensure the legality of a single case record. The aim for all rehabilitation professionals should be to have a single case record system for best patient care. However, although this may be ideal, the multiple providers of home based care may make it difficult to implement. An example of a day hospital record developed in this way over two years is included as appendices I–V at the end of the book.

Stage 1 Agreed assessment pro-formas held in a central record. Interdisciplinary discharge plan and record held in central record.
Stage 2 Agreed patient/team goals recorded on a single sheet.
Stage 3 All intervention evaluation recorded on a concurrent record.
Stage 4 Single interdisciplinary record.

REFERENCES

Arnadottier, S.A. and Mercer, V.S. (2000) Effects of footwear on measurement of balance and gait in women between the ages of 65 and 93 years. *Physical Therapy*, 80(1), 17–27.

Baumberg, L., Long, A. and Jefferson, J. (1995) *International Workshop: Culture and outcomes*, Barcelona, 9–10 June, European Clearing House on Health Outcomes, Leeds.

Berg, K.O., Wood-Dauphinee, S.L., Williams, J.I. and Maki, B.E. (1992) Measuring balance in the elderly: validation of an instrument. *Canadian Journal of Public Health*, 83, 7–11.

Bergquist, T.F. and Jacket M.P. (1993) Awareness and goal setting with traumatically brain injured. *Brain Injury*, 7(3), 275–282.

Bowling, A. (1997) *Research Methods in Health*, Open University Press, Buckingham.

Campbell, H., Hotchkiss, R., Bradshaw, N. and Porteous, M. (1998) Integrated care pathways. *British Medical Journal*, 3(6), 133–137.

Collen, F.M., Wade, D.T., Robb, G.F. and Bradshaw, C.M. (1991) The Rivermead Mobility Index: a further development of the Rivermead Motor Assessment. *International Disability Studies*, 13.

Conradie, G. (1997) *Outcome Measurement Grid*, Royal College of Speech and Language Therapists Bulletin, London.

Department of Health [DoH] (1998) *Saving Lives: Our healthier nation*, Cm 4386, The Stationery Office, London.

DoH (2000) *The NHS Plan*, The Stationery Office, London.

Enderby, P. (1997) *Therapy Outcome Measures: Speech and language pathology*, Singular Publishing Group, London.

Enderby, P. (1998) *Therapy Outcome Measures: Physiotherapy, Occupational Therapy, Rehabilitation Nursing*, Singular Publishing Group, London.

Fairfield, G. and Long, A. (1996) *A Review of Stroke Outcome Measures*, UK Clearing House on Health Outcomes, Leeds.

Finlay, O. (1994) Communication Chart. *Physiotherapy*, 80(3), 173.

Gill, T.M., Williams, C.S., Richardson, E.D. and Tinetti, M.E. (1996) Impairments in physical performance and cognitive status in predisposing factors for functional dependence among nondisabled older persons. *Journals of Gerontology*, Series A, Biological sciences and Medical sciences, 51A(6), M283–288.

Henwood, M. (1994) *Hospital Discharge Workbook: A manual on hospital discharge practice*, Department of Health, London.

Hodkinson, H.M. (1972) Evaluation of a mental test score for assessment of mental impairment in the elderly. *Age and Ageing*, 1, 233–238.

Johnson, M. (1997) Outcome Measurement: towards an interdisciplinary approach. *British Journal of Therapy and Rehabilitation*, 4(9), 472–477.

Kiresuk, T. and Sherman, R. (1968) Goal Attainment Scaling: a general measure of evaluating comprehensive mental health programs. *Community Health Journal*, 4, 443–453.

Le Roux, A. A. (1993) TELER, the concept. *Physiotherapy*, 79(11), 755–758.

Mahoney, F.I. and Barthel, D.W. (1965) Functional Evaluation: the Barthel Index. *Maryland State Medical Journal*, 14, 61–65.

Royal College of Physicians and British Geriatric Society [RCP/BGS] (1992) *Standardised Assessment Scales for Elderly People*, RCP and BGS, London.

RCP (2000) *National Clinical Guidelines for Stroke*, Intercollegiate Stroke Working Party, Royal College of Physicians, 11 St Andrews Place, London, www.rcplondon.ac.uk

Reid, A. and Chesson, R. (1998) Goal Attainment Scaling: is it appropriate for stroke patients and their physiotherapists? *Physiotherapy*, 84(3), 136–144.

Rodgers, H., Curless, R. and James, O.F.W. (1993) Standardized functional assessment scales for elderly patients. *Age and Ageing*, 22, 161–163.

Roper, N., Logan, W. and Tierney, A. (1996) *The Elements of Nursing, A model for nursing based on a model of living*, 4th edn, Churchill Livingstone, Edinburgh.

Rothstein, J.M. and Echternach, J.L. (1986) Hypothesis-oriented algorithm for clinicians. A method for evaluation and treatment planning. *Physiological Therapeutics*, 66(9), 1388–1394.

Rudd, A., Goldacre, M., Fletcher, J., Wilkinson, E., Mason, A., Fairfield, G. *et al.* (1999) *Health Outcome Indicators: Stroke*. Report of a working group to the Department of Health, National Centre for Health Outcomes Development, Oxford, p. 117.

Schut, H.A. and Stam, H.J. (1994) Goals in rehabilitation teamwork. *Disability and Rehabilitation*, 16(4), 223–226.

Scottish Executive (2000a) *Our Joint Future – the report of the Joint Future Group*, Department of Health and Community Care, Edinburgh.

Scottish Executive (2000b) *Our National Health – A plan for action, a plan for change*, Department of Health, Edinburgh.

Shah, S., Vanclay, F. and Cooper, B. (1989) Improving the sensitivity of the Barthel Index for stroke rehabilitation. *Journal of Clinical Epidemiology*, 42, 703–709.

Sheik, J.I. and Yesavage, J.A. (1986) Geriatric Depression Scale; recent evidence and development of a shorter version. In: *Clinical Gerontology: A guide to assessment and intervention* (ed. Brink, T.L.). Haworth Press, New York.

Smith, R. (1994) Validation and reliability of the Elderly Mobility Scale. *Physiotherapy*, 80(11), 744–747.

Spirduso, W. W. (1996) *Physical Dimensions of Ageing*, Human Kinetics, Champaign, IL.

Squires, A., Rumgay, B. and Perombelon, M. (1991) Audit of Contract Goal Setting by physiotherapists working with elderly patients. *Physiotherapy*, 99(12), 790–795.

Squires, A. and Wardle, P. (1988) To rehabilitate or not? In: *Rehabilitation of the Older Patient* (ed. Squires, A.J.), Chapman & Hall, London.

Sutherland, S. (1999) *With Respect to Old Age: Long term care – rights and responsibilities*, A report by the Royal Commission on long-term care, The Stationery Office, London.

Wade, D.T. (1999) Outcome measurement and rehabilitation. *Clinical Rehabilitation*, 13(2), 93–95.

World Health Organisation [WHO] (1999) *International Classification of Impairment, Disability and Handicap*, WCC World Health Organisation Collaborating Centre, The Netherlands.

Young, A. and Dinan, S. (1994) Fitness for older people. *British Medical Journal*, **309**, 331–334.

9 PSYCHOLOGY AND THE REHABILITATION OF THE OLDER PERSON

Marie Donaghy and Elizabeth Baikie

AIMS OF THE CHAPTER

The purpose of this chapter is to highlight issues relevant to rehabilitation and to discuss approaches informed by a psychological perspective that are intended to help professionals to be more effective in rehabilitation. Problems of patient distress, bereavement and loss, difficulties of motivation, issues around sexuality, and a range of psychological problems, for example memory impairment, confusion, depression and anxiety, can make it very difficult to achieve what the team, older person and carer believe is best. Aspects of psychology can inform those involved in the rehabilitation of older people in order to maximise their input to the patient and outcome from the rehabilitation process.

INTRODUCTION

The term rehabilitation is familiar to lay people and health-care professionals alike, with the expectation that it will lead to an improvement in function, for example increased mobility, and a return to as normal a level as possible. However, the complex nature of the process, the links between mental well-being and physical impairment, individual differences in motivation, and how it relates to changing a person's behaviour may be less well understood by the recipient, carers, health and social care professionals.

Following illness or disability the older person undergoing rehabilitation will be adjusting to possible losses, which may include coming to terms with one or more of the following: impairment, disability, alterations to health, mood status and outlook on life in general (Ormel *et al.*, 1997). For some people this creates ambivalence towards rehabilitation. For example, the 86-year-old woman, recently widowed and unable to live at home independently, may question the value of improving function when the prospect of independent living is unlikely. It therefore seems reasonable to expect that aspects of psychology can inform those involved in the rehabilitation of older people in order to maximise their input to the patient and outcome from the rehabilitation process.

With the emphasis on partnership, which emphasises patient choice, it is important that the older person is engaged in the decision-making process. This may be difficult, however, owing to a lack of understanding of the advantages of change, or because it does not seem to fit with their beliefs about what is wrong with them. For example, in Chapter 3, false beliefs about stroke were described, which include that recovery occurs at the same speed as the illness occurred; rest is needed until recovery occurs; recovery is the result of tablets; and that exercise is bad for the affected side.

The importance of working with the individual to agree aims and procedures, in order to facilitate the desired outcomes is emphasised throughout. The
content of this chapter focuses on the application of psychological principles to
the rehabilitation of the older person, highlighting, where relevant, key theory
and practice.

KNOWLEDGE OF PSYCHOLOGY

There is scope for all health care personnel to apply knowledge from psychology
to health care, which can be construed in terms of different levels of psychological expertise, some of which are common to all health-care personnel, for
example communication. In addition, specific skills, requiring a period of training
and supervision, may be utilised by various professionals, and these include
counselling and cognitive behavioural approaches. Complex psychological problems require the breadth and depth of skills that come from a detailed knowledge
of, and training in, psychology applied to health care, and remain the domain
of psychologists. This will most likely be a clinical psychologist, but in some
settings teams may have access to a health psychologist or a counselling psychologist. However, only a few problems occurring within the rehabilitation of older
people require the direct input of a psychologist. This chapter will focus on the
skills that are either common to health and social care professionals or that can
be acquired following some training.

THE PSYCHOLOGY OF AGEING

In this section we will explore the psychology of ageing in relation to the
following: cognition and associated memory problems; personality and emotions;
pain reduction; motivation and adherence to treatment plans; and sexuality in
later life. It is, however, useful to start with a general overview of what we
mean by the psychological aspects of ageing.

Normal ageing has been found to affect cognitive, emotional and interpersonal behaviour (Kempen *et al.*, 1997) and illness or trauma may exacerbate
one or more of these processes. Psychological effects of ageing are both real in
terms of everyday experience, and in terms of many people's attitudes and
expectations, for example the belief that ageing, frailty and global mental deterioration go hand in hand. These changes need to be taken into account to
optimise the results of rehabilitation with older people, thus planning the right
approach is a challenge to both the team and older people themselves. It is
hoped that this chapter will dispel some of the myths and assumptions about
the behaviour of older people for example, that the person is not trying, is not
motivated or is attention seeking. Adaptation of rehabilitation when necessary
is not ageist – it is age-appropriate (see also Chapter 6).

While the plethora of research on the physiological changes associated with
the central nervous system (CNS) and ageing has provided some explanations
for changes observed in perception, memory, speech and language (Mera, 1997)
(see also Chapter 17), there is a need to place these changes within the context

of the life span and societal change, in order to consider the experience of the individual. Ageing of the individual may be viewed as the final stage of human development and is part of a continual process of change. As such it is difficult to determine when middle age stops and old age begins.

Much of the literature on ageing tends to focus on one direction of change, typically a decline in function. This emphasis, however, tends to obscure the actual magnitude of change. For psychological changes, the magnitude tends to be a relatively small proportion of the absolute level of function; the personal experience of normal ageing is therefore one of continuity. For many, age differences (what you observe if you compare today's younger with today's older people) are more pronounced than age changes (what changes are observed if you follow the same individuals over their life span). Not surprisingly, it is much easier to study age differences, using so-called cross-sectional designs, rather than age changes. The latter demand longitudinal study over many years, at least in humans. There are relatively few research projects that have so far been able to yield such data. Age differences are magnified by differences in upbringing and other experiences that are common to whole generations and societies. Thus today's 80 year old will, for example, have had very different opportunities of education, work and travel from today's 30 year old. To understand the effects of true ageing, we must make allowance for this.

The task for the health professional working with an individual patient is to distinguish between changes that are due to normal ageing and those resulting from illness and psychological factors. Evidence from functional neuro-imaging experiments suggests that some brain changes seen with age may be compensatory, with greater activity seen in some task relevant brain areas when compared to younger adults (Grady and Craik, 2000). Some skills remain relatively unchanged, for example retaining crystallised intelligence (the amount of knowledge acquired over time), compared to fluid intelligence (the ability to solve novel problems). This tends to show a decline in most if not all people, for example changes in working memory (necessary for reasoning and comprehending) and attention span (Palladino and De Beni, 1999). Increases in reaction time have also been frequently reported (Craik and Salthouse, 2000). One widespread finding is that differences between individuals increase with age (Fairweather, 1991). Such age changes usually refer to the average for a group of people; some will show a lot of change, others much less. This means that predicting someone's ability on the basis of age alone is much less accurate in later life. Often for a given psychological function the 'best' older people will be doing as well as the average younger person, the 'worst' are however doing very much worse (Holland and Rabbitt, 1991). Understanding of the individual's previous ability level and educational attainment is important, particularly when assessing mental function, for example using the Mini Mental State Examination (MMSE) (Folstein et al., 1975).

Cognition

There is strong evidence that memory changes occur with normal ageing (Vanneste and Pouthas, 1999; Craik and Salthouse, 2000). However, although there is a general trend of decline in memory with the widely held view that this is attributable to changes in the speed by which information is processed in the CNS, the extent of the loss is probably much less than people imagine, including older people themselves. Where there is marked memory loss this is usually associated with altered pathology in the CNS as can be seen in the dementias (Peterson, 2000).

Memory is often thought of as the mental function most susceptible to ageing. This may be because normal ageing has been confused all too readily with dementia, with memory loss being the hallmark of this condition. Working memory declines slightly. Whereas in young adulthood, we can remember about seven to nine items or chunks of information, we might find this reduced to six to eight by our late seventies. This itself has few implications for most everyday life. Long-term memory is the name given to the brain's permanent store for information, and similarly shows a tendency to decline, but the extent of this depends very much on the nature of the task. Our ability to recall stored information without prompting shows a clear decline on average, but recognition memory is much less affected. Therapists can therefore use recognition memory in rehabilitation rather than free recall.

Older people can benefit greatly from being encouraged to use strategies to improve memory. These strategies include using a diary and notice board to ensure important appointments are not forgotten (Maylor, 1996). Research supports the use of an eight session cognitive enhancement programme, with non-dementia patients requiring assistance with living, to improve everyday memory such as arranging appointments and delivering messages (McDougall, 2000).

An understanding of the different aspects of memory will enable the health professional to plan an appropriate rehabilitation programme with the individual. There are various aspects of memory to consider, including autobiographical memory (the recall of personal events from the past), semantic memory (the recall of facts and information), prospective memory (the ability to remember to do something in the future) and, of course, the difference between verbal and visual memory. For a full discussion on these aspects, see Gruneberg and Morris (1992). Patients are constantly surprised that they can remember things from their childhood but have an unclear recall of last week's events.

In an interesting series of experiments (Cohen and Faulkner, 1989) quality of memory was found to alter with age. It appears that older people make different kinds of errors when remembering what has happened. The difference between their memories for what they have done and for what they have thought of doing is more marked. They are less likely to be accurate about the latter. They seem to be more likely to make the error of remembering something they thought of doing as being something they actually did. The effects are quite subtle but can have very real practical consequences.

One example of quality of memory in rehabilitation is when the patient and the therapist may give significantly different accounts of what happened on a home assessment visit, possibly affecting agreement on the goals in a treatment plan. If the patient recalls that he or she did something, which in fact was only discussed, this may be no more than a normal ageing phenomenon, not the sign of a dementia. The individual going on a home visit for OT assessment, may be anxious to pass the test in order to be discharged from hospital. This may affect memory recall, however this is likely to be counteracted to an extent by the familiarity of their own home and kitchen.

Another example might be the taking of medicines where the consequences of the 'thought it/did it' discrepancy can be profound. It is important to emphasise that these normal age changes in memory will be exacerbated by illness, distress or other difficulties. Interestingly, adherence with medication has been found not to be related to health status but to self-efficacy and the confidence in ability to successfully remember to take the medication (Gould et al., 1997). Confidence can be facilitated through positive feedback when medicine is correctly taken.

Changes are also found in thinking and language (the ability to recognise letters and words and extract meaning from phrases). The most pervasive change seems to be the speed of information processing, which consistently shows decline with ageing. Both simple tasks, such as choice reaction time, and more complex ones such as processing language, show greater age effects when speed and complexity are involved (see also Chapter 17). Put another way, slowing things down a little and making them easier helps everybody, especially older people. Again, this has very practical implications for the way in which we present information, especially in unfamiliar and stressful situations such as being a patient in hospital.

Changes in the speed by which information is processed also reduces the ability to divide attention between two tasks, increases risk of errors and slows down performance. It is important for health-care professionals to be aware that noise and distraction caused by other activity on the ward, day hospital or department, will greatly reduce the ability of the patient to concentrate on a particular instruction or task. Other more pronounced changes are found in Alzheimer type dementia where there is a progressive loss of semantic memory, manifested by progressive language deficit and marked changes in attention span.

Personality and emotions

A number of studies exploring the relationship between personality and health demonstrate a link with dimensions of personality such as neuroticism and extroversion (Mathews and Deary, 1998). In working with individuals, it may be more helpful to consider psychological factors and their behavioural consequences, for example, anxiety and health beliefs. Personality factors, according to Resnick (1999), have been linked to personal goals, fears and beliefs influencing both motivation and actual behaviour, all of which are amenable to change. These are all aspects that can be influenced by health-care professionals. Improved motivation has been linked to having clear and realistic goals, humour where appropriate, and encouragement, feelings of control and a reduction in negative beliefs (Resnick, 1996). Examples might be the belief that they will not succeed or the expectation that they should have a daily bowel movement.

Any changes in personality in later life are more likely to be the result of other factors such as changes in health status and social circumstances, and social contacts and income, than due to the effect of ageing alone. How you feel about your age and how you view your disposable income have been found to be associated with how content you are in later life. There have been many studies of constructs, such as social comparison, life satisfaction, emotional well-being, morale, social support and happiness in later life (Power *et al.*, 1988). The good news is that most older people are actually happy most of the time. Research findings suggest that the way in which individuals address existential concerns has profound implications for physical and mental well-being (Wong and Fry, 1998). Depression is noticeable among older people in the hospital setting, especially after bereavement of a spouse where the feeling may be 'why bother'. However, depression and loneliness in older people has been found to be uncommon, and where it is present it has been linked to poor health, poverty and family or other interpersonal difficulties (Fees *et al.*, 1999). Although social support has been found to be useful in facilitating better health outcomes in older people (Bisconti and Bergeman, 1999), there is some inconsistency in the literature. Dunbar *et al.* (1998) highlight, in their review of the topic, the fact that social support may cause feelings of inequity resulting in increased psychological distress. One way of minimising this is to help the recipient to consider how they can repay the person giving the support, for example this may be in providing emotional support or undertaking small favours. Health-care professionals are in a position to reduce feelings of inequity by encouraging the recipient to look back at when they provided support for others. This may be important to maintain personal autonomy.

Pain and fear

Despite many older people having potentially painful conditions they have been found to under-report pain (Klinger and Spaulding, 1998), and the authors recommend that assessment of pain should be undertaken routinely during clinical examination. In the past, older people with cognitive impairment have not been given the same level of pain medication as cognitively intact individuals (Kaasalainen *et al.*, 1998). The reasons for this are unclear, but it may simply be due to poor communication between the individual and health-care staff. The need for effective communication is crucial between older people and the team, especially pharmacists (see Chapter 20C), to facilitate appropriate interventions (McCormick *et al.*, 1996). Pain may result in withdrawal from activities, refusal to co-operate, low mood state and altered behaviour, and such observations can be easily labelled as personality and emotional change. It is therefore important that it is recognised and treated. Pain may produce fear of an activity, for example transferring from the bed to a chair. Fear and pain are linked; while fear and anxiety can increase pain and prevent or limit activity, distraction can reduce it. When patients have cognitive impairment causing language problems, they do not always report pain, and staff may be unaware of this. It may be evident in behaviour, however, e.g. restlessness, or holding self in a different way, thus staff need to be vigilant in noting such changes in behaviour.

Older people who have fallen several times while walking may understandably become afraid of doing so again when they move. They may, as a result, refuse or be reluctant to rise to stand, to transfer or to attempt to walk. These tasks should be broken down into components, each one building on the other, for example rising to stand, standing balance, walking with assistance. Understanding the individual's fears and taking cognisance of their beliefs about their ability to complete the task successfully is crucial. The traditional placing of a walking aid in front of the person may provide sufficient reassurance to some, while others may initially require a more familiar and solid looking form of standing support. In some cases, the back of a readily available dining chair fills the space in front of the patient and offers solid visual reassurance. In neither case should the patient be encouraged to pull themselves out of the chair by using the aid, but push down on the chair arms to facilitate a safer and kinaesthetically more normal movement.

Older people may also show fear of falling when being moved on the bed. Reassurance and careful physical handling can minimise this fear, allowing the person time to adjust to any changes in position. The view of the floor when rising from the bed or when descending down stairs may create anxiety and loss of confidence. This effect can be reduced by the use of positioning when assisting the person. For example, when rising from the bed by positioning him or herself close to the bed and level with the person's head the assistant can block the view of the floor. Similarly the patient's fear of descending the stairs can be minimised if the assistant steps down first, facing the patient. When tackling the feared behaviour, gradually the person can slowly build confidence. All those involved in the individual's care should integrate ideas and recommendations from different team members to minimise difficulties so that they can be used consistently. Any lapse in continuity of approach may undo any hard won progress. Expert advice should be sought early (see Chapter 15).

Physiotherapists are often faced with the necessity of carrying out movements that can cause pain. Following a recently repaired hip fracture, surrounding muscles may be sensitive and pain-killing drugs are usually necessary before treatment. The progression of treatment following fractures may need to be unusually slow until the pain subsides – although responsive to the patient's needs, this may compromise performance indicators against national pathway guidance (see also Chapters 1 and 8). An empathetic approach to people's fears and anxieties is likely to increase participation in treatment regimens during rehabilitation.

Motivation and adherence

Poor motivation during rehabilitation is an issue that often confronts health-care professionals and carers, and it is important to gain some insight into the possible reasons for this. It may be linked to any of the following – fear, pain, anxiety, depression, irrational health belief, an awareness of the inability to function as before. The attitude and behaviour of others may aggravate this through lack of empathy, accusations of being a 'difficult patient', 'attention seeking', 'not trying' or over-protectiveness with resultant loss of self-esteem and personal autonomy. Once the reasons for the lack of motivation are understood then motivation can be facilitated through the use of appropriate task oriented goals. The older person taking part in a rehabilitation programme should, wherever possible, be actively involved in setting out their goals, which should be realistic in expectation, include a time frame, and a clear outcome that is measurable (see Chapters 8 and 13–20).

Getting older people motivated into undertaking a rehabilitation task or adhering to a regimen is one challenge, while the other is to sustain motivation over a longer period of time, particularly when the person is not being supervised and after discharge from the stimulation of the relevant service. A useful model for approaching adherence issues is to take into account the gap between what the person knows or perceives, and current versus optimal level of functioning. This immediately implies that we need to know both about the likely prognosis and choices of treatment and outcomes, and what the individual and family expect. The task is to bring these as far as possible into alignment (see also Chapter 5). At most stages of rehabilitation, the focus is on improving the level of function or adapting the environment to give the maximum amount of independence. We also need to take account of how the person sees their future and what they want. This is particularly important because there can be a gap between these, which results in unnecessary pessimism or unrealistic optimism. Rehabilitation is best achieved by taking a positive approach, focusing on skills rather than failures. This approach increases the person's self-efficacy, that is the belief that the outcome of treatment can be successfully achieved. Older people who participate in regular physical activity are motivated by the belief that they will benefit from the outcomes of exercise and that they have control over the decision to exercise (Resnick and Spellbring, 2000).

It is equally important for both health-care professionals and the older person to be able and willing to recognise when the goals of rehabilitation change. Generally, in the early stages of a programme, the emphasis is on encouragement and enhancing motivation. We need the person to believe that all the hard work we are going to recommend to achieve the agreed rehabilitation goals will, in the end, be worth it. The message is something like 'work hard and you will improve'. Often at a later stage we have to modify the goals to work to maximise independence within what may be very serious limitations. The message here is 'lets see how we can help you live with your disability' to enjoy a certain quality of life. This involves adjustment and feelings of loss. This change is very often not explicit, and certainly the person may not agree to these different goals.

There is therefore a dilemma in that at one stage we are asking the person to put in much effort, when in reality it may be very hard to predict how independent he or she will eventually become. Sometimes this is inherent in the nature of the illness (stroke outcome is known to be particularly hard to predict) or it may be because there are subsequent additional health (for example, problems with a hip prosthesis) or social (for example, a recent bereavement) problems.

Where there is only a rough idea of the likely outcome, the tendency is to err on the side of optimism when predicting for the individual – also responding to the need of professionals to feel of value, whatever the hopelessness of the situation. If the person wants to go home the team will try to enable this and provide as much support in the community as possible but realisation of this goal is not always feasible. Members of the team also have to learn to let go and to appreciate when their input is no longer tenable. Successful goal negotiation is a highly skilled competence for professionals in the speciality (see Chapter 8).

Sexuality in later life

A knowledge of sexuality, e.g. sexual needs, sexual expression and sexual identity, is an important part of care of the older person, if we adhere to the philosophy of treating the 'whole' person. Mood disorders, physical illness, acquired disability, medication, consequences of surgery and various treatments can all affect sexual functioning. The sexual consequences may be direct, e.g. impaired erectile function, or indirect, by reducing sense of sexual attractiveness and self-esteem. These factors have major implications for rehabilitation and treatment, and are of particular relevance for health-care professionals.

The older person may be reluctant to raise their intimate concerns and seek help for sexual problems, but certain tasks within rehabilitation may put them in focus and also make it easier for them to be discussed in relation to certain Activities of Daily Living. Thus a treatment plan to improve mobility may (potentially) open up a discussion on movement difficulties and therefore implications for comfort during sexual intercourse. Dressing practice, relaxation training and bathing may act as similar triggers. Discussion prior to and after a home visit to a spouse provides the opportunity to discuss not only how the person coped with cooking and toileting, but also their concerns about adjusting at home. These examples noted above serve as opportunities to provide holistic care but depend on the health professional's comfort with their patients' sexuality, as well as their own. It may be that the intimacy, physical closeness and privacy of these tasks facilitate deeper self-disclosure and therefore the opportunity to discuss sexual feelings. It is not unheard of, however, for older people not to be asked about their sexual feelings and relationships, simply because they are over 65 years of age. The reluctance to discuss sexual issues with an older patient may be explained by a belief that older people are neither sexually active nor interested in being so; the age gap between health professional and older person, which could range from 6 to 70 years (59-year-old therapist treating a 65-year-old patient or 22-year-old therapist treating a 92-year-old patient). The difficulty may be in coming to terms with the fact that sex is not only for the young and attractive. There may be unconscious identification of the older person with the professional's own parent or grandparent and therefore a resistance to see the older person as a sexual being. This may expose the health professional's own discomfort with sexuality.

Our knowledge of sexuality in general and sexual aspects of illness and disability has increased significantly since the pioneering work of Masters and Johnson (1996, 1970). Interest in sexuality in later life has somewhat lagged behind, but recently practitioners have started to research issues relating to sexuality and dementia – the latter often being seen by health professionals as problem behaviour. Oppenheimer (1997) cites several studies in her review of sexuality in old age, which report figures of sexual activity in people over 60 years of age. Spence (1991) summarises the findings on sexuality in later life. These include the following: older people continue to be sexually active; sexual interest declines with age; older men show greater sexual interest than older women; the physiological changes that occur with ageing do not account for the changes in sexual functioning; sexual dysfunction is not directly related to age.

Although the apparent intimacy and physical closeness of certain tasks can facilitate a helpful discussion with the older person, sometimes this can be a negative experience for staff. When touch is used with a person who is cognitively impaired, e.g. to facilitate movement or demonstrate exercise, aid behaviour such as dressing or washing, provide comfort or aid spatial orientation, it may be sexually arousing and/or be misinterpreted in the function it is serving. When cognitively intact older people make sexual statements or act inappropriately towards staff, common reactions include embarrassment, disgust or use of humour. In order to deal effectively with the situation, the health professional needs to understand what is underlying the behaviour and, if necessary, to assert him or herself tactfully to maintain appropriate boundaries. In the case of dementia, sexually inappropriate behaviour may be due to one or more of the following reasons and so would entail a different response:

- the patient misidentifies the staff member as their spouse (most commonly male patient and female member of staff), particularly if they believe they are younger than they actually are;
- the older person misinterprets the staff member's use of touch;
- a combination of disinhibition and attraction towards the staff member; expression of need, e.g. to urinate (opening trouser flies or lifting skirt up); normal behaviour, usually carried out in private, being displayed in public, e.g. masturbation.

SPECIFIC SKILLS RELATED TO PSYCHOLOGICAL CARE

Having a knowledge of the psychological changes and the problems commonly associated with ageing, for example life events, enables health-care professionals to provide strategies to enhance individual care. A key skill for all health-care professionals is good communication and this has already been alluded to in regard to active listening skills and is discussed in Chapter 17. In addition to the requirement for all staff to have good communication skills, there are a number of areas of psychological care in the rehabilitation of older people, where any appropriately trained member of the team can provide effective help. The areas we will discuss will be grief and loss, disability counselling and breaking bad news. Within this section we also discuss depression and suicidal intent, highlighting when specialist psychological skills may be required. We have also included carers in this section, as we recognise that they have specific skills that both inform, and can be informed by, health-care professionals' knowledge (see also Chapter 12).

Grief and loss

Like many other psychological problems in rehabilitation, grief is not unique to older people. Experiencing the death of someone close can happen at any age. What is more likely to be the experience of older people is the cumulative effect of several bereavements, and the chance that the loved one lost may have been close to that person for a very long time. There is good evidence that the risk of depression in older people increases with the multiplicity of problems (Schumacher *et al.*, 1997). One of the most important of these is the loss of someone close. The relationship may be one that has lasted for many decades. Older people are likely to be in their 70s, at least, before celebrating 50 years of marriage. That duration may make it very difficult to adjust to the loss but may also indicate a good relationship. How one adapts to loss compared to grief is also influenced by the quality of the relationship. For example, where the partner has also been undertaking a carer role the loss may mean the individual has a greater physical upheaval, as they no longer have the support they require to live independently.

Typical grief reactions have been well described and include phases of numbness or shock (characterised by absence of feeling or disbelief that the loss has occurred), acute grief (characterised by crying, pining and pangs of grief) and assimilation (gradually adapting to life without the loved one). In a multi-cultural society, awareness of the differences between ethnic groups in dealing with bereavement should be understood, particularly by staff dealing first hand with the loss.

Adjustment can be a lengthy process and does not follow a straightforward progress through clearly defined stages or time sequence. This is most obvious when anniversaries and other stimuli can evoke acute grief some months or even years after the loss or other losses, for example loss of a friend or an animal. Most people who suffer a bereavement do not need grief counselling; they will adapt to the loss given time and the support of those around them. However, specific counselling may be helpful for complex grief where adjustment is impaired. Factors such as the circumstances of the loss, the quality of the relationship and other life stresses, for example a hip fracture, and the availability of support, all affect the risk of impaired adjustment, that can lead to feelings of 'why bother' and 'no one to live for'. Targeting those at higher risk is the best strategy (Parkes, 1992).

Disability counselling

The reactions to disability may be similar to those of bereavement. This is especially so in the case of sudden loss of function, such as that following a stroke, or losing a limb through amputation. One important difference is that disability often follows very serious illness and, in the acute phase, life itself may be threatened. The point at which it becomes appropriate to focus on psychological issues will vary considerably from patient to patient. It is very often helpful to be guided by the patient's reaction to therapy, for example the person feels they are not making any progress with their therapy, expressing feelings of hopelessness. Difficulties in adjustment are often manifested as 'problems of motivation' or episodes of acute distress.

Psychological problems are often not raised by the patient directly with the doctor, they are in practice more likely to emerge during an OT or physiotherapy session, during discussions about family care input, or when the patient has intimate personal care, such as having a bath. There are parallels with other areas where the patient's willingness to disclose problems is inversely proportional with the perceived status of the staff member; the consultant physician is therefore at the low end of likely confidants. Often the familiar environment of a home assessment visit may be the best place to start addressing important personal issues. A good team enables those involved to share the relevant information, taking into consideration issues of confidentiality, and can identify the best person to help with each type of problem.

Other patients, relatives, and indeed other patients' relatives, are all potential sources of support, although they can also be the source of misleading advice. Comment or advice given with the best of intentions can create problems when they do not fit with that person's unique circumstances, for example, in the case of depression, the suggestion that it is all in the person's mind.

This means that it is always important to try to keep in touch with the older person's view of their situation and to understand how they see their progress. After lengthy rehabilitation even eventual discharge can be quite threatening. The personal implications of disability can vary widely. Where there is sudden enforced role change, for example, there is likely to be more distress over and above the actual level of disability.

Breaking bad news

Both bereavement and disability are situations in which the professional can find themselves being the bearer of bad news or being asked some very searching questions. It is a fact of health and social care that the least experienced spend the most time with service users, and it is to these people in one-to-one situations that often quite personal concerns are addressed. The patient may have plucked up the courage to raise their concerns with some difficulty, and only one opportunity for a response may exist. The response must be honest, and consistent with what other team members might offer if asked – regular team meetings should provide the background knowledge needed. Where issues are sensitive, confidentiality is important, but where appropriate the issue should be discussed with the team to prepare any member (from professional to support worker) for another approach on the subject.

Usually we think of these challenges as being associated with terminal illness, especially cancer. However a question such as 'Do you think I will be able to go home?' or 'Do you think I will ever walk again?' can be just as challenging. Like communication in general, it is still only recently that it has been recognised that such skills can be taught. There are, however, several examples of applying social skill analysis to such situations, although so far this has been aimed mainly at medical staff.

When necessary all professionals need to be able to break bad news, that is tell patients something that may alter their expectations of the future. An example in occupational therapy might be having to say that it will not be possible to adapt someone's home enough or to provide enough care for them to go back to living there. These are very much 'bad news' from the patient's perspective. The manner of telling is important; the use of voice, tone, speed of information giving, phrasing that gives recognition to the person's understanding, feelings and expectations, for example 'I know this is a blow for you, that you are longing to go home but...'. It is *essential* that there is consistency in what is being said and that the statement is evidence based as far as is possible, fully agreed with the team and documented for the information of staff not present.

Mortality, depression and suicidal intent

Coming to terms with the process of dying, fear of pain and discomfort, possible fear of dying alone, concern about those left behind, and religious beliefs regarding the after life, is quite properly seen as a common psychological task for older people and especially for those whose health has been impaired. We know that older people suffer from depression (Silveira and Ebrahim, 1998; Zimmerman *et al.*, 1999), and we know that this is a treatable distress. Suicide rate among older people is at least as high as those in the middle years of life, however, the rates for attempted suicide are much lower; parasuicide is not a typical phenomenon of later life. Taken together these suggest that we should take very seriously expressions of suicide intention in older people, since attempt is likely to be successful. Therefore if the older person is expressing the desire to end their life, staff should not rely on just providing reassurance, but sensitively check out feelings of why, and how.

Conversely, just to complicate matters, older people may express the wish to die without suicidal intent. Typically they may say something to the effect that they are fed up with living and they will be glad when their time has come and they can join their partner. This is particularly so in those whose health is failing, including some who are receiving rehabilitation. Such patients may have a very clear idea of having had a full and interesting life, and have come to terms with the fact of their mortality. This, however, is a passive wish to die and not an active desire to end their own life.

Distinguishing between these is clearly important and certainly one of the ways of using specialist psychological skills. One of the important differences is that those who are feeling 'enough is enough', but who are not depressed can still find much in the present and in the immediate future to look forward to. They have undiminished interests, particularly in such common priorities as family and friends, but because of their disability, may need alternative ways of pursuing their interests.

There have been a number of attempts to devise simple screening tests for depression in older people and these should be readily available in all rehabilitation settings. They can take no more than a few minutes to complete and provide a rational basis for deciding who would benefit from further investigation. Examples of these are: the Geriatric Depression Scale, GDS (Yesavage *et al.*, 1982); Hospital Anxiety and Depression Scale (HAD) (Zigmond and Snaith, 1983); Beck Depression Inventory (BDI) (Beck and Steer, 1979). For a comprehensive review of these scales and others see McDowell and Newell (1996).

CASE STUDY SUSAN HUNTER – PSYCHOLOGICAL ASSESSMENT

In some settings various members of the team, for example nursing, medical, occupational therapy and speech and language therapy staff, routinely carry out screening for assessments of mood and cognition, using one of the above tools. If these results are suggestive of difficulties, a referral might be made to a psychologist. These results may be related to staff observations that this person is weepy and detached. Relevant factors to consider are: recent widowhood; mild hypothyroidism could have implications for cognitive function; there may be depression post stroke as a result of the extent of the damage; or a combination of factors. In planning a rehabilitation programme for Susan Hunter, her mood and her level of cognitive functioning in negotiating goals has to be considered. Susan Hunter's perception of available social support is also important. Her son and daughter could be involved in the planning of the care, taking cognisance of relevant hobbies and interests. It is important to take into account changes in social contact, and to consider whether these have declined. Does the loss of the carer support and/or depression mean that she has cut down on the number of social contacts? In this particular case the psychologist needs to be involved in order to assist the team in identifying the relevant crucial psychological factors that are contributing to her current presentation in order to inform the planning of appropriate treatment goals and implementing rehabilitation. To this end the psychologist in the team will be working with other team members, such as the occupational therapist and the physiotherapist, to assist in the consideration of appropriate treatment goals to be discussed and agreed with Susan Hunter.

CARERS' NEEDS

Carers provide essential support during rehabilitation of their older person. However, their role is not an easy one; the degree of perceived control over the care giver's situation appears to be important and may be used as an indicator of carers who need assistance to provide care (Szabo and Strang, 1999). Such assistance may be provided by the team dealing with the cared-for person, or by a different team depending on local arrangements and personal need. The provision of day centre support to the cared for is also important to carers' well-being and has been found to reduce the impact of negative consequences on life satisfaction and social interactions for carers of older people (Lorensini and Bates, 1997) (see Chapter 12).

SUMMARY

The evidence from research and clinical practice highlights the complexity and diversity of psychological changes that occur with normal ageing and disability. It challenges negative, ageist attitudes that suggest change is universal, demonstrating both the dynamic nature of change and the influence of context. This evidence, combined with the authors' experience gained from working with older people, highlights the special challenge associated with the rehabilitation of the older person. We have attempted to demonstrate how members of the health-care team can apply many of the skills informed by psychology theory and practice, with appropriate support from a psychologist working from one of the following perspectives; clinical psychology, health psychology or counselling psychology. There is sufficient evidence in the literature to indicate that when these skills are applied within the rehabilitation setting the quality and effectiveness of care will be improved.

REFERENCES

Beck, A.T. and Steer, R.A. (1979) *Beck Depression Inventory Manual*, Psychological Corporation, Harcourt Brace Jovanovitch, New York.

Bisconti, T.L. and Bergeman, C.S. (1999) Perceived social control as a mediator of the relationships among social support, psychological well-being, and perceived health. *Gerontologist*, 39(1), 94–103.

Cohen, G. and Faulkner, D. (1989) The effects of ageing on perceived and generated memories. In: *Everyday Cognition in Adulthood and Late Life* (eds Poon, L.W., Rubin, D.C. and Wilson, B.A.), Cambridge University Press, Cambridge.

Craik, F. and Salthouse, T. (eds) (2000) *The Handbook of Ageing and Cognition*, 2nd edn, Lawrence Erlbaum, Mahwah, NJ, pp. 293–357.

Dunbar, M., Ford, G. and Hunt, K. (1998) Why is the receipt of social support associated with increased psychological distress? An examination of three hypotheses. *Psychology and Health*, 13, 527–544.

Fairweather, D.S. (1991) Ageing is a biological phenomenon. *Reviews in Clinical Gerontology*, 1, 3–16.

Fees, B.S., Martin, P. and Poon, L.W. (1999) A model of loneliness in older adults. *Journals of Gerontology: Series B: Psychological Sciences and Social Sciences*, 54B(4), 231–239.

Folstein, M.F., Folstein, S.E. and McHugh, P.R. (1975) Mini Mental State: a practical method for grading the cognitive state of patients for the clinician. *Journal of Psychiatric Research*, 12, 189–198.

Gould, O., McDonald, M. and King, B. (1997) Metacognition and medication adherence: How do older adults remember? *Experimental Ageing – Research* **23**(4), 315–342.

Grady, C.L. and Craik, F.I. (2000) Changes in memory processing with age. *Presse Medicine,* **29**(15), 849–857.

Gruneberg, M. and Morris, P. (1992) *Aspects of Memory, Volume 1: The Practical Aspects,* Routledge, London.

Holland, C.A. and Rabbitt, P. (1991) The course and cause of cognitive change with advancing age. *Reviews in Clinical Gerontology,* **1**, 81–96.

Kaasalainen, S., Middleton, J., Knezacek, S., Hartley, T., Stewart, N., Ife, C. *et al.* (1998) Pain and cognitive status in the institutionalized elderly: perceptions and interventions. *Journal of Gerontological Nursing,* **24**(8), 24–31.

Kempen, G.I.J.M., Brilman E.I. and Relyveld, J. (1997) Adaptive responses among Dutch elderly: The impact of eight chronic conditions on health-related quality of life. *American Journal of Public Health,* **87**, 38–44.

Klinger, L. and Spaulding, S.J. (1998) Chronic pain in the elderly: is silence really golden? *Physical and Occupational Therapy in Geriatrics,* **15**(3), 1–17.

Lorensini, S. and Bates, G.W. (1997) The health, psychological and social consequences of caring for a person with dementia. *Australian Journal on Ageing,* **16**(4), 198–202.

Maylor, A.E. (1996) Older people's memory for the past and the future. *Psychologist,* **9**(10), 456–459.

Masters, W.H. and Johnson, V.E. (1966) *Human Sexual Response,* Churchill Livingstone, London.

Masters, W.H. and Johnson, V.E. (1970) *Human Sexual Inadequacy,* Churchill Livingstone, London.

Mathews, G. and Deary, I.J. (1998) *Personality Traits,* Cambridge University Press, Cambridge.

Maylor, A.E. (1996) Older people's memory for the past and the future. *Psychologist,* **9**(10), 456–459.

McCormick, W.C., Inui, T.S. and Roter, D.L. (1996) Interventions in physician-elderly patient interactions. *Research on Ageing,* **18**(1), 103–136.

McDougall, G.J. (2000) Memory improvement in assisted living elders. *Issues in Mental Health Nursing,* **21**(2), 217–233.

McDowell, I. and Newell, C. (1996) *Measuring Health: A guide to rating scales and questionnaires,* Oxford University Press, New York.

Mera, S.L. (1997) *Pathology and Understanding Disease Prevention,* Stanley Thornes, Cheltenham.

Ormel, J., Kempen, G.I.J.M, Penninx, B.W.J.H., Brilman, E.I., Beekman, A.T.F. and Van Sonderen, E. (1997) Chronic medical conditions and mental health status in older people: Disability and psychological resources mediate specific mental health effects. *Psychological Medicine,* **27**, 1065–1077.

Palladino, P. and De Beni, R. (1999) Working memory in ageing maintenance and suppression. *Memory and Cognition,* **27**(6), 948–955.

Parkes, C.M. (1992) Bereavement and mental health in the elderly. *Reviews in Clinical Gerontology,* **2**, 45–51.

Peterson, R.C. (2000) Mild cognitive impairment: transition between ageing and Alzheimer's disease. *Memory,* **1**, 37–49.

Power, M.J., Champion, L.D. and Aris, S.J. (1988) Development of a measure of social support: The Significant Others Scale. *British Journal of Clinical Psychology*, 27, 349–358.

Resnick, B. (1996) Motivation in geriatric rehabilitation. *Journal of Nursing Scholarship*, 28(1), 41–45.

Resnick, B. (1999) Motivation to perform activities of daily living in the institutionalized older adult: can a leopard change its spots? *Journal of Advanced Nursing*, 29(4), 792–799.

Resnick, B. and Spellbring, A.M. (2000) Understanding what motivates older adults to exercise. *Journal of Gerontological Nursing*, 26(3), 34–42.

Schumacher, J., Wilz, G. and Brahler, E. (1997) Influence of dispositional coping strategies on physical complaints and life satisfaction in the elderly. *Gerontology Geriatric*, 30(5), 338–347.

Silveira, E.R. and Ebrahim, S. (1998) Social determinants of psychiatric morbidity and well-being in immigrant elders and whites in east London. *International Journal of Geriatric Psychiatry*, 13(11), 801–812.

Spence, S.H. (1991) *Psychosexual Therapy: A cognitive-behavioural approach*, Chapman & Hall, London/New York.

Szabo, V. and Strang, V.R. (1999) Clinical scholarship. Experiencing control in caregiving. *Journal of Nursing Scholarship*, 31(1), 71–75.

Vanneste, S. and Pouthas, V. (1999) Timing in aging: The role of attention. *Experimental Ageing Research*, 25(1), 49–67.

Wong, P.T. and Fry, P.S. (1998) *The Human Quest for Meaning: A handbook of psychological research and clinical applications*, Lawrence Erlbaum Associates, Mahwah, NJ.

Yesavage, J.A., Brink, T.L., Rose, T.L., Lum, O., Huang, V., Adey, M. *et al.* (1983) Development and validation of a geriatric screening scale: a preliminary report. *Journal of Psychiatric Research*, 17, 37–49.

Zigmond, A. and Snaith, R.P. (1983) The Hospital Anxiety and Depression Scale. *Alta Psychiatrica, Scandinavica*, 67, 361–370.

Zimmerman, S.I., Smith, H.D., Gruber-Baldini, A., Fox, K.M., Hebel, J.R., Kenzora, J., Felsenthal, G. and Magaziner, J. (1999) Short-term persistent depression following hip fracture: a risk factor and target to increase resilience in elderly people. *Social Work Research*, 23(3), 187–196.

10 REHABILITATION SETTINGS

Susan A.R. Hawkins

AIMS OF THE CHAPTER

This chapter will discuss the settings in which activity may take place to meet the needs and aim of rehabilitation. It will describe the different challenges that each of these venues presents to clinicians in terms of the delivery of efficient, effective and safe treatments, as well as the need for assessing the risks associated with treating people in different settings. Attention is given to the fact that rehabilitation may be required for older people following acute or chronic illness; that most will receive treatment for an acute condition in a district general hospital (DGH) or a teaching hospital, although some can be cared for in their own homes or in local community or cottage hospitals, or day hospitals; and that rehabilitation may equally be required for chronic conditions where community based settings may be more appropriate. The chapter describes the various settings for rehabilitation of older people – inpatient or outpatient treatment at a hospital; at a day hospital, their own home, day centre, residential home, intermediate care unit, nursing home, hospice or facility for those who are homeless.

The author states that the challenge to the team is to deliver efficient, effective and equitable treatment in whichever setting. To do so they must take into account the effect that the setting has on both the older person and the staff involved, as well as other people with whom the older person comes into contact. Attention is drawn to the strengths and weaknesses of each setting that may affect service delivery and present challenges to the team in their delivery of care. The importance of an awareness of the social and psychological impacts of the different settings, the staff and capital resources, the role and purpose of the 'unit' in which treatment is provided, and the role and workload of staff contributing to the interdisciplinary team, is emphasised, in order to allow the team to deliver treatment to the best of their ability.

CHOICE OF SETTING

Kramer (1997) describes the relationship between length of stay and treatment settings. Rehabilitation facilities provide more intensive rehabilitation for shorter lengths of stay, whereas subacute nursing facilities (such as community hospitals) provide lower intensity rehabilitation for slightly longer lengths of stay. When placement is being debated, the needs of the individual patient should be considered alongside the economic imperatives.

Most rehabilitation services in the UK are provided by health services in hospital settings, the potential for other settings, such as intermediate care facilities, is undergoing development in line with the National Service Framework for Older

People (see Chapter 6). There is currently a paucity of specialist rehabilitation units (Nocon and Baldwin, 1998).

Hospital settings

Many older people, following an acute illness that has required admission to hospital, require a period of rehabilitation to maximise their functional recovery. This rehabilitation can start in the very acute phase of the illness, with maintenance work and activities that reorientate ill and confused patients to normal function. When the acute illness has improved, a more detailed, individual programme of rehabilitation should be implemented. This rehabilitation can be delivered in the acute hospital or community/cottage hospitals or, in some areas of the UK, in specifically designed rehabilitation units/intermediate care units. Some people recover sufficiently from their acute episode to go straight home and have ongoing treatment at a day hospital or at their local health centre, or they may have domiciliary treatment in their own homes.

Ambulatory care – day hospital

The day hospital is an outpatient health-care facility in which interdisciplinary assessment, treatment and rehabilitation are available for a full or part of a day for older people living in the community. The day hospital can facilitate earlier discharge after inpatient treatment and postpone or prevent admission to hospital. It offers a flexible and responsive resource as part of an integrated service spanning both primary and secondary care. The day hospital should have close links with community and hospital rehabilitation teams to enable patients to receive rehabilitation in the most appropriate environment. Most elderly people who attend day hospitals have stroke disease, arthritis and other musculo-skeletal disorders and falls.

Community settings

As well as the clinical treatment settings of the acute hospital, community or cottage hospitals, day hospitals or nursing homes, the team may also be called upon to provide rehabilitation in a community setting. Older people can live in numerous different types of accommodation. They can live in their own home, their families' homes, sheltered accommodation, warden-controlled flats, residential homes, prison or be homeless, living in either temporary low cost accommodation or on the streets.

Home

With an expansion or redeployment of outreach services, rehabilitation can take place in the patient's home, whether it be their own home, residential unit or nursing home. The availability of domiciliary services allows for a much greater degree of flexibility. The community physiotherapist and occupational therapist work in the older person's own home environment and this is more relevant to his or her everyday existence. Domiciliary programmes also give health and social care professionals access to the carers, family or paid staff involved with the individual.

Day centre

Day centres are provided by the local authority for social care. A programme of activities together with lunch and transport are usually provided. Day centres have to date been little used by health-care staff for ongoing rehabilitation after discharge from hospital or day hospital, the main contact being initial education of staff in the individual's abilities and care. The space, availability of care assistants and the wide range of users could make day centres a useful facility in a community rehabilitation programme. Some already provide basic equipment such as tilt table and parallel bars, which may be essential in a rehabilitation package but inappropriate in a home setting.

Intermediate care

There has been a recent growth of interest in schemes described as intermediate care, although its definition is as yet rather vague. It has been described as a range of services designed to facilitate transition between hospital and home; and from medical dependence to functional independence, where the objectives of care are not primarily medical, the patient's discharge destination is anticipated, and a clinical outcome of recovery is desired. Others have described these facilities as services that do not require the resources of a general hospital, but are beyond the scope of the traditional primary care team. There is often an assumption that it is not medically led and it should include components of rehabilitation, convalescence and respite. The term intermediate care encompasses a wide variety of practices in different facilities (Table 10.1), but there is no universally agreed definition of this form of care delivery.

Table 10.1 Forms of intermediate care

- Hospital at Home schemes
- Community Assessment and Rehabilitation schemes
- Social Rehabilitation schemes
- Step Down Rehabilitation units
- Nursing homes
- Hospital hotels
- Nurse-led units in various settings
- Therapist-led units in various settings
- Rapid response rehabilitation and support teams

Step down rehabilitation units are one form of intermediate care facility. They were initially set up in response to the high bed pressures that acute hospitals find themselves under, particularly during the winter months. Patients are admitted to them for short lengths of stay to have high intensity rehabilitation in settings that facilitate independence. They follow structured programmes designed by the interdisciplinary team following assessment and full involvement of the patient/carer (see Chapter 8), and implemented by trained and supervised health-care or rehabilitation assistants. Patients are encouraged to 'fend for themselves' in a safe, supervised environment. Help is provided if necessary, but the enablement ethos that pervades these settings ensures that where possible patients are encouraged to be independent in all activities.

To facilitate rehabilitation being included as an integral and initial part of any care assessment and to keep open the possibility of a return home the government, in the National Plan (Department of Health [DoH], 2000), have put a three-month waiver on older people having to use the asset of their own home in the means testing of residential care funding. This gives rehabilitation time to have its effect before any irreversible decisions on long-term care are taken. Further investment is also being provided for the provision of aids and adaptations, and new guidance on fairer charging for home care services to help those that wish to return to their own homes (DoH, 2000).

Staffing profiles vary enormously, but intermediate care facilities probably encompass a core mix of nurses, rehabilitation therapists, social service staff and family doctors. The evidence base for the efficacy of intermediate care is lacking. Although these units may appear to be an effective way of delivering rehabilitation, it is important that while using them elderly disabled people should not be denied access to appropriate inpatient diagnostic or therapeutic facilities. This type of provision may only be available in secondary care hospitals, and the balance should be to allow access to them while ensuring that older people do not remain in hospital longer than they need (British Geriatrics Society, 2000).

Residential homes

Residential homes provide temporary or permanent accommodation for older people. Residents may receive means tested help with the fees. The range of services provided and levels of support offered vary considerably in quality and quantity. They range from meal provision and recreational activities to assistance in most aspects of ADL. The role of residential homes has changed greatly over recent years, with increasingly more frail residents being admitted to them. The levels of support provided has had to increase, but residential homes are not able to provide nursing support. Temporary or minor nursing care can be provided by community nursing services or by GP practice nurses, but if the level required is more than this the resident may be asked to move to a nursing home. Some residential homes are 'dual registered', providing residential and nursing home beds and therefore a continuum of care if necessary. The changes to the regulation of care homes will lead to single care homes with increasing support and nursing care being provided.

Homeless

Crane (1999) draws attention to the barely visible but increasing number of older people who are recorded as homeless, the majority living in basic bed and breakfast or other low cost accommodation such as mobile homes or house-boats. The majority are male and have lived in this type of accommodation long term; the minority are women who are more likely to have become homeless at an older age. The main causes of homelessness are social change, personality disorders or previous institutional living, with homelessness often triggered by an economic or social crisis such as widowhood or family dispute.

Biologically, homeless people are 20 years older than their chronological age (Crane, 1999), with older women more likely to have problems associated with mental health and men those associated with alcohol. All are at risk of infec-tions, circulatory and musculo-skeletal problems; rough sleepers are at further risk of hypothermia and foot problems resulting from continuous walking in poor footwear.

Access to health care is compromised by stigmatisation, especially in primary care and A&E departments. The homeless are a group who often have multiple problems, poor compliance and their transient accommodation can make contact and follow up difficult. Where ongoing care is needed, the accommodation in which it is provided may be unsuitable and street care almost impossible. Pioneering examples show what can be achieved, particularly in primary care, occupational therapy to improve independent living (Mobsy, 1996; Mitchell and Jones, 1997), physiotherapy for aids to mobility, podiatry to improve foot health and mobility, and social work to refer people for advice or advocacy around issues of benefits, housing and possibly addiction services.

Nursing homes

Nursing homes provide long-term accommodation for older people who need high levels of personal and nursing care, and are unable to live supported at home or in a residential home (O'Brian and Topping, 1995). Kramer (1997) explains that nursing homes may or may not have an orientation towards rehabilitation, depending on the volume of people they treat who have the potential for recovery, their remit, and on the availability or access to rehabilitation clinicians. As with residential care, nursing home places may be subsidised by local authorities. The NHS Plan (DoH, 2000) makes reference to the use of nursing homes for rehab-ilitation of NHS patients (see Chapter 1), and further detail is awaited. To date, the input of rehabilitation staff and equipment has been sporadic and dependent upon local, variable and inconsistent agreements, traditional practices and good-will. Successful change of use will be dependent on appropriate space, equipment, staffing and above all philosophy of care.

Hospices

Hospices offer services for patients who have passed the curative stage of their illnesses and require palliative care. Hospices have moved away from offering services for the dying, to the active management of, and symptom control for, any patient diagnosed with a terminal condition. In line with this, they also offer respite care and rehabilitation as required, particularly with a view to returning and maintaining people at home.

PHYSICAL AND PSYCHOLOGICAL CONSEQUENCES OF THE SETTING ON REHABILITATION

In all of these treatment settings the team need to consider physical factors that will affect the intervention, such as the amount of space that is available to carry out the proposed activity and what equipment is available. How much time they have available to assess and treat the older person, or how much assistance they can access for more complex situations, will also affect the treatment session. As well as these considerations, staff need to have awareness of the psychological impact of the treatment setting upon the older person and how this might affect their ability or desire to co-operate with treatment.

Physical considerations

When preparing to provide rehabilitative health care, staff need to assess the available space to determine whether it is sufficient safely to carry out the proposed assessment and treatment. Hospital bed spaces are notoriously small and restrictive of many forms of functional assessment. The team may consider it necessary to move some furniture out of the way, or move the patient to another location. This may be the physiotherapy gym, or the occupational therapy assessment bedroom/kitchen. While treating someone in a residential setting or at home, space also needs to be considered. Staff should ask themselves whether it is necessary to move some furniture and, if so, whether the patient will consent to it being moved.

Physical rehabilitation generally involves the use of space and equipment, for example to practise Activities of Daily Living (ADL) or to facilitate exercise. Different treatment settings affect the availability of such equipment; a hospital may have a gym full of exercise equipment that a physiotherapist can use, while none may be available in the patient's home, stretching the ingenuity of the therapist to adapt household items for use or facilitating access to local leisure facilities. However, an occupational therapist may find all that he or she needs is available in the patient's home to practise all aspects of personal activities of daily living (PADL) and domestic activities of daily living (DADL), but may have limited access to such equipment in a residential home. The nurse, doctor and podiatrist are more likely to have equipment designed for domiciliary use, to take it with them to community settings and have it to hand in clinical environments.

Financial considerations

Health care outside of an institution is sometimes perceived as a cheap option due to the savings on *capital* costs. Although the caseload norm of staff who have traditionally worked in the community, such as GPs, community nurses and social workers is accepted, that of clinicians moving from a tradition in institutions to respond to community demands has been largely overlooked – the transference of similar caseload being conveniently assumed. This erroneous assumption has at last been acknowledged by the Audit Commission (2000).

Squires's (1993) Service Input Profile (see Figures 10.1 and 10.2) shows the empirical level of input of representative professionals along the hypothetical patient career from hospital to home. Figure 10.1 shows the input over time; typically this is intensive medical and nursing input on admission, changing places with therapists input as needs change over time.

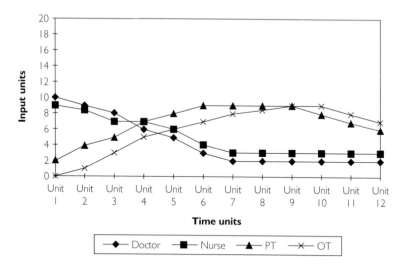

Figure 10.1 Rehabilitation input/venue gap

(*Squires, 1993*)

Figure 10.2 shows what occurs, in this example to physiotherapy therapy demand, when the hypothetical patient is discharged – often just at the time of increasing therapy need.

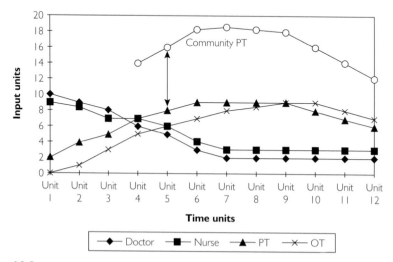

Figure 10.2 Rehabilitation input/venue gap

(*Squires, 1993*)

The time constraints of travel and the social requirements of being a visitor in the patient's home mean that in effect the therapy input is at least doubled for the same patient at the same point in their care but in a different venue. When this factor is multiplied by the number of disciplines likewise affected, the need to cost a complete episode of care becomes apparent, as does the need to share skills appropriately. Not only will such calculations have to be balanced against capital savings, but also against the availability of increasingly scarce skilled staff who make up the interdisciplinary team.

In a further study (Squires *et al.*, 1997), using the example of physiotherapy, but adaptable for other disciplines, it became clear that the potential caseload that can be carried is continuously but unconsciously calculated by all practitioners. The type of venue within the community affects case load and can be weighted by site (Table 10.2). For example, a patient's own home will have less access to equipment or competent help and, in this example, the physiotherapist requires the time, knowledge and capacity to deal on the spot with what he or she finds – a fall, deterioration or even death. Consequently treatment in a patient's 'own home' carries a high weighting.

Table 10.2 Weighting of treatment sites for physiotherapy

Site	Example	Weighting
Serviced site	Day hospitals, outpatients	Low
Supported accommodation	Residential and nursing homes	Medium
Own home	Private residence and sheltered housing	High

(Squires et al., 1997)

The case mix in the community will usually be based on the population content of a geographical area. At any one time it will consist of a mix of patients receiving physiotherapy inputs, such as assessment, rehabilitation and/or monitoring in line with their personalised care plan. The potential caseload will be dependent on the number and intensity of inputs (case complexity); stage of care; travel (per case); and venue (responsibility weighting).

In this study, 1,000 physiotherapists working with older people were asked to calculate what is realistically achievable while meeting national quality standards. The results are shown in Table 10.3.

It should be noted that, for example on a 'serviced site', a physiotherapist has the capacity for 5 assessment *inputs* or 10 rehabilitation *inputs*, etc.; the number of *inputs* will depend on the severity of the case so that 4 cases might absorb the 10 assessment *inputs*, and the assistant support in this situation would expand the *inputs* available between the members of staff to 16. Assessment *inputs* are not altered by assistant availability, the skills and knowledge base for assessment being integral to the specialised training of the graduate physiotherapist.

Table 10.3 Average case weighted inputs (not cases) per three-hour physiotherapy session

	Assessment		Rehabilitation		Monitor		Mixed
Serviced site	5	or	10 (16)	or	20 (26)	or	9 (12)
Patient's home	3	or	7 (8)	or	14 (15)	or	6 (7)
Residential/ nursing home	5	or	10 (13)	or	20 (24)	or	9 (11)

(Where helper support is appropriate increased inputs are shown in brackets.)
(Squires et al., 1997)

Carers

When available, family members may be the key to successful rehabilitation (see also Chapter 12). They can provide much of the care and stimulation that older people require to achieve some level of independence. Carers should be involved along with the older person in setting treatment goals and designing and implementing care plans; and must be willing and able to contribute (Mulley, 1994; Kramer, 1997). They should have their own needs taken into consideration; and should be trained in the elements of care that they agree to become involved in, with written or video information for ongoing reference. Earlyexplanation and instruction can avoid problems with over-protection or unrealistic expectations.

In return for asking family members to contribute towards the rehabilitation of their older relative, team members need to be aware of the responsibility they owe to carers. There are well-documented sequalae to being a carer; these can include tiredness, depression, family disruption and back problems. Professionals need to provide instruction, support and respite care where necessary to help avoid these problems.

Communication

The setting can affect how often interdisciplinary team (IDT) members have the opportunity to meet with each other and to coordinate the rehabilitation service that they are providing. Efficient coordination of service delivery is essential for effective rehabilitation, to focus all clinicians on the same, agreed goals, and to prevent unnecessary duplication of effort between the team (see also Chapters 4, 7 and 8). Where the setting precludes easy communication and coordination, systems need to be in place for team members easily and effectively to communicate with each other. This can be achieved via patient/client-held records, community case conferences, or regular team meetings. Technological developments such as e-mail and telephone or video conferencing may be valuable communication tools in certain settings to facilitate efficient goal directed rehabilitation. The welcome development of nurse and therapy specialists and consultants should improve coordination and communication in elderly care (Department of Health, 2000).

Resource considerations

Some staff will require the assistance of another person to make the treatment session safe or more effective. For example, an occupational therapist treating a heavy patient with a dense stroke may need the assistance of another occupational therapist, or an experienced occupational therapy assistant. This additional help might not be available in some settings, and although other team members may have some supportive skills in providing specialist assistance, it may lead therapists to question whether they can give an effective, safe treatment or whether the patient would be more appropriately treated elsewhere. How such information is communicated to colleagues will largely influence the ultimate decision. A patient with simple mobility problems who requires the assistance of two people to build up confidence in mobilising, may be effectively treated in a residential home, if assistance from staff in the home and training, supervision and monitoring of progress is available. Such input should enable ongoing encouragement of the individual at least to maintain their progress.

The closer an activity can be made to resemble normal function, the easier it will be for a patient to perform. People draw on their memory of previous activities to access movement engrams (Horn, 1991; Merzenich and Sameshima, 1993) and achieve what is required. Some settings facilitate the assessment, treatment and practice of functional activities because they can be incorporated into everyday life. For example, a person who has limited mobility is more likely to reach the toilet regularly in his or her own home than in an unfamiliar hospital ward. Likewise, when assessing competence in a kitchen, an occupational therapist will get a more realistic picture of ability if he or she is working with the person in their own kitchen, rather than in an assessment kitchen in a rehabilitation unit. The degree to which an activity can be made 'normal' will also help compliance and performance when people are confused. A person may well be able to eat a meal while sitting at a table with cutlery laid out normally. However, they may be unable to eat one sitting up in bed with the meal on a tray and the cutlery in a plastic bag wrapped with a serviette, affecting function as well as nutritional intake. Appropriate settings can promote the normalisation of function.

These considerations are outlined in Table 10.4 overleaf. The lists are not exhaustive and the same setting in two different locations may be able to provide for completely different levels of intervention, as a result of the levels of staffing or the systems in place. Team members should be aware of these differences and consider the impact they may have on their ability to treat older people in different rehabilitation settings.

Psychological considerations

When considering rehabilitation in a variety of settings it is necessary to think not only about the physical aspects of the delivery of treatment, but also about the psychological ones. Older people may be 'residing' in an unfamiliar setting at the time of treatment, or in familiar settings with unfamiliar things happening to them. The degree to which a person feels in control of a situation is directly related to the extent they can, or are willing to, co-operate with the

Table 10.4 Physical considerations in various rehabilitation settings

Setting	Space	Equipment
Acute hospital	Very limited unless gym or ADL flat available	Lots and specifically designed
Community or cottage hospital	Very limited unless gym or ADL flat available	Lots and specifically designed
Day hospital	Tend to be well set up, usually with access to gym and ADL flat	Lots and specifically designed
Rehabilitation unit	Tend to be well set up with treatment area and ADL flat	Lots and specifically designed
Own home	Limited by furniture but more amenable to adjustment	Limited and needs adapting from everyday items, but relevant to individual and tasks
Carer's home	Limited by furniture but more amenable to adjustment	Limited and needs adapting from everyday items
Residential home	May be reasonable, but can impinge on other clients, for example shared bedrooms	Some, often provided by clinician but may be limited and need adapting from everyday items
Nursing home	Can be reasonable, but can also be very limited, depending on design of the home	Limited. May be provided by clinician but often needs adapting from everyday items
Hospice	Depends on design of the unit but often reasonable because designed to be like home not hospital	Some, provided by the unit but may be limited and need adapting from everyday items

Clinician time and coordination	Assistance for clinician
Very limited. High levels of coordination and regular opportunities to meet other MDT members	As required from therapy assistants or limited from busy nursing staff
Can be limited in bigger hospital. High levels of coordination and regular opportunities to meet other MDT members	As required from therapy assistants or limited from nursing staff
Often more time available. High levels of coordination and regular opportunities to meet other MDT members	As required from therapy assistants
Often more time available and additional staff dedicated to rehabilitation. High levels of coordination and regular opportunities to meet other MDT members	As required; all staff have rehabilitation philosophy and training
Contact time can be limited but more time for practice, especially if family or carer available to assist/supervise. Coordination between MDT members can be difficult	Variable, dependent on staff availabilit (some assistants work in the community); assistance may be available from family
Contact time can be limited but more time for practice, especially if family or carer available to assist/supervise. Coordination between MDT members can be difficult	Variable, dependent on staff availability (some assistants work in the community); assistance may be available from family
Contact time can be limited but more time for practice, especially if residential staff available to assist/supervise – staff time can be very limited. Coordination between MDT members can be difficult	Generally limited. Residential home staff busy with own routines and may lack rehab ethic. May have community therapy assistant to help
Can be limited but some time for busy practice if staff available to assist/ supervise – staff time can be very limited. Coordination between MDT members can be difficult	Generally limited. Nursing home staff with own routines and may lack rehab ethic. May have community therapy assistant to help
Contact time can be limited but more time for practice, especially if family, volunteer or carer available to assist/ supervise. High levels of coordination and regular opportunities to meet other MDT members	Variable, dependent on staff availability; may have community therapy assistant, or assistance may be available from hospice staff

intervention. If the older person feels that they have some control over the situation, or that their views are being incorporated into the treatment planning and goal setting, they may feel more empowered to participate (see also Chapters 4, 8 and 9). Hence, compliance and therefore outcomes are automatically enhanced.

Some settings are much more likely to disempower older people than others. In hospital older patients, although not discouraged from wearing day clothes, often feel that the wearing of nightclothes is more appropriate. This may stem from past experience of hospitals (wearing nightclothes and being in bed was the expected norm), or from a need to legitimise their illness and hospital admission. It is often associated with the adoption of the 'sick role'. Similarly, many older people remain highly deferential to staff and feel that they must stay by their beds in case the doctor wants to see them or tests have been arranged for them (see also Chapter 5). Unfortunately, this 'hospitalisation' precludes normal activity. It leads to the patient becoming disempowered and losing autonomy, and with it the desire to be functionally independent. Many, who were previously mobile and independent, feel tied to their bedside and do not continue to mobilise and keep active, which can lead to diminished function, exercise tolerance, mobility, flexibility, strength and confidence. There is the hope that newer cohorts of older people will feel more empowered, but this may, however, make staff feel uncomfortable. Training may be required to help staff develop empowerment skills and to address their anxieties (see also Chapters 4 and 5).

As well as being psychologically disempowering, loose-fitting pyjama trousers that fall down, or nightdresses with open backs, or so long that a patient slips on them can make patients reluctant to mobilise and maintain independence. Appropriate clothing should include secure, well-fitting footwear. Shoes are often not brought in with a patient to hospital, or worn even when present, with many patients and staff heedless of the dangers of mobilising in loose-fitting, shiny-soled slippers, bare feet or only socks (see also Chapter 18). 'Normal attire' worn in different settings can directly and indirectly impact on the effectiveness of rehabilitation.

The problems associated with 'hospitalisation' are diminished, but not eliminated, in other institutional settings such as residential homes or rehabilitation units. Unfortunately they can become very deeply ingrained, which can be a particular problem in the rehabilitation of older people recently discharged from hospital who may have lost the ability, the autonomy or desire to function independently.

Another problem associated with caring for older people in an institutional setting, such as a hospital or a residential home, is that the institution often imposes its own routine on to the older patient. Someone who is used to rising at 10a.m. to a leisurely breakfast may be completely disorientated by the routine of an acute hospital ward where patients are woken by the night shift before they leave at 7a.m. Their breakfast is provided for them at 8a.m. to be cleared away by 9a.m. If they are disorientated by this they may be unable to co-operate with treatment until late morning. Other problems associated with the institutional setting can include distress at being surrounded by other, more ill, confused or 'older' patients, sadness at being separated from loved ones, including pets, loss of individuality and agitation or tiredness from disturbed sleep and excess noise (Mulley, 1994) or light.

When considering function, and trying to minimise the psychological disturbance of illness, the 'team' needs to endeavour to normalise all activities. Consider the facilities for an older person to make a cup of tea or a snack for themselves in the different settings. How would they feel if they were permitted some level of autonomy in functional activity? Bear in mind, also, the added rehabilitation benefits of making a meal for themselves rather than have one brought to them.

The team ought to be aware of the familiarity of a place or an activity to an older person when designing and carrying out a rehabilitation programme. Unfamiliar places, faces or activities can significantly distract the older person. So much more might be achieved from the same person at home, because they have more control and are less frightened by their surroundings, and have memory of successfully functioning in this environment (Bainbridge, 1995).

Familiarity can also help gain adherence to a programme. When a speech and language therapist is assessing a patient who is having difficulty swallowing, they might have more success getting them to eat something familiar cooked at home than mass-produced hospital food. Likewise, a patient may be more likely to continue with an exercise programme that is associated with normal activities, such as purposefully walking up stairs, rather than doing step ups on a box.

Fear can be disabling in unfamiliar environments. An older person who manages to stay mobile at home by walking around the furniture may become immobile in some settings because of a fear of open spaces and lack of furniture close enough to move around. Different floor types can exacerbate these fears; consider someone at risk of falling when walking on shiny linoleum or someone with a shuffling neurological gait trying to walk on carpet. These factors need to be recognised when assessing people in unfamiliar settings.

Availability of a patient advocate is essential in rehabilitation settings. The person who assumes this role has an important place in ensuring that the patient gets what they need and want, and has goals set that pertain to their own individual desires and needs. Kramer (1997) found that one of the greatest predictors of volume of therapy services received by an individual was the availability of an able and willing advocate (see also Chapter 4).

These psychological considerations are summarised in Table 10.5.

Rehabilitation culture

There are many definitions of rehabilitation: Brody and Pawlson (1990), describe it as 'The maintenance and restoration of physical and psychological health necessary for independent living and functional independence'. Considerable health gain can be achieved from successful rehabilitation, restoring function for older people and facilitating their return to independence. Kramer (1997) cautions against clinicians becoming too focused on improvements in physical

Table 10.5 Psychological considerations

Setting	Functional activities	Familiarity
Acute hospital	Little call for, opportunity, or available equipment, to practise PADL and DADL. Patients often disempowered, may remain in nightclothes all day. May not even walk to the bathroom	Unfamiliar and very frightening high-tech surroundings. All staff unfamiliar and generally not there long enough to build trusting relationships
Community or cottage hospital	More emphasis on dressing and PADL but still little call for, opportunity, or available equipment, to practise DADL. Independent mobility encouraged	Unfamiliar but more low-tech and less frightening surroundings. All staff unfamiliar. Patient may be there long enough to build trusting relationships
Day hospital	Independence in mobility and PADL encouraged but still limited opportunity to practise DADL	Unfamiliar but more low-tech and less frightening surroundings. Patient morein control because come in and out from home each day
Rehab unit	Lots of encouragement to be independent in PADL, DADL, and mobility. More equipment available and patient access to kitchens, etc.	Unfamiliar but still more low-tech and less frightening surroundings. All staff unfamiliar. Patient may be there long enough to build trusting relationships
Own home	Lots of function-based activities; equipment readily available	Familiar, own surroundings, own equipment, own routine
Carer's home	Depends on integration with the family and their preparedness to allow their older relative to use DADL equipment. Generally lots of function-based activities; equipment readily available	Familiar. More ownership of surroundings but not own. Unfamiliar equipment, may have own routine imposed by clinician
Residential home	Independence in PADL and mobility encouraged but often limited facilities for residents to continue independent DADL	Generally familiar, known staff, own or familiar furniture
Nursing home	Depending upon the ability of the patient independence in PADL and mobility is encouraged. Facilities are limited for residents to continue independent DADL	Generally familiar, known staff, less of own furniture but home should be familiar
Hospice	Lots of encouragement to be independent in PADL, DADL, and mobility. More equipment available and patients have access to kitchens, etc.	Unfamiliar, but designed to be more homelike, so should be less frightening than hospital. Often have opportunity to develop trusting relationships
Provider and imposed	Patient – nil. Family – nil. Although not disallowed Patient often feels	Nurse

Day and routine led by	Autonomy and clothing	Advocate
	disempowered to wear own clothing; or feels the need to wear nightclothes to legitimise illness. Generally in slippers	
Provider more patient involvement but still imposed	Patient – nil. Family – increasing. Wearing of day clothes encouraged but because of accidents and laundry facilities may be hospital-provided day clothes. Generally in slippers	Nurse or family
Patient at home, provider in unit. Imposed while on unit	Patient – some. Family – some. Patient wears own day clothes and shoes	Nurse, family, or SS's care manager
Some degree of patient control but often imposed by provider	Patient – increasing. Family – some. Patient wears own day clothes and shoes	Key worker or family
Patient, but appointment often imposed by clinician	Patient – more. Family – more. Patient wears own day clothes, but often wears slippers	Family or SS's care manager
Patient or family (not always in harmony) but appointment often clothes, but often wears	Patient – some. Family – increasing. Patient wears own day slippers	Family or SS's care manager
Some degree of patient control but often imposed by provider	Patient – more. Family – some. Patient wears own day clothes; laundry facilities should be provided on site; might wear slippers or shoes	Key worker or family
Provider and imposed	Patient – decreasing. Family – some. Patient wears own day clothes, laundry facilities should be provided on site, generally wears slippers	Key worker, nurse, or family
Patient, but appointment may be imposed by clinician	Patient – more. Family – some. Patient wears own day clothes; might wear slippers or shoes	Key worker, or family, or nurse

and functional outcome measures. It is more pertinent to acknowledge the older person's perception of the effectiveness of the treatment in restoring them to their desired level of function and social interaction, rather than one imposed upon them by clinicians. The focus of care must remain user centred, and should be tailored to the individual's needs and wishes (Mulley, 1994). It should incorporate strategies to provide them with both attitudinal as well as physical changes.

Barriers to successful rehabilitation

Many professionals and agencies are involved in the provision of rehabilitation services to older people. A core list might include doctors, nurses, therapists, health visitors, community nurses, social service social workers or care managers, link workers, and other commercial and voluntary agencies. As explained in Chapter 7, members of this potentially huge team require effective coordination if rehabilitation is to be cost- effective. Hospital rehabilitation at its most organised can provide for a well coordinated communicative team, working to common goals agreed with the patient and relatives. The team will have developed the relationships necessary through regular informal 'corridor' contact (see also Chapter 7). Rehabilitation provision outside the hospital system provides challenges to team coordination and integration of provision, because of the spread and geographic distribution of providers, and the legal, social and commercial requirements of different agencies. The government's Clinical Standards Advisory Group (1998), in their report on 'Community health care for elderly people', draws attention to:

- poor coordination of discharge plans
- lack of interagency collaboration
- lack of attention to the rehabilitation needs of older people
- inequities in provision of services.

The Audit Commission (2000) report on rehabilitation services for older people concluded that they showed disorganised not organised care. Team members involved in the rehabilitation of older people should endeavour to streamline their provision to ensure effective sharing of information and joint decision-making regardless of the setting in which it is delivered, and of the agencies involved. A number of pilot projects exploring closer co-operation between health and social services are being evaluated. It has to be remembered that combining services and ensuring that they work collaboratively are quite different issues, and effective change management techniques will be needed if these two distinct cultures and their different political frameworks are to be successfully joined.

Staff attitudes

Historically, rehabilitation of older people has been seen as the poor cousin to the more glamorous rehabilitation of younger age groups. Positive staff attitudes to rehabilitation, raising the profile of the speciality through the work of its pioneers (see Chapter 1) (Stewart and Hawker, 1999; Williams, 1999), and an increasing recognition of the potential for older people to maximise function and independence (Chapter 2) have meant that rehabilitation with older people has improved its position within health service delivery. However, negative attitudes still need addressing and challenging, and staff need to have a commitment to rehabilitation and full treatment inputs for older people so that they can achieve this maximisation of function (Kramer, 1997). This will only be achieved within conducive environments with a focus on service and staff development.

Resistance to change in ability

The life of a carer can often be fully occupied by caring for the 'disabled' person. Caring can become a major, if not the only, role that they have. Rehabilitation aims to increase the level of function that a disabled person can achieve independently. With increasing independence comes a decreasing reliance on the carer and a possible increase in natural risk such as falls and scalds from resumed activities. This decreasing reliance ought be seen as a positive move for both the older person and their carer. If the carer's life, however, revolves around caring, they may find the older person's increasing independence threatening. It may lead to a change in the balance of power and influence within the household, changing roles for each person, and it may have economic implications regarding the amount and type of benefits that come into the home. Team members need to be acutely aware of these factors. They need to take into account the possibility that changes in the relationship between carer and cared for, if not managed well, can become obstructive to rehabilitation. Time needs to be spent listening to the carer; educating them not only in how they can promote independence for the older person, but also how they can manage their own independence and increasing freedom. Financial advice may be required and team members should know where this can be obtained.

As always, there should be good communication and co-operation with the carer, as well as the older person, when planning and implementing rehabilitation programmes. How well they both adapt and respond to changes in levels of function, will depend largely on the level of involvement and influence they feel they have had in the decisions being made or whether they feel that they have been imposed upon them (Mullins, 1996).

RISK ASSESSMENT

It is important when working in a variety of different rehabilitation settings that team members are aware of the risks associated with each.

Within a hospital or rehabilitation unit, specialist equipment should be available for the performance and assessment of exercises and ADL tasks. In some community settings, specially manufactured rehabilitation equipment may not be available. A therapist may, for example, choose to use the bottom step in someone's house to perform step-up exercises as a precursor to stair climbing; or, in an attempt to 'normalise' treatment activity, they may specifically choose everyday equipment such as the older person's own kettle. In both instances the clinician must be able to perform a competent and thorough assessment to identify the risks present. They must do this at every treatment encounter in order to eliminate or minimise risks. Where it is not possible to eliminate risk, team members must inform themselves, their colleagues and the older person of the risks and be prepared for dealing with them.

To assess risk factors, particulary manual handling risks while encouraging function, mobility and transfers, the clinician needs to consider the load/patient, the environment, the equipment to be used, the tasks to be performed, and the individual performing them (Royal College of Nursing and National Back Pain Association [RCN/NBPA], 1997), whether staff or carer.

The load/patient

What is the size of the patient and their weight distribution?
A 60-kilo patient could be tall and thin or short and fat. The clinician should assess whether this will alter the ability to manoeuvre them or safely handle them if they stumble.

How able is the patient?
The 60-kilo patient may be very able and mobile or they may be quite immobile and disabled. This will alter the risks associated with treatment and there should be awareness of how it would do so.

Moving and handling the patient involves some degree of risk to the clinician. It should be determined whether the handling about to be performed is necessary. Could the patient help more than they are being asked to, or could a piece of equipment be used to reduce the risks?

What is the mental state of the patient?
They may be relaxed and co-operative, confused and uncooperative, or anxious and unable to take in any instructions that are given to them. This will affect how safe they are moving around or handling hot saucepans. The risk involved must be assessed and managed appropriately.

Is the patient medically stable or have they ongoing co-morbidities that might affect the treatment session?
They may have unstable angina, or COPD, or debilitating osteoarthritis in their knees. This will have a bearing on what and how much the patient can do. This must be established during the initial assessment and considered when planning interventions.

The environment

The amount and sufficiency of space the activity will take should be known. The area should be cleared of all unnecessary items. The floor surface should be assessed to see whether it is slippery, whether the carpets are worn or rug edges raised, and minimise the risks of the patient, carer or clinician tripping or slipping. The area should be well lit, ventilated and warm enough for the person exercising or practising ADL tasks.

The equipment

Any furniture used as part of the treatment must be stable and the correct height. Competency in using the correct manual handling equipment by either team member or carer must be assured. Infection risks associated with the equipment that it is proposed to use must be ascertained. Kitchen appliances used must be safe, with attention paid to knotted electrical flexes, bare wires or malfunctioning thermostats.

The task

Establish first whether the task is necessary – could the same result be achieved differently, with fewer risks involved? The patient should be able to follow instructions accurately. If not, can they be made easier by also training a carer, giving written instructions or can the task be simplified? The patient should be capable of taking on board safety instructions and incorporating them into their treatment and daily activities. If not, their activities need to be altered or their safety ensured, with the assistance of other people or outside agencies.

Staff responsibility

All clinicians have an obligation to keep themselves up to date with mandatory training in manual handling and cardiopulmonary resuscitation. They need to be aware of their own physical capabilities and health status, and that of any others who may be assisting in the treatment session. Appropriate clothing should be worn to enable tasks to be performed safely. It should allow unrestricted movement, with securely fitting footwear that must be non-slip and able to provide adequate foot protection.

SUMMARY

Whenever assessing, treating or instructing an older person or their carers in any rehabilitation setting, team members should ask themselves whether they are doing something that involves unnecessary risk of injury or harm to self or others. It is not possible to eliminate all risks but those risks that remain must be minimised and procedures must be in place to manage problems if they arise. Staff should familiarise themselves with the safety procedures, methods of raising the alarm and location of first aid facilities in the areas in which they need to work. By doing so in all rehabilitation settings, safe, successful practice will be ensured.

REFERENCES

Audit Commission (2000) *The Way to Go Home: rehabilitation and remedial services for older people*, Audit Commission Publications, Abingdon.

Bainbridge, L.A. (1995) Cognition and learning. In: *Physiotherapy with Older People* (eds Pickles, B., Compton, A., Cott, C., Simpson, J. and Vandervoort, V.), W.B. Saunders, London.

British Geriatrics Society, (2000) *Compendium of Giudelines: D4 Intermediate Care*, British Geriatrics, Society, London.

Brody, S. and Pawlson, L. (1990) *Ageing and Rehabilitation*, 2nd edn, Springer, New York.

Clinical Standards Advisory Group (1998) *Community Health Care for Elderly People*, The Stationery Office, London.

Crane, M. (1999) *Understanding Older Homeless People*, Open University Press, Buckingham.

Department of Health (2000) *The NHS Plan*, The Stationery Office, London.

Horn, G. (1991) Learning, memory and the brain. *Indian Journal of Physiotherapistology and Pharmacology*, 35(1), 3–9.

Kramer, A.M. (1997) Rehabilitation care and outcomes from the patients' perspective. *Medical Care*, 35(6), JS48–57.

McCormack, B. (1998) Community care for elderly people (editorial). *British Medical Journal*, 317, 552–553.

Merzenich, M.M. and Sameshima, K. (1993) Cortical plasticity and memory. *Current Opinions in Neurobiology*, 3(2), 187–196.

Mitchell, H. and Jones, D. (1997) Homelessness: a review of the social policy background and the role of occupational therapy. *British Journal of Occupational Therapy*, 60(7), 315–319.

Mobsy, I. (1996) A guide to the responsibilities of occupational therapists and their managers in regard to homeless people who use their services. *British Journal of Occupational Therapy*, 59(12), 557–560.

Mulley, G.P. (1994) Principles of rehabilitation. *Reviews in Clinical Gerontology*, 4, 61–69.

Mullins, L.J. (1996) *Management and Organisational Behaviour*, 4th edn, Pitman Publishing, London.

Nocon, A. and Baldwin, S. (1998) *Trends in Rehabilitation Policy*, The King's Fund, London.

O'Brian, K. and Topping, A.U. (1995) Institutional health services. In: *Physiotherapy with Older People* (eds Pickles, B., Compton, A., Cott, C., Simpson, J. and Vandervoort, V.), W.B. Saunders, London.

Royal College of Nursing and National Back Pain Association (1997) *The Guide to Handling of Patients; Introducing a safer handling policy*, 4th edn, RCN and NBPA, London.

Squires, A. (1993) Key issues for purchasers and providers in hospital, day hospital and community rehabilitation services for older people. In: *A Unique Window on Change: The Annual Report of the Director of the NHS Health Advisory Service for 1992–1993*, HMSO, London.

Squires, A., Hastings, M. and Smalls, M. (1997) Physiotherapy with older people: calculating staffing need. *Physiotherapy*, 83(2), 58–64.

Stewart, M. and Hawker, M. (1999) Early rehabilitation. *AGILITY – Commemorative 21st Anniversary issue; AGILE – Physiotherapy with Older People*, Chartered Society of Physiotherapy, London.

Williams, B. (1999) History of geriatric medicine in the United Kingdom. *AGILITY – Commemorative 21st Anniversary issue; AGILE – Physiotherapy with Older People*, Chartered Society of Physiotherapy, London.

Williams, J.I. (1991) *Calculating Staffing Levels in Physiotherapy Services*, Pampas Publishing, Rotherham.

PART Three

THE PRACTICE OF REHABILITATION

11 THE ROLE OF THE PRIMARY CARE GROUP OR TRUST

Chris Drinkwater

AIMS OF THE CHAPTER

This chapter describes how the creation of Primary Care Groups and Trusts (PCGs and PCTs) has the potential to maximise the principles of a primary care led and collaboratively developed and provided health and social care service, of which older people will be the main beneficiaries. The author identifies that a need exists to build on to the strengths of local experience the knowledge and capacity for rehabilitation and consistent quality of provision to take full advantage of the opportunities that await.

INTRODUCTION

The introduction to this chapter in the last edition of this book referred to the *Priorities and Planning Guidance* for the NHS 1996/97 (NHS Executive, 1995) and identified two medium-term priority areas, which would have a significant impact on the rehabilitation of older people. These were to:

- work towards the development of a primary care-led NHS, in which the decisions about the purchasing and provision of health care are taken as close to patients as possible; and
- ensure in collaboration with local authorities and other organisations that integrated services are in place to meet needs for continuing health care and to allow elderly, disabled or vulnerable people to be supported in the community.

These statements are as true today as they were in 1995. The major difference is that there have been significant changes in policy and practice, and the development of a number of levers, which should ensure that these priorities are delivered.

The most important change has been the creation of Primary Care Groups (PCGs) (Local Healthcare Co-operatives in Scotland and Local Health Groups in Wales), with some of these becoming first wave Primary Care Trusts (PCTs) in April 2000. These are new organisations, which were first proposed in the December 1997 White Paper for England, *The New NHS: modern, dependable* (Department of Health [DoH], 1997). PCGs in their most developed form take devolved responsibility for managing the budget for health care in their geographic area, acting as part of the Health Authority, while PCTs are freestanding bodies accountable to the Health Authority for commissioning care, and for the provision of community services for their population. In both cases they consist of a grouping of general practices, typically serving a population of around

100,000. The White Paper specified that whatever functions these groups took on, they would all be required to:

- be representative of all the GP practices in the group
- have a governing body that includes community nursing, social services and a lay representative, as well as GPs drawn from the area
- take account of social services as well as Health Authority boundaries, to help promote integration in service planning and provision
- abide by the local Health Improvement Programme (see below)
- have clear arrangements for public involvement including open meetings
- have efficient and effective arrangements for management and financial accountability.

THE DEVELOPING ROLE OF PCG/Ts

As the number of PCTs increase, GPs and primary health-care teams, instead of just influencing the purchasing and provision of services for older people, will become directly responsible for commissioning and delivering these services. This will mean a shift from a demand-led service (for example, winter pressures) to a more proactive, planned and managed service. It will require a more systematic approach to local assessment of needs and the ability to work effectively with a range of providers in order to ensure that high quality services are delivered as close to patients and as cost-effectively and efficiently as possible. One possible way of ensuring that this happens would be to develop a five-tier model of care, which focuses on the inter-dependence of generalist and specialist health and social care providers.

Tier 1: Core primary care with continuity and a user sensitive approach as key values, but also including health promotion, disease prevention and early identification.

Tier 2: Specialist interventions delivered by primary care practitioners within community settings. This tier is about increasing the level of skills and competencies within primary care settings and it could for instance include appropriate trained community nurses and therapists taking on care management responsibilities.

Tier 3: The functions that need to be delivered at this level are:

- local needs assessment
- coordination of locality services across the PCG/T
- development, maintenance and use of effective information systems
- quality control of systems using information feedback loops, service users' views, best available evidence and formal evaluation; and
- development of professional, inter-professional and inter-agency education and training linked to personal, professional and practice development plans.

If this is going to be done effectively, it requires a Clinical Director (not necessarily a doctor) for Old Age Services for the PCG/T.

Tier 4: Interventions delivered by trained and accredited specialists, who will usually cover a number of PCG/Ts, possibly within a Health Authority or sub-regional area. Where the service is delivered is less important than the fact that the approach is specialist rather than generalist and the focus is on the management of more complex cases. These specialists will also need to provide a support function to Tier 3, in order to ensure consistency and common approaches across PCG/Ts.

Tier 5: This is essentially about acute admissions and specialist functions that require central capital plant of one sort or another.

Unfortunately, though describing a model is easy, making sure that it is implemented and has an effect on the care of people such as our case study of Susan Hunter (see Chapter 8) is much more difficult.

WHY PRIMARY CARE-LED REHABILITATION?

Before considering how services might best be delivered in primary care, it is worth exploring whether this is a change for change's sake, a change in order to control expensive secondary care costs or whether it might have definite benefits for patients. The strengths of primary care in respect of the care and rehabilitation of older people are as follows:

- There is a registered list of patients, which means that the size of the population can be identified and the likely level of need predicted.
- There is a relatively accessible service, with continuity of care, often over many years. This can result in high levels of trust and confidence; an important motivator in rehabilitation.
- There is an understanding and knowledge of patient and family dynamics and relationships. Problems in this area are often a cause of readmission following rehabilitation in hospital.
- There is an ability to balance therapeutic optimism and realistic pessimism. The common caricature is the GP who is perceived to blame all problems on old age. This conveniently ignores the fact that growing old is often about coming to terms with functional disabilities for which there is no magical solution, although there may be suitable coping strategies, and that inappropriate intervention can be harmful.
- There is greater sensitivity to patient autonomy, if only because the patient is within the familiar environment of their home or local practice, rather than in an alien hospital bed or clinic.
- There is core knowledge within the team about the medical, nursing and preventive care of older people in the community.

These are all potential strengths and the fact that these strengths are not always used or developed is also the greatest weakness of primary care-led rehabilitation of older people. Other weaknesses include:

- competing demands on time from other areas of work
- lack of resources of accommodation and finance to deliver enhanced community-based services
- lack of knowledge of the norms with a multi-cultural community, which may impact on traditional rehabilitation (see also Chapter 3)
- a broader resource issue of dis-economies of scale: delivering services in patients' homes and in GPs' surgeries may be more expensive than delivering services from a central site (see also Chapter 10)
- increasing pressure from ever-earlier hospital discharge, which may overload the system and result in breakdown
- lack of appropriate knowledge and skills within the practice team about care of older people and more particularly about rehabilitation; undergraduate and postgraduate training for GPs in these areas is often very limited
- lack of appreciation of the increasingly knowledgeable and assertive cohorts of older people and their carers (see also Chapter 5)
- poor but improving links with social services (see also Chapter 19)
- failure to involve carers, on whom much responsibility will be placed, as part of the decision-making process (see also Chapter 11)
- conflicts around professional power and autonomy that result in referrals for treatment rather than assessment by an autonomous colleague
- wide variations between practices in the type of service that they offer.

This last point is illustrated by the fact that the balance sheet of strengths and weaknesses varies from practice to practice. This variation is one of the major clinical governance challenges for PCG/Ts (see also Chapters 1 and 6).

WHAT SORT OF SERVICE SHOULD PRIMARY CARE BE DEVELOPING?

The best way of addressing this is to take a systems approach and to look at the critical transitions, as patients such as our case study, Susan Hunter, move through the system.

CASE STUDY SUSAN HUNTER'S PRIMARY CARE

- Could or should her cerebro-vascular event have been prevented, thus avoiding the need for entry into care?

- Was there a rapid and skilled interdisciplinary assessment with early intervention, production and implementation of an effective care plan agreed with Susan Hunter?

- Are appropriate arrangements in place to ensure effective discharge from hospital?
- What services need to be in place to maintain function and to prevent re-entry to care?

Prevention
From what we know of Susan Hunter's previous social and medical history, a number of opportunities for prevention can be identified, which may have a significant impact on the relative success or failure of rehabilitation following her cerebro-vascular event. These can grouped under physical, psychological and social factors.

Physical factors
Susan Hunter is a non-insulin dependent diabetic who has had a right total hip replacement for osteoarthritis. Her diabetes and her osteoarthritis suggest that she is likely to be overweight. Diabetes, particularly if poorly controlled, and obesity are risk factors for stroke (Ebrahim, 1988). They are also causal factors for high blood pressure, which is the commonest preventable cause of stroke (Ebrahim, 1988). The final significant factor is maintenance of physical activity, which is likely to be poor because of her osteoarthritis. Good evidence exists that maintenance of physical activity protects against stroke (Shinton and Sagar, 1993). Evidence also suggests that maintenance of physical activity improves mobility, and reduces pain (McKeag, 1992) and the risk of falls in patients with osteoarthritis (O'Loughlin et al., 1993). Good baseline physical fitness also contributes to successful rehabilitation.

The primary health-care team, therefore have a significant role to play in hopefully either preventing or delaying the onset of Susan Hunter's stroke. Ideally this should include the following elements:

- regular monitoring with formal annual review of her diabetes – this should include measurement of her weight and blood pressure, with appropriate advice and treatment when necessary
- regular medication review to reduce the risk of drug interactions and to improve compliance – a significant number of patients with known high blood pressure are inadequately treated (Smith et al., 1990)
- provision of lifestyle advice about physical activity and diet.

Psychological factors
The major issue to address here is Susan Hunter's recent bereavement. Loss of a spouse in later life is associated with high levels of psychological morbidity, and with physical morbidity and mortality (Clayton, 1974). There is evidence that Susan Hunter was depressed prior to her stroke – recent loss of appetite and weight loss, and that she has become more depressed following her stroke – weepy and withdrawn. Some primary care teams offer routine bereavement visits, which provide an opportunity to assess how an individual is coping and if necessary to mobilise support in terms of family, friends, local churches and the voluntary sector such as Cruse or Age Concern. On some occasions anti-depressants

may be indicated, but often the most difficult factor to cope with is lack of the will to live, which is frequently articulated by the bereaved as a positive wish to die and to join the deceased (see also Chapter 9). Not surprisingly this is likely to have an adverse effect on rehabilitation.

Social factors

It is a truism to say that social isolation is bad for your health. The important thing for Susan Hunter is to try and ensure that her bereavement does not become part of a downward spiral of increasing social isolation. Since her husband's death, the carer support has been withdrawn so there is less incentive for her to keep up with her hobbies of bowling and the local church groups. There are also risks that increasing depression and withdrawal drive away her immediate family and friends. Continuing support and encouragement to maintain social links can be very important at this time, and good social links and networks are also an important motivator, in what can sometimes be a slow and frustrating process of rehabilitation (Walker et al., 1997).

Need for assessment and care

In Susan Hunter's case, even if prevention of her stroke has failed, attention to her physical fitness and psycho-social circumstances will hopefully have resulted in a better baseline position for rehabilitation. However, once a stroke of this severity has occurred, the priority will be admission to hospital, preferably to a specialist Stroke Unit, as there is good evidence that early admission to a Stroke Unit reduces both mortality and long-term morbidity (Stroke Unit Trialists' Collaboration, 1997), for interdisciplinary assessment, appropriate intervention and the development of an agreed care plan. The key issues to be determined are:

1 Is she likely to recover sufficiently to be able to live independently in her own home with some support?

2 Does one of her relatives wish to offer her a home and, if so, are they fully aware of the implications of such an offer?

3 Is she likely to require continuing nursing care and placement in a nursing home?

The general practice/primary care perception of this process is that insufficient account is often taken of the knowledge held by GPs and community nurses about family and social circumstances. The other difficult area is balancing the sometimes conflicting views of the patient, their relatives and the professionals (see also Chapter 4). Maintaining patient autonomy and choice in these circumstances can be very difficult. The patient may wish to go home. The professional assessment suggests that the risk is too great and the relatives are ambivalent. In these circumstances liaison with general practice is essential and sometimes a trial of home treatment is required so that the patient can find out themselves whether or not it is a feasible option.

Discharge from hospital

Ever earlier discharge home or to residential or nursing home care is increasingly common because of the pressure on acute medical beds. This inevitably reduces the margin of error, making it even more important to get the care plan right and in place before the patient is discharged. Failure at this point usually results in readmission or inappropriate placement in residential or nursing care. One of the most common and often overlooked reasons for failure is the difficulty of transferring functional ability in a hospital setting to functional ability in a community setting. The patient in the hospital bed has been rehabilitated, is desperately keen to go home and puts on a wonderful performance. The hospital team are desperate to clear beds to admit waiting admissions. The carer at home is anxious, uncertain and sometimes over-caring, which results in dependence rather than independence. The GP and community nurse are concerned about the carers' ability to cope. The pre-discharge home assessment visit goes some way to addressing this issue, but too often the focus is on functional and instrumental issues rather than on patient/carer psychology and psychodynamics. Unless these issues are addressed, if necessary by providing additional support, then the result is usually failure.

Other issues that are important for good discharge practice include:

- good rapid communication systems between secondary and primary care, which should include information about what the patient and their carer have been told
- rapid provision of aids and appliances and, if more complex household adaptations are required (provision of a stairlift for example), following appropriate assessment and an agreed plan and timescale for doing this, together with equally efficient maintenance when needed
- agreement on a continuing home-based rehabilitation package and clear identification of the person responsible for providing the package
- good communication between providers of health and social care, either through a key worker or a care manager
- an agreed mechanism for reviewing the care package after a certain time or in response to changing needs.

Clearly a number of different professionals need to be involved in the process, but the key issues concern good communication with patients and carers and between members of the team (see also Chapter 7). To some extent this is about ensuring that good systems are in place and that they are regularly reviewed, but the more important issue is often about attitudes and values as barriers to better inter-professional working. In the long term, the best way of tackling this is likely to be through working together, learning together and mutual respect at the level of a PCG/T.

Maintenance of function

The final part of the system is about maintaining the gains achieved through rehabilitation. From a primary care perspective, this is often an area that is overlooked. The common pattern is rehabilitation and discharge followed by a gradual decline in function, which at some stage triggers the need for a further intensive episode of rehabilitation. If anything, this is becoming more of a problem, with targeted and costed brief interventions becoming the purchasing norm. This makes it very difficult to develop a service that contains a costing for a regular review and support visit, which is focused on educational reinforcement of patient and carer and maintenance of morale. The fact that chronic visiting of house-bound patients remains a part of primary care attests to the value that patients and their carers place on this sort of service, despite the fact that it is often resented by GPs, who see it as social visiting where nothing medically useful takes place. It is just such visits that can identify early need for team input, and whether such visits need to be undertaken by the GP or another suitably skilled professional requires debate and evaluation.

The other important area where maintenance of function is a major problem, and which is likely to have implications for patients such as Susan Hunter, is nursing home care. There are four reasons for this. First, placement in a nursing home is often seen as an end point, providing professionals with an opportunity to withdraw and concentrate on the next case. Second, this group is likely to contain the most physically frail and vulnerable patients who will inevitably have the greatest difficulty maintaining their functional status. Third, although regular reassessment should be part of all nursing home care packages, this is usually the area that is abandoned if there is increasing pressure in other parts of the system, such as discharge arrangements, and also offers a perverse incentive. Fourth, there is variable access by nursing homes and their residents to therapy services dependent on the status of the home and availability of resources (Royal College of Physicians, 2000). Hopefully, some of these issues will be resolved by the NSF for Older People (see also Chapter 6).

A COMMUNITY REHABILITATION SERVICE

The previous sections of this chapter have discussed recent changes in the infrastructure of primary care and have explored how primary care should be meeting the needs of patients such as Susan Hunter. This section will try and pull these strands together and look at how PCG/Ts could begin to develop community rehabilitation services. This is an agenda that is becoming increasingly important because of proposals in the NHS Plan (DoH, 2000), which state that PCG/Ts will have to set up Intensive Rehabilitation Services to help older patients regain health /independence after illness/surgery. They are also charged with establishing recuperation facilities in nursing homes, one-stop services and integrated home care teams. In addition, there are also proposals to establish Care Trusts, which will provide integrated health and social care, with some of these in place by the end of 2001.

One possible model is to develop community care of the elderly teams, which would function across PCG/Ts. These would be multidisciplinary teams with a full range of core professionals: nursing, medical care of the elderly, physiotherapy, occupational therapy, speech and language therapy, podiatry, dietetics and social services, with access to other disciplines as relevant. Other possible additions to this team could include general practice input to build bridges with other GP practices and medically led services, and psychology input to provide support around the behavioural and motivational issues that can occur when providing community care to dependent and disabled people (see also Chapter 9).

Such a team would operate at what has already been described as Tier 3, and would be responsible for the coordination of services for older people across the PCG/T. The advantage of this approach is that it would begin to break down inter-professional barriers and would ensure better communication between the different professionals who are involved in the delivery of complex care packages. This approach would also simplify and improve interdisciplinary assessment, as well as improving access to a range of therapists by primary health-care teams. In the longer term this sort of team could also begin to enhance knowledge and skills in primary care teams, and residential and nursing homes through educational and audit approaches. There would also be the potential to foster better links with the voluntary sector, including carer support, and to address important issues of health promotion, illness prevention and early intervention for older people.

SUMMARY

The number of older people with complex problems who live in the community is increasing. Many of these people live alone and informal care is problematic because the main carer is often elderly, and social expectations and traditions around family support are changing. Against this background, national policy for both health and social services has been to move away from institutional care to integrated services, which allow vulnerable people to be supported in the community. The other main policy change has been the development of PCG/Ts serving local populations of around 100,000 people. These bodies will ultimately have responsibility for commissioning and delivering community based services for older people.

These changes leave PCG/Ts in a unique position to establish local Community Care of the Elderly Teams, which would consist of an interdisciplinary group of autonomous professionals who would be responsible for community based assessment of older people. They would also be able to coordinate local services and to ensure their quality and consistency within a framework of national standards.

REFERENCES

Clayton, P.J. (1974) Mortality and morbidity in the first year of widowhood. *Archives of General Psychiatry*, **30**, 747–750.

Department of Health [DoH] (1997) *The New NHS: modern, dependable*, Cm 3807, The Stationery Office, London.

DoH (2000) *The NHS National Plan*, The Stationery Office, London.

Ebrahim, S. (1988) *Clinical Epidemiology of Stroke*, Office of Health Economics, London.

McKeag, D.B. (1992) *The relationship of osteoarthritis and exercise. Clinical Sports Medicine*, **11**, 471–487.

NHS Executive (1995) *Priorities and Planning Guidance for the NHS: 1995/96*, EL(95)68, Department of Health, Leeds.

O'Loughlin, J.L. Robitaille, Y., Boivin, J.-F. and Suissa, S. (1993) Incidence of and risk factors for falls and injurious falls among community-dwelling elderly. *American Journal of Epidemiology*, **137**, 342–354.

Royal College of Physicians [RCP] (2000) *The Health and Care of Older People in Care Homes*, RCP, London.

Shinton, R. and Sagar, G. (1993) Lifelong exercise and stroke. *British Medical Journal*, **307**, 231–234.

Smith, W.C., Lee, A.J., Crombie, I.K. and Tunstall-Pedoe, H. (1990) Control of blood pressure in Scotland: the rule of halves. *British Medical Journal*, **300**, 981–983.

Stroke Unit Trialists' Collaboration (1997) Collaborative systematic review of the randomised trials of organised inpatient (stroke unit) care after stroke. *British Medical Journal*, **314**, 1151–1159.

Walker, K., MacBride, A. and Vachon, M.L.S. (1997) Social support networks and the crisis of bereavement. *Socal Sciences and Medicine*, 7(11), 34–41.

FURTHER READING

Rummery, K. and Glendinning, C. (2000) *Primary Care and Social Services: Developing new partnerships for older people*, Radcliffe Medical Press, Oxford.

12 WORKING WITH CARERS

Jill Manthorpe and Helen Alaszewski

AIMS OF THE CHAPTER

The carers of older people are the largest group of informal supporters and the care they provide is likely to be progressively intensive. The needs of carers providing care at home have been recognised over the past ten years, and current trends in policy emphasise the 'empowerment' of service users and carers. This chapter considers the social and legal impact of caring, and questions whether carers are 'empowered' service users.

Carers assumed a status of their own during the last decades of the twentieth century. Prior to this they were generally referred to as kin or family, if at all. Largely invisible, those providing care to disabled people at home received little recognition, particularly in terms of their own needs for financial, practical or emotional support. There have since been several developments at policy and service level, which have undoubtedly put carers on the agenda. In this chapter we shall draw on some of these and make some observations relevant to carers of older people in particular. We shall also discuss the case of Susan Hunter to reflect on how her own experience of caring for her late husband impacts on her own expectations and the possible, but not easy or automatic, transformation of her family into a caring support system for her.

CARERS OF OLDER PEOPLE

This group of carers forms the largest and most disparate group of stakeholders in health and social care. The people they care for may have physical or mental health problems (sometimes both). Carers of older people are most likely to be spouses and to have their own health problems (Moriarty, 1999). Their needs are not always recognised and although they generally take on this role for shorter periods of time than, for example, parents of children with disabilities, the care they provide is likely to be progressively intensive. Moriarty (1999) argues that this group have different needs from younger carers due to their own vulnerabilities and reports that their preference is to have support within the home, particularly with more physically demanding tasks. There are substantial differences in the levels of services provided between carers, although overall most support goes to people who live alone (Parker and Lawton, 1994). Nonetheless, the Department of Health [DoH], in *Caring for People* (DoH, 1989), reports that married disabled people are only one-third as likely to receive a home help as a single disabled person. This may relate to our case study, Susan Hunter's, experience (see Chapter 8). Myers and MacDonald (1996) suggest that some older people are reluctant to seek information but would rather have an advocate (see chapter 4) or an expert who can take control for them. Susan Hunter, as a spouse carer, may have had little contact with services and low expectations of their support.

If, as research indicates, older people's needs are likely to be overlooked and they are not a priority for receipt of the types of services they need, the relationships of their carers with professionals, whether as carers or service users, and involvement in decision-making, are likely to be limited. Walker and Warren (1996) maintain that carers' requests for services are not always successful and that in relation to formal services they feel frustrated and a sense of 'powerlessness to effect changes to provision with: limited opportunity for contact with service providers and organisers'.

Many would like sufficient help on a regular but flexible basis, but frequently their only contact is through changes in circumstances such as hospitalisation. It is against this background that Susan Hunter's possibly low expectations may be explained.

Current trends in policy emphasise the 'empowerment' of service users and carers. In the next section we explore the conflicting pressures on professionals when seeking to provide such support (see also Chapter 4).

PROFESSIONALS SUPPORTING CARERS OF OLDER PEOPLE

Carers who provide 'a substantial amount of care on a regular basis' have a legal right to assessment of their needs as part of the Community Care Assessment, under the Carers Recognition and Services Act 1995. Professionals (usually social workers) are required to assess needs, share decision-making and provide information, but they are also gatekeepers; rationing or restricting access to social care services. Myers and MacDonald (1996) describe such professionals as 'neutral advisers' who are aware of the limited choices available and the eligibility criteria governing access. However, Twigg (2000) argues that some professionals are reluctant to lose the status and power that goes with assessing and determining levels of service, and that they continue to display features of institutional culture. Practitioners are required to 'support safety and minimise risk', while 'maximising autonomy and self-determination' (Braye and Preston-Shoot, 1995). The position for professionals is therefore a difficult one of trying to balance the needs of service users and carers (which are not necessarily in accordance) against the background of restricted resources and performance measures of waiting time and responsiveness.

Current debates emphasise partnerships in care between health and social care agencies and stress the need for good communication. The Social Services Inspectorate (1998), which examined support for carers, while citing some areas of good practice, identified a whole range of issues that were unsatisfactory. They report a similar sense of frustration (in para 1.8) as Walker and Warren (1996) in relation to formal services. Carers have to repeat information to different professionals and this often results in delays in service provision. Carers' perceptions are that health and social care agencies work separately, are uncoordinated and when they do communicate it is not effective (paras 4.6–4.10). Of particular relevance to rehabilitation, the Audit Commission (2000) found long delays in obtaining equipment for users and carers following assessment. It was noted in Chapter 1 that home nursing equipment is provided by the NHS, and aids for home independence by Social Services – where integration of these services has occurred, there has been the opportunity to improve coordination and reduce delays. The evidence suggests that, in spite of policies that are user and carer oriented, the service being delivered does not reach current expectations of older people, let alone the anticipated raised expectations of the future (see Chapter 5).

ROOM FOR IMPROVEMENT

Twigg (2000) argues that there is a lack of 'ideological focus' in service development for older people. She suggests this is because policy-makers are reluctant, due to the large numbers and needs of older people, to develop a rights based framework, as for example, normalisation in services for people with learning disabilities. This lack of focus may however be attributable to the lack of homogeneity of this group of carers. Uniform models of rehabilitation will probably fit neither all older people nor their carers (see also Chapter 4), hence the current move from standardisation to personalisation with its probable short-term costs but long-term benefits. Easterbrooke (1999) suggests:

> *The focus should be far more on fitting the treatment, care and support around older people's lifestyles, rather than an older person experiencing a lifestyle that could be restricted by illness, disability and service responses.*

Following this call for flexibility, she makes a number of recommendations including 'staff who can work across organisational and professional boundaries', a prominent feature of the NHS Plan (DoH, 2000). It will also be increasingly necessary for staff to be able to work with both users and carers.

POLICY DEVELOPMENTS

Despite the variation in carers and their experiences, policy has tended to be simplistic in demanding 'support'. For example, the White Paper *Caring for People* (Department of Health, 1989) placed as the second most important objective of community care policy the need 'to ensure that service providers make practical support for carers a high priority'. Perhaps because this was so generalised, reviews of the NHS and Community Care Act 1990 have been less than impressed by developments in this field. Henwood and Wistow (1999), for example, point to the Department of Health's 'awarding' of two stars (out of a maximum five) for progress (in its view) in respect of carers. The NHS Plan (DoH, 2000) is more specific and acknowledges that its plans for developing rehabilitation services will necessitate support for carers: here, though, this is quantified as an extension of respite care services for 75,000 further carers (para. 15.14).

It is appropriate to listen to carers to learn what they consider to be both the aims of support services and the best way of delivering such services. Drawing on research among groups of carers, Qureshi *et al.* (1998) established a set of outcomes desired by carers. These would help contribute towards improvements in carers' quality of life and may be summarised as:

- freedom to have a life of their own
- maintaining their own health and well-being
- preventing social isolation
- delivering peace of mind.

Such aims are useful measures against which to set out existing or planned services. They are explicitly focused on carers and thus avoid the 'grey areas' where services are provided in the expectation that they might help carers. Thus, providing a place at a day centre for Susan Hunter, in order to provide her family with a break, might be relevant unless the timing fails to fit in with the family's routine, they worry about her happiness there and, along with Susan Hunter, they find the 'break' is not particularly useful. Fine-tuning of carers' support services will be one key criterion in successfully engaging them in the rehabilitation process.

Qureshi and her colleagues (1998) learned that carers were very concerned about the way services were delivered to them. Carers placed emphasis on:

- 'having a sense of shared responsibility'
- 'having a "say"'
- being 'confident in services'.

These characteristics again provide a useful framework for the evaluation of any care plan. Because they can be related to individuals and their families, they can be applied to the unique circumstances of each case. Arising from Nocon and Qureshi's (1996) earlier work is the aim, again derived from research into carers' perceptions, that generally they desire a 'normal life' as far as possible. Some will want to continue in employment, to enjoy a social life or to carry out other family responsibilities. Services should promote such capacity for reasons of offering effective support to carers, and reducing their strain and distress. In many circumstances such support will confirm the desires of the person receiving care. However, in some cases it will not. We might imagine, for example, that there might be pressure on Susan Hunter's daughter-in-law to provide a range of practical and personal care. She might have 'only' a part-time, lowly paid job ... it might be better for everyone if she gave this up and claimed Invalid Care Allowance ... it might, but it would need to be carefully considered, particularly from the daughter in law's short-term and long-term perspective: is it her main social outlet; how does it affect her future employment and pension prospects and her own position in old age?

Identifying and resolving possible conflict between carers and disabled people is one key aspect of professional roles. They may be able to offer a perspective from outside an emotionally charged family atmosphere. Much debate in respect of possible conflict centres around risk. There is evidence from a variety of sources (for example, Reed, 1998) that older people's abilities to take risks may be constrained by family and professionals alike. Rehabilitation, by its very nature, often involves taking risks and one element of the professional task is to support those taking risks in order to achieve desired ends, such as independence, activity and social interaction. Providing support to carers, for example, may entail involving them in the risk assessment and risk management processes (with the consent of the service user). Carers' anxiety or guilt may be one key to the slow progress being made once a person is being 'looked after' at home (see also Chapter 4).

Occupational therapists, in particular, may have a key role in resolving conflict between carers and the older person. There is a balance between patients' needs and desires and those of carers. They should recognise their obligation to take these into consideration under the Carers (Recognition and Services) Act 1995, but avoid being directed by carers. This legislation gives carers the right to request an assessment of their own needs, if the person they care for is also being assessed. Obviously any evidence of carer stress or abuse of, or by, the older person needs to be responded to as a priority. For Susan Hunter, therefore, part of her rehabilitation may well include explaining to her well-meaning (hopefully) family that she should attempt certain activities, however slowly. A useful handbook is available for patients and their family to guide them through all stages of recovery (Rudd *et al.*, 2000).

For some carers this is possibly a source of concern. The use of carer support groups is one way in which carers can share such feelings and learn from each other. Some groups are specific to conditions, such as stroke or dementia; others are general but may also offer a social, educational or quasi-therapeutic network (Twigg, 2000). While carers' groups are well established in most localities, less common but growing in number are Carers' Centres, offering a resource for carers that may provide professional or voluntary advice, information or activities. Such centres will increasingly provide access via the Internet to the latest information with which carers can pursue the interests of their dependant – confidently challenging professionals from an informed base. One key task for professionals is to introduce carers to such local networks and ensure resources to enable them to participate if it is their wish.

CARERS' STRATEGIES

It is widely acknowledged that support for carers developed over the past decade somewhat haphazardly and unevenly. Parker (1999) attributes this to the continuing ambiguity of services – Are they to help users or carers? – and to the strains of responding to rising expectations (see also Chapter 5) and levels of needs within 'essentially static' resources. She considers that consultation with carers varies widely; that there remain major unmet needs for information; that many carers do not receive copies of care plans (making monitoring or complaining impossible); and that carers' own support servicesare unpredictable in extent and quality. The NHS Plan, like many other policy documents such as the Long-Term Care Charter, seeks to address these continual complaints.

To some extent this failure of the new system of community care to make 'support for carers a high priority' could have been predicted. The system was built on a theory that targeting services on those most in need would be the best use of resources. Individuals such as Susan Hunter, with active, willing and available (in theory) family members are not in the highest priority bands for service receipt. Parker also observes that while support for carers might have been uneven within social care it was generally more accepted than within the health service. As she notes this may be attributable to the 'culture' of the NHS, to its history of 'border skirmishes' with other practitioners and agencies, and to the major upheavals affecting all parts of the NHS (see Chapter 1).

Nonetheless, Parker identifies some positive developments. She considers that the 'culture of assessment has taken carers on board'. While the Carers (Recognition and Services) Act 1995 may not have produced much resource, this too has confirmed the legitimacy of carers as the proper focus of professional attention and service development. In a research project focusing on 4 local authorities and the experiences of 51 representative carers, Arksey et al. (2000) found half the carers interviewed did not even fully realise they had been assessed. Nonetheless, most were highly satisfied with the services provided – although problems with flexibility, reliability, lack of staff continuity and transport problems were mentioned. This unqualified satisfaction of people dependent on goodwill is a feature of public services and further explored in Chapter 5. Further, a number wished for more emotional support for themselves and a minority considered financial advice would be helpful. It appears therefore that the Act has opened further the door in respect of carers. Many carers, at least, will have heard of the legislation and their higher expectations for themselves may be one crucial spur to service development.

Finally, in this section we briefly mention the Carers' National Strategy (HM Government, 1999). Introduced by Prime Minister Blair, this document refers to carers as 'among the unsung heroes of British life' and represents a 'substantial policy package'. One key theme is the support of those carers in employment; another is the continued development of short-term or respite provision. As we shall now see these may be highly relevant to Susan Hunter and her family.

This may be an expensive time for all concerned. While Susan Hunter may be responsible for charges incurred in respect of home care services or equipment (deposits or hire) (see also Chapter 18), her family may well find that they too will face further expenses in respect of travel, extra shopping or specific purchases. For some families these place additional pressures on stretched budgets. Like Susan Hunter, help may be rejected if it incurs a charge. Alternatively, it may be accepted and monitored like any other commercial provision.

CASE STUDY Caring for susan hunter

During her rehabilitation, it is possible that her family will share Susan Hunter's uncertainty. Each of them will be affected, possibly, in different ways. We have already noted that gender expectations may affect how the family envision providing care, if this is needed. In any event the family, as well as Susan Hunter, may find the level of support provided to her at home gives rise to a series of questions about the sharing of tasks and responsibilities between the family and formal services. To some extent, the care plan should help set out the optimum position: it should include details of the routine, of the contact numbers and of the opportunities to monitor and review progress. The family should be informed and involved if Susan Hunter wishes. They may be advised in advance of the arrival of equipment or carry out agreed preparations round the home to make life comfortable and practical. All family members may have views about the extent to which the home begins to resemble a hospital ward and may make decisions that stress the familiarity and comfort of the environment above factors of convenience or logic. Such a process presumes Susan Hunter is happy to have her family fully informed and involved. In some instances this may not be so and a sensitive approach will be needed to work with the family, possibly coordinated by a member of the social work team.

One key element in the family system is the new roles that will follow on Susan Hunter's discharge from hospital. Prior to her illness, Susan Hunter appears to have been independent: indeed like many older people she may have contributed to her family by offering child-care, regularly or in emergencies, some help with household tasks or social support. Now, on the receiving end, her changing role may impact on her family's perceptions of her. They may see her in need of care or protection and resist professional advice to encourage independence. If such plans have not been developed with full involvement, equipment may remain unused or services rejected that appear directive or unnecessary. Even if there has been full involvement, unanticipated pressures may lead to the same outcome. At its extreme, relatives may exert their power over disabled older people to such an extent that it becomes abusive. With the growing awareness among professionals of issues around elder abuse, professionals should be alert to families who deny the rights of the older person. Such rights, of course, extend not only to personal protection but also to access to rehabilitation or services more generally.

We noted earlier how the Carers' National Strategy identified caring and employment as an area where there was much room for policy development and good practice at local level. In the case of Susan Hunter, while there may be pressures for individuals to leave employment, there might be other factors at play that enable carers to stay in employment. These might include, for example, provision to take time off work, to work flexibly or to attend appointments. Some employers have developed policies permitting leave or reduced commitment. Others have developed information and support through human resources departments or provide access to telephones or alarm services. It may also be useful to consider research findings in respect of shared living arrangements. While this remains a minority option, over 10 per cent of older women aged 80 or more live with a son or daughter, often once a significant illness or event has precipitated a search for an alternative home. Healy and Yarrow (1997) report that such arrangements, while not to everyone's liking, seem to work well possibly because both parties are generally aware of the risks and enter such arrangements in a prepared and practical frame of mind. For Susan Hunter, we are not aware if this is an option and such deliberations may be one of the private sides of family life to which few professionals have access. Such a move represents one of the options open to Susan Hunter: it may be however that her desire to remain in her own home is prominent.

Finally, we have discussed the issue of caring in respect of family alone. While the great majority of informal care is provided to older people by family members, other individuals such as friends or neighbours may well offer valuable social and practical support. Much depends on individuals' networks, and the capacities and willingness of those involved. However, research shows that many older people derive great benefit and pleasure from maintaining their social identity. Wenger (1994), for example, points out that friends provide companionship and emotional support, but may also be available for emergency help and are likely to be dependable. In some rare instances, friends may be similar to family or kin. Neighbours, too, may provide low level but helpful support, particularly if the relationship is positive and long-standing. While neither groups may be appropriately classified as carers for individuals such as Susan Hunter, they may be valuable in enhancing her morale and motivation. Sensitive care plans will make room for the maintenance of social contacts.

CARERS AND REHABILITATION

Involving carers in rehabilitation is a necessary part of the process. Few models of good practice exist however. Rehabilitation is largely conceived of as a professional task: involving the patient and expert, while carers conceive of themselves as lay people, able to provide ordinary, commonsense support. It is clear, however, that many carers learn and exercise skills that are highly developed, and that professionals often do invoke their active participation in the rehabilitation process. Carers can also contribute skills to the repertoire of the professional through their experience of having to solve practical problems.

Existing information based on carers' expressed priorities and views may offer some ways forward. In the first instance, carers have expressed a need for information; some of this should be specifically designed for carers – ideally written by them or based on their own experiences. 'Carer to carer' seems to be an approach that works well at information as well as interpersonal levels. Secondly, carers may need support in managing their own feelings about rehabilitation and the dilemmas they might encounter. It is possibly a mistake to represent this as a linear and uncomplicated process, for carers are likely to be among the first to realise that their relative may not value rehabilitation or may hold strong views about the messages being given by professionals. This would indicate that the patient has not been, or has not been capable of being, a true partner in the plans. Thirdly, some carers will want to be members of the rehabilitation team – helping to carry out set activities, providing monitoring and liaising between professionals and agencies, although for some enthusiasm may exceed capability. But some will not and indeed their own poor health may make this difficult. They will want instead to remain as family members and to concentrate on the relationship or, indeed, their own lives.

All these factors suggest that Susan Hunter's family may be a resource for the professionals involved in her care or they may choose another route. The labelling of all family members as carers can be optimistic and inaccurate. In our discovery of carers we may have gone too far and should perhaps consider asking family members if this is a correct picture of their relationship.

Summary

We end this chapter with a brief commentary on future developments planned to support carers. These include the extension of direct payments to older people. Such payments are only in respect of work performed by *non* family members for the reason that this should prevent abuse. This has not been widely welcomed by older people who may prefer their relatives' care than that of neighbours, friends or strangers. Family members, equally, may resent the suggestion that they are more likely to be exploitative than anyone else and that their contribution will again be taken for granted.

Vouchers or systems that enable disabled people to purchase specific care services from accredited care providers are a further way of offering some choice and flexibility to disabled people and their families, and were introduced for older people in 2001. A parallel voucher system for carers operating in a number of areas may enable them too to extend choice over the type of service, such as short-break care, they prefer. This might permit more appropriate responses to individual circumstances. For example, in the case of Susan Hunter, should her disability continue and worsen, or the ability of her main carer diminish, her carer(s) might wish to use a voucher to purchase overnight care from an agency whose staff Susan Hunter knows and trusts.

We are therefore entering a world in which some service responses to carers are enhancing their ability to care. Instead of simply providing a replacement, when crisis or breakdown occurs, services should aim to work with carers, to maintain quality of life for all concerned. Clearly this is the ideal and for many carers there will continue to be a gap between what support is available and their own needs. This will place demands on professionals to try to advocate on behalf of carers. Within rehabilitative or intermediate services, carers may become used to a high or reasonable level of support and assistance. Once this level of service stops, however, carers may feel let down and burdened, and this emphasises the need for clear explanation throughout at both planning and implementation stages. Practitioners working in this area need to acknowledge that when 'official' treatments or interventions are over, it will most likely be carers who will carry on their work. How competent and confident carers feel about this role will depend to some extent on the quality of the handover from 'recuperation' to continuing support.

REFERENCES

Age Concern (1999) *Turning your Back on Us: Older people and the NHS*, Age Concern England, London.

Arksey, H., Hepworth, D. and Qureshi, H. (2000) *Carers' Needs and the Carers Act: An evaluation of the process and outcomes of assessment*, Social Policy Research Unit, York.

Audit Commission (2000) *Fully Equipped*, The Audit Commission, London.

Braye, S. and Preston-Shoot, M. (1995) *Empowering Practice in Social Care*, Open University Press, Buckingham.

Department of Health [DoH] (1989) *Caring for People: Community care in the next decade and beyond*, Cm. 849, HMSO, London.

DoH (2000) *The NHS Plan: A plan for investment, A plan for reform*, Cm. 4818–1, The Stationery Office, London.

Easterbrooke, L. (1999) *When We are Very Old: Reflections on treatment, care and support of older people*, The King's Fund, London.

Healy, J. and Yarrow, S. (1997) *Family Matters: Parents living with children in old age*, The Policy Press, Bristol.

Henwood, M. and Wistow, G. (1999) Clarifying responsibilities and improving accountability? In: *With Respect to Old Age* (ed. Sutherland, S.), The Stationery Office, London, Research Volume 3, Chapter 1.

HM Government (1999) *Caring about Carers: A national strategy for carers*, The Stationery Office, London.

Moriarty, J. (1999) Older people. In: *Rights, Needs and the User Perspective: A review of the National Health Service and Community Care Act 1990* (eds Balloch, S., Butt, J., Fisher, M. and Lindow, V.), National Institute for Social Work, Joseph Rowntree Foundation, London.

Myers, F. and MacDonald, C. (1996) 'I was given options not choices': Involving older users and carers in assessment and care planning. In: *Developing Services for Older People and Their Families* (ed. Bland, R.), Research Highlights in Social Work 29. Jessica Kingsley, London.

Nocon, A. and Qureshi, H. (1996) *Outcomes of Community Care for Users and Carers*, Open University Press, Buckingham.

Parker, G. (1999) Impact of the NHS and Community Care Act (1990) on informal carers. In: *With Respect to Old Age* (ed. Sutherland, S.), The Stationery Office, London, Research Volume 3, Chapter 4.

Parker, G. and Lawton, D. (1994) *Different Types of Care, Different Types of Carer: Evidence from the General Household Survey*, Social Policy Research Unit, HMSO, London.

Qureshi, H., Patmore, C., Nicholas, E. and Bamford, C. (1998) *Overview: Outcomes of social care for older people and carers*, Social Policy Research Unit, York.

Reed, J. (1998) Care and protection for older people. In: *Risk, Health and Health Care* (ed. Heyman, B.), Arnold, London, pp. 241–251.

Rudd, A., Irwin, P. and Penhale, B. (2000) *Stroke at Your Fingertips*, Class Publishing London.

Social Services Inspectorate (1998) *A Matter of Chance for Carers: Inspection of local authority support for carers*, Department of Health, London.

Twigg, J. (2000) The changing role of users and carers. In: *The Changing Role of Social Care* (ed. Hudson, B.), Jessica Kingsley, London.

Walker, A. and Warren, L. (1996) *Changing Services for Older People: The Neighbourhood Support Units innovation*, Open University Press, Buckingham.

Wenger, G.C. (1994) *Support Networks of Older People: A guide for practitioners*, Centre for Social Policy Research and Development, Bangor.

13 THE PHYSICIAN'S ROLE

Brian Owen Williams

AIMS OF THE CHAPTER

Within secondary care (acute hospital), the physician has the responsibility for the medical management of the patient and may take a coordinating role in the overall management of their care. Referral will usually have been made from a general practitioner for specialist advice in the management of the patient and the physician's skill is in the diagnosis of disease. This chapter considers the full clinical assessment and discusses the medical management of the patient, especially the case study. The requirements for clinical governance of clinical effectiveness, audit and risk management are considered.

INTRODUCTION

The consultant physician is responsible for the medical management of the patient in secondary care settings and shares ethical responsibilities with the other members of the team. He or she must ensure that the salient medical and social facts about the patient are shared with the team, is responsible for diagnosis of disease, instigation of drug regimens and ensuring that autonomous colleagues are notified regarding the need for any specialist assessments. The physician must then ensure that he or she is regularly informed about the patient's progress.

Before rehabilitation can take place, a full interdisciplinary assessment should be performed (Audit Commission, 2000) (see also Chapter 8), the physician contributing the medical assessment and diagnosis of disease.

MEDICAL ASSESSMENT

Diagnosis of disease

Accurate medical diagnosis is imperative to inform the patient, carers and health-care team about prognosis. Full clinical examination is essential. Special attention must be paid to the neurological and musculoskeletal systems with respect to impairment affecting mobility, to the cardiorespiratory systems in relation to limitation of exercise tolerance and to the gastrointestinal system for changes in nutritional state. Elderly patients may have restricted ability to take part in active rehabilitation programmes and may require careful goal planning to regain functional ability. Vision and hearing should be assessed, as minor deficits can be compensated by simple measures (see also Chapter 20).

These screening procedures (Table 13.1) should be undertaken by the most appropriate team member (See also Chapters 6 and 8).

Table 13.1 Physical screening

Cardiovascular	Heart rate, lying and standing blood pressure, signs of heart failure
Respiratory	Airflow obstruction
Blood	Anaemia or metabolic disorder
Locomotor	Bone or joint disease, foot disorders
Neurological	Muscle weakness, sensory deficits
Gastrointestinal	Abdominal masses
Genitourinary	Causes of urinary incontinence
Endocrine	Thyroid abnormalities
Vision	
Hearing	
Skin integrity	

The results from the screening should then be pooled for team consideration. Diagnoses may be further elucidated with appropriate laboratory tests or radiological imaging techniques. Anaemia will require investigation and biochemical abnormalities, e.g. hypokalaemia or calcium disorders should be corrected. Cardiovascular disease may require further investigation by electrocardiography, chest radiography and echocardiography. Respiratory disease is best elucidated with chest radiography and pulmonary function tests. Remediable conditions should be treated before the final rehabilitation plan is prepared for discussion with the patient/carer.

Mental state

A detailed evaluation of the patient's mental state is as important as an accurate physical diagnosis. Acute and chronic confusion and depression are important barriers to successful recovery (see Chapter 9).

Nutritional status

Nutritional deficiencies are common problems in older people in ill health. Obesity is probably the principal problem and this is often very difficult to manage. Weight reduction is often elusive in many older people. Following nutritional screening the advice of the dietician may be required (see Chapter 20A). Gross malnutrition will require correction and lesser degrees of subnutrition may be associated with reduced calorie and protein intake and vitamin deficiencies. Excess alcohol may be a contributory factor.

Drug therapy

A comprehensive assessment must include special attention to current or proposed drug therapy and the pharmacist has an important role to play in assessment, advice on adverse drug reactions and the promotion of adherence to the drug plan (see Chapter 20C). Changes in drug therapy may be appropriate as many older people are required to take large numbers of prescribed medications. Powerful drugs may be replaced by milder drugs, for example diuretics. Courses of antibiotics should not be unduly prolonged. Sedatives and hypnotics should be kept to a minimum and cardioactive drugs should be rationalised whenever possible. Additional drugs may be indicated for the acute illness or other underlying problems, for example treatment of heart failure or arthritis.

Older people are more susceptible to the unwanted effects of drugs than their younger counterparts and older people are frequently admitted to hospital as the result of side-effects of prescribed drugs. Adverse drug reactions are often produced, particularly by diuretics, pyschotrophic agents, digoxin, non-steroidal anti-inflammatory drugs and anti-Parkinson's medication. Any sudden change in functional status should lead to a close scrutiny of current drug therapy. Careful rationalisation of the patient's drug regimen is a major part of effective rehabilitation and simple rules for prescribing are as follows:

- Is a drug required at all?
- Is the choice of drug correct?
- Is the dosage correct?
- What are the potential adverse drug reactions?
- Do they outweigh any possible benefits?

All non-essential drugs should be discontinued. In the run up to discharge from hospital the irreducible number of drugs should be determined, and patient ability to self-medicate should be assessed and improved where necessary. Aids to adherence may be indicated, for example dosette boxes.

Functional assessment

The premorbid functional activity of the patient is best assessed by the appropriate rehabilitation therapists (see Chapters 15, 16 and 17) and fed back to the team for discussion.

Social and environmental factors

Assessment of the patient's social and environmental circumstances will be undertaken by the social worker (see Chapter 19) and/or the ward nurse (Chapter 14) and occupational therapist (Chapter 16), depending on local arrangements and ease of access. This should include the view of carers who will be increasingly key to implementation of ongoing rehabilitation (see Chapter 12).

Goal setting

Once all the numerous aspects of the patient's problems are to hand, the relevant team member will need to facilitate a way forward to which all parties, particularly the patient and carer(s), are in agreement. This move away from paternalism to partnership can be a challenge to professionals who must be increasingly adept in communicating their vision, rationale and concerns to their colleagues, patient and carers, so that the eventual agreed choice is fully informed, accepted and enthusiastically implemented, audited and reviewed (see also Chapter 4).

After adequate investigation and treatment of the acute episode in hospital, a frail older person might be best managed within a rehabilitation area. The demands of acute medical wards for critical care procedures and high technology interventions can prevent adequate time being available to meet rehabilitation needs. If adequate and coordinated rehabilitation is neglected, then the avoidable result may be of a bed-fast, immobile, dependent older person who will require long-term institutional care.

BED REST

Frail, elderly people with additional acute medical conditions may require bed rest.

The issue of bed rest in rehabilitation environments is always contentious and is worthy of consideration. Bed rest is appropriate in certain circumstances (Table 13.2), but it should be actively prescribed and supervised to avoid the inevitable adverse effects of prolonged immobility.

Table 13.2 Indications for bed rest

• Fever	• Reduced conscious level	• Acute infection
• Bleeding	• Acute confusion	• Acute arthritis
• Shock	• Severe pain	• Acute myocardial infarction
• Dehydration	• Deteriorating clinical state	• Pulmonary embolism
• Vomiting/ diarrhoea	• Terminal care	• Heart failure

Prolonged, unnecessary bed rest affects muscle strength, joint contractures and balance, can cause pressure sores and may induce a natural reluctance to get out of bed. This must be managed firmly but sympathetically, the team using the experience to improve practice and prevent recurrence where possible.

INTEGRATION

In recent years geriatric medicine has become increasingly integrated with acute care. This can reduce the available time of the geriatrician to elderly rehabilitation and long-term care patients. Increasing demands on geriatric medicine to manage patients within acute care, and those attending A&E departments, in addition to the need for faster throughput of patients, causes conflicting pressures on the service and patients may be discharged from acute to community care without full consultation with the team. This results not only in lost rehabilitation opportunity but also the frustration of team members, carers, other agencies involved and the increasingly assertive patients themselves when they are discharged without having had the benefit of a full, coordinated, interdisciplinary assessment and treatment plan to meet their needs. Doctors and therapists in particular will receive immediate feedback from their community colleagues on such ill-prepared discharges, reducing the reputation of the unit.

Rehabilitation

Rehabilitation is an integral part of the work of geriatricians, neurologists, stroke physicians and other specialists dealing with acute and chronic medical conditions, and the Audit Commission (2000) emphasises that rehabilitation services require the close involvement of geriatricians. General practitioners and the primary care team are applying the principles of rehabilitation to the disabled patient at home and with laboratory facilities available are able to access appropriate investigations. If the primary care team is supported by appropriate nurses and therapists, then a family doctor with suitable training and experience in rehabilitation can ensure key worker coordination of a home-based programme when hospital admission is unnecessary, nearly complete or the patient chooses to remain at home (see also Chapter 11).

Rehabilitation after acute illness, surgery or injury follows a journey of care. The aim is to restore optimal function (see Table 13.3).

Older people often require longer than younger people to recover from acute illness, e.g. acute infection or head injury, and this principle should be recognized by the rehabilitation team to avoid undue pessimism about progress.

Limitations of rehabilitation

Table 13.3 Rehabilitation after acute illness

•   Treatment of acute event
•   Prevention of complications of event or treatment
•   Physical rehabilitation
•   Provision of aids to daily living
•   Resettlement

The limitations of rehabilitation must be recognised by the rehabilitation team, older people themselves and their carers (Table 13.4). The most obvious are those of persistent severe physical disability and mental impairment.

The original illness may progress, or intercurrent illness may supervene, for example, pneumonia or stroke. A sudden or more often gradual setback in progress towards functional recovery may suggest a new impairment, e.g. silent myocardial infarction or the development of depression. Setbacks may be precipitated or aggravated by inappropriate medication or adverse drug reactions.

The patient's motivation may be difficult to assess and may be adversely affected by staff–patient interrelationships. An institutionalised patient may feel that it is pointless to co-operate with the rehabilitation team, especially if the severity of the disability has been overemphasised and the likelihood of recovery played down or ignored. Diminished self-esteem may adversely prejudice the potential for the achievement of independence.

Table 13.4 Limitations to rehabilitation

* Severe physical disability
* Gross sensory deficit, e.g. visual impairment
* Dementia
* Depression
* Learning disorder
* Poor motivation
* Loss of confidence
* Intercurrent illness
* Inappropriate medication
* Inadequate rehabilitation resources

COORDINATION AND LEADERSHIP

Rehabilitation is a continuous, multi-faceted process and requires multiple inputs and skills (Squires, 1994). These are rarely available in one professional and the interdisciplinary team approach is required. There is therefore a need for careful coordination of services, organisation and communication.

The hospital consultant generally ensures coordination of the work of the rehabilitation team in secondary care settings, for example hospital wards and at the day hospital, increasingly through a key worker. In future, responsibility for coordination may pass to a nurse or therapy consultant (Department of Health, [DoH] 2000) in appropriate situations.

Usually, but not always, the consultant has overall responsibility for the leadership of the rehabilitation team, that is the facilitation of a culture conducive to the objectives of the team. Leadership and management style will influence participation of team members at meetings/ward rounds and the appropriateness of subsequent goal setting and care management to meet the patients' needs.

The new personal responsibility of all clinical staff for clinical governance (CG) (DoH, 1998) requires each member to ensure that interventions carried out are appropriate, of a suitable standard and follow best practice. Coordination of clinical governance for a team may rest with the CG lead, or team leader. The coordinator will facilitate clinical audit and research activity and take an overview of the service development in the area, for example:

* audit activity
* ensure local guidelines and care pathways
* research activity and implementation of research findings into clinical practice
* performance issues for good practice (Health Advisory Service standards, British Geriatrics Society/Inter-collegiate standards, local standards)
* Governance issues, e.g. Clinical Risk Management; Critical Incident Analysis
* outcome measures.

In hospitals there are continuing and accelerating pressures to reduce the length of inpatient stay, but clearly *successful* earlier discharge from hospital can only be achieved if patients can manage to function in their own homes or supported accommodation. Focused and timely rehabilitation is of crucial importance and will reduce unnecessary residential and nursing home placements (Millard, 1999). The value of rehabilitation is increasingly being recognised and many systematic reviews show evidence of positive clinical effectiveness (Table 13.5), but others present equivocal or negative results (Nocon and Baldwin, 1998).

Systematic reviews support the evidence base for rehabilitation successes in comprehensive geriatric assessment, stroke and cardiac disease in older patients. Equivocal results have been observed in rehabilitation after femoral neck fractures and simple, single interventions in various conditions (Sinclair and Dickinson, 1998).

Table 13.5 Evidence of positive clinical effectiveness of rehabilitation

Problems	Diagnoses	Client groups
Back pain	Stroke	Frail older people
Incontinence	Coronary heart disease	Surgical patients
	Chronic respiratory disease	Patients with mental health problems
	Diabetes mellitus	

(Sinclair and Dickinson, 1998)

Stroke is due to vascular pathology, mostly cerebral infarction, and is the third most common cause of death in the developed world. Ten per cent of those with ischaemic stroke die within 30 days of onset and of the survivors 50 per cent will have some degree of disability after six months. Recently published National Clinical Guidelines for Stroke (Rudd *et al.*, 2000) form a useful basis for the management of Susan Hunter.

CASE STUDY SUSAN HUNTER – PHYSICIAN'S NOTES

Case history: Susan Hunter (D.O.B. 13.8.19)

Acute Left Hemiplegia

Organised stroke care has been shown to be effective and patients fare better when they are managed by experts in a facility responsive to their complex needs (Langhorne *et al.*, 1993). Lives are saved and disability is reduced and this effect may be sustained (Indredavik *et al.*, 1997). These beneficial effects are at least partly due to rehabilitation, as more rehabilitation is sometimes associated with better functional outcomes (Langhorne *et al.*, 1996). Stroke rehabilitation is often described as a 'black box' intervention because the content of the process is often not clearly defined. The package of care is complex and provided by an inter-disciplinary team (Young, 1996) (Table 13.6).

Table 13.6 Elements of stroke rehabilitation

- Information provision
- Counselling
- Exercise therapy
- Personal care therapy
- Swallowing therapy
- Speech and language therapy
- Leisure therapy
- Mood modification
- Secondary prevention

Acute medical care

Susan Hunter should be admitted directly to a stroke unit and managed by an interdisciplinary team of stroke specialists. This organised stroke service should comprise inter-disciplinary care, involvement of family and carers in the rehabilitation process, and education of staff, patients and carers (Stroke Unit Trialists' Collaboration, 1997).

Acute medical assessment usually confirms the clinical diagnosis of stroke and brain imaging should be performed to detect intracerebral or subarachnoid haemorrhage or exclude other causes of stroke syndrome, e.g. tumour. Brain imaging, e.g. CT scan, should be performed within 48 hours of the onset but should be performed urgently if head trauma is suspected or if there is a clinical deterioration in the patient's condition.

Susan Hunter's comorbid impairments should be assessed and particular attention should be paid to her diabetic control (blood sugar levels and Hb A1C) and her known hypothyroidism (serum TSH level).

Acute medical treatment

Special supportive care, including airway protection, should be implemented if her conscious level is reduced. Bed rest should be maintained in accordance with the criteria described in Table 13.2. Pyrexia, hyperglycaemia and dehydration should be corrected. Aspirin should be prescribed as soon as possible if cerebral haemorrhage has been excluded, anticoagulation with Warfarin may be indicated in atrial fibrillation and thrombolytic therapy with tissue plasminogen activator (tPA) should be considered in the small number of patients who can be treated within three hours of the onset of stroke symptoms in a specialist centre.

Secondary prevention

- In the acute phase, lowering the blood pressure may aggravate ischaemic damage, but if hypertension persists for over one month it should be treated.

Tight blood pressure control in the presence of diabetes is advisable.
* Long-term anticoagulation with Warfarin is indicated if atrial fibrillation is present.
* If not on Warfarin all cerebral infarct patients should receive daily aspirin or an alternative antiplatelet agent.
* Carotid endarterectomy should be considered in patients with carotid artery area stroke and minor or absent residual disability.
* Cholesterol lowering statin agents should be considered for all stroke patients with a past history of myocardial infarction and a serum cholesterol over 5.00 mmol/litre.

Prudent advice on lifestyle modification should include:

* stopping smoking
* balanced diet with reduced salt and fat intakes
* moderation of alcohol intake
* weight reduction in morbid obesity
* physical exercise if possible.

Physical rehabilitation

Appropriate therapists should be involved at the earliest phase of the stroke illness. Any of the current exercise therapies practised within a neurological framework will improve function (Rudd et al., 2000) If Susan Hunter has symptomatic spasticity in her arm she may obtain benefit from anti-spastic agents combined with her physical treatments. Botulinum toxin may provide symptomatic relief and functional improvement (Rudd et al., 2000).

Susan Hunter has three identifiable barriers to recovery, i.e. low mood, probable osteoarthritis of her right knee and persistent urinary incontinence. Her low mood, loss of appetite and weight loss may relate to her recent bereavement and she might respond to antidepressant drugs. Her knee pain could respond to analgesics or non-steroidal anti-inflammatory drugs, orthotic management and/or physiotherapy. The urinary incontinence merits further investigation including urodynamic screening (see also Chapter 20d), although it may be irremediable as the result of the extensive anterior circulation infarction.

Close supervision of her drug regimen is important as she may require a combination of the following: thyroxine, analgesics, antidepressants, antihypertensives, anticoagulants, antiplatelets, cholesterol lowering agents and oral antidiabetic agents.

SUMMARY

There is widespread agreement that rehabilitation for older people is clinically effective, but there is growing concern that an erosion of rehabilitation facilities in acute care hospitals may not be compensated by adequately funded, developed and coordinated services in the community at large (Young *et al.*, 1998) (see also Chapters 2 and 10). Rehabilitation is a crucial element in the journey of care of elderly ill people and restoration of health and function should be the principal objectives of the health-care team.

REFERENCES

Audit Commission (2000) *The Way To Go Home. Rehabilitation and Remedial Services for Older People*, Audit Commision, Abingdon.

Department of Health [DoH] (1998) *A First Class Service*, The Stationery Office, London.

DoH (2000) *NHS Plan*, The Stationery Office, London.

Indredavik, B., Slordahl, S.A., Bakke, F., Rokseth, R. and Haheim, L.L. (1997) Stroke unit treatment: long term effects. *Stroke*, **28**, 1861–1866.

Langhorne, P., Williams, B.O., Gilchrist, W. and Howie, K. (1993) Do stroke units save lives? *Lancet*, **342**, 395–398.

Langhorne, P., Wagenaar, R. and Partridge, C. (1996) Physiotherapy after stroke: more is better? *Physiotherapy Research International*, **1**, 75–88.

Millard, P. (1999) *Nursing Home Placements for older people in England and Wales. A national audit 1995–1998*, Department of Geriatric Medicine, St. George's Hospital Medical School, London.

Nocon, A. and Baldwin, S. (1998) *Trends in Rehabilitation Policy*, The King's Fund, London.

Rudd, A.G., Wade, D. and Irwin, P (2000) The national clinical guidelines for stroke. *Journal of the Royal College of Physicians of London*, **34**, 131–133.

Sinclair, A. and Dickinson, E. (1998) *Effective Practice in Rehabilitation*, The King's Fund, London.

Stroke Unit Trialists' Collaboration (1997) Collaborative systematic review of the randomized trials of organised inpatient (Stroke Unit) care after stroke. *British Medical Journal*, **314**, 1151–1159.

Young, J. (1996) Rehabilitation and older people. *British Medical Journal*, **313**, 677–681.

Young, J., Robinson, J. and Dickinson, E. (1998) Rehabilitation for older people. At risk in the new NHS. *British Medical Journal*, **316**, 1108–1109.

14 THE NURSING ROLE

Ronnie McGovern

The major goal of rehabilitation is to enable individuals to achieve and maintain a maximal level of function and independence. Attaining that goal depends on the participation of many members of the rehabilitation team, including the client, significant others, and various professionals. The nurse is essential to that team.

(Association of Rehabilitation Nurses, 1996)

AIMS OF THE CHAPTER

The nursing profession makes up the largest group of professionals involved in health care both in the community and hospitals. This chapter discusses the development of nurse skills in the field of rehabilitation along with nursing models of care delivery. The nurse in hospital provides 24-hour care during which they are expected to continue the patients' planned intervention programme. They have to develop their skills in all areas of rehabilitation, while maintaining their own significant role in specialist areas of tissue viability, pain management and facilitating team communication. The role of the nurse in the care planning for the case study is reviewed.

The role of nursing in differing fields is still widely debated, none more so than in the fields of rehabilitation and elderly care. According to the latest government data, there are 300,000 nurses and 150,000 health-care assistants employed in the NHS across all specialities in both hospital and community services (Department of Health [DoH], 2000). When most people consider the nursing role in rehabilitation, the perception is that it still occurs only in hospitals. The reality is that, while this is possibly where traditionally the greatest concentration of nurses exists, the wider community settings available have a great deal to offer. Therapists are moving out into the community as patients stay for a shorter time in hospital. Community nursing also needs to develop service delivery patterns over 24-hour periods to support this move. This chapter will consider the role nursing plays in these areas.

THE ROLE OF NURSING

The unique function of the nurse is to assist the individual, sick or well, in the performance of those activities contributing to health or its recovery (or to a peaceful death) that he would perform unaided if he had the necessary strength, will or knowledge. And to do this in such a way as to help him gain independence as rapidly as possible.

(Henderson, 1969)

Henderson's definition of nursing clearly identifies the key rehabilitation aims and the role of nursing to be those of assisting the individual to be as independent as possible. Thirty years after this was written, perhaps now should be added 'assisting *where necessary*'. Henderson has been identified with the term 'basic nursing care' and much debate has surrounded these three simple, yet professionally binding words. Central to this debate is that to 'care' for a patient or client has negative connotations in rehabilitation theory. It infers nurses doing things for and to the patient. This is opposed to the central theme of nurses enabling and empowering the patient to care for themselves as far as possible. Williams (1993) indicates that the term 'basic nursing care' has maligned the nursing profession as 'essential nursing is what we practice'.

The uniqueness of nursing practice has to be in the holistic approach, which encompasses care provided from essential nursing care, through facilitation and enablement within rehabilitation, to teaching and health promotion for patients and their carers. Nursing is the profession that will be available to the patient throughout the 24 hours in a day. While other professions have developed specialist roles (many originally from nursing, for example, physiotherapy), nursing retains the key role in overseeing the continuing practice of new/revised functional skills, specialist areas of tissue viability and pain management, and facilitating team communication. The nurse has the pivotal role in ensuring that the appropriate screening tests are carried out and alerting specialist staff when more detailed problem analysis is required.

THE NURSING ROLE IN REHABILITATION

A King's Fund (1998) report has identified that the primary objective of rehabilitation involves restoration (to the maximum degree possible) either of function (physical or mental) or of role (within the family, social network or workforce). Wade (2000) considered that nurses working with the older person had difficulty in defining their role. Nurses may feel threatened by the greater role clarity of other professionals in the team.

Young *et al.* (1999) found the International Classification of Impairment, Disability and Handicap (ICIDH-2) (World Health Organisation, 1999) (see Chapters 4 and 8) to be of value in helping nurses to find the balance between disease modification and maximising independence. Anecdotal evidence, from discussion with groups of nurses involved in rehabilitation, indicates that we as a profession target the 'disability' (activity) aspects and generally do very well in this regard, but do not do so well in dealing with 'handicap' (participation). The author suggests that this is strongly linked to the concepts of 'basic nursing care' because that is what we know and have understood as our role. This parternalistic rather than facilitatory approach may be ascribed to past experience of a medically dominated approach to hospital based rehabilitation (Young *et al.*, 1999), but like the majority of other professions, nursing is moving to psycho-social and more autonomous models of care.

Today, the core feature of rehabilitative nursing practice is in re-enabling the older person (and families and carers) to adjust to changes brought about by injury or disease processes (Royal College of Nursing [RCN], 2000), focusing on what the patient can and has the ability to do.

The RCN Rehabilitation Nursing Forum Philosophy (1994) states that rehabilitation nurses believe that:

- they should be building on their knowledge base and participating in research relevant to rehabilitation
- rehabilitation should commence at the onset of illness
- an interdisciplinary approach is essential if rehabilitation based on goal planning is to achieve the best outcome for the client and family
- effectiveness and continuity in rehabilitation can only be achieved through the provision of a 24-hour/7-days-a-week interdisciplinary service
- clients are people with individual personalities and needs, who have a role to play in educating nurses and other professionals in rehabilitation
- communication is vital to the rehabilitation process
- clients have a right to privacy, dignity and a right to say 'no'
- recreation, leisure and social interaction are important aspects of rehabilitation
- clients are entitled to have a high standard of care from a named registered nurse and named therapists
- a framework is needed to assess, plan and evaluate care, which should be developed in partnership with the client and family
- a health promotion focus is necessary to enable them to concentrate on health and wellness rather than disability and illness
- education should be ongoing and must cater for the specialist needs of rehabilitation for staff, clients and relatives.

This is a good base for nursing practice and can be shared by all members of the team.

KEY THEMES IN REHABILITATION NURSING

Historically the role of nursing in 'geriatrics' is closely interlinked to that of geriatric medicine. Nolan *et al.* (1997) claim that nursing became a series of tasks that other professionals did not want as part of their roles. They then cite Evers (1991) who indicated that this led to patients being subjected to 'aimless residual care'. This would occur in units where there is lack of focus on the patient and where roles and boundaries are considered more important.

In exemplar units where everyone knows their contribution, there is no competition, appropriate overlaps and cover exist, and there is clear communication between different groups. This aimlessness of care is absent and replaced by patient focused team work (see Chapter 7). Themes in the rehabilitation nurse's role in such situations have been suggested by Smith (1999) as:

- technical expert and provider of holistic nursing care
- psychological support

- educator of patients and carers and other team members
- coordinator of patient's care plan
- team worker
- evaluator of the care plan
- communicator with all members of the team – patient, relatives, carers.

Waters (1996) categorised the role of rehabilitation nursing as falling into three areas:

- General Maintenance Work
- Specialist Functions, and a
- Carry-on Role.

General Maintenance Work was the term given to 'basic nursing care', such as enabling the patient in areas such personal hygiene, oral hygiene, eating and drinking, and including the environment and atmosphere within the ward or home. Specialist Functions were the often-critical areas of continence promotion and the prevention, detection and treatment of pressure damage. The Carry-on Role was indicative of the 24-hour-a-day/7-days-a-week unique role of nursing when nurses assume or take on support roles of other team members. This role is about supervising the continuing practice of what the patients have been taught by other disciplines. Patients can only be re-educated by practising new patterns and techniques until they become familiar.

It is essential, in any rehabilitation setting, that good communication systems are in operation for 24 hours a day, 365 days per year (or all working hours). Rehabilitation interventions are the responsibility of all staff working with the patient. Specialist staff will provide specialist interventions within their professional and legal remit (for example nursing, physiotherapy, occupational therapy, chiropody), and all members of the team will carry out the routine practice of different skills and endurance activities, maintaining continuity of progress, on aspects for which they have been trained.

Where changes in movement patterns, behaviour and function have been advised, only practice throughout the day will enable a relearning and incorporation into normal activity. The nurse in rehabilitation of older people has a key role in monitoring the changes in the patient's functional activity over the 24-hour period.

The British Geriatrics Society [BGS] and RCN (1975) considered that 'remedial therapy' was an integral part of the patient's day and should not be sporadic in nature. They also recognised that the nurse was uniquely placed to continue the rehabilitation process for that part of the day when no therapists were available. In 1987 Waters considered 'that part of the day' to be 'about twenty-three-and-a-half hours for five days a week and twenty-four hours at weekends'.

Sadly, nothing seems to have altered 15 years later to fund therapists to provide care beyond their core hours, although there will always be exceptions. Changing the perception that rehabilitation is only occurring when the patient 'is being treated' is a key task for rehabilitative nursing.

The RCN (1997) highlight five nursing functions, which are essential in re-enabling the older person. These are Supportive, Restorative, Educative, Life-enhancing and Team functions:

Supportive functions include psychological, emotional and social support. Adaptation to change and empowerment. This will also include nursing practices in relation to the rehabilitation of elderly people from ethnic minorities, which can play a major part in individualised re-enablement care packages (see Chapter 3).

Restorative functions are primarily focused on improving functional ability and independence such as in washing and dressing. It also includes improving the patients' quality of life and preventing any loss of functional ability.

Educative functions of the nursing role are not just geared towards the patient or carers but to other professionals within the team. The promotion of continence, self-medication and health issues, such as smoking, diet and alcohol, all fall within the nursing remit supported by others in the team.

Life-enhancing functions include pain management and appropriate diet and fluid intake. Despite many older people having potentially painful conditions they have been found to under-report pain.

Team functions include the management of the ward or home environment. It also includes the key features of communication and coordination described in the named nurse role below.

REHABILITATION NURSING MODELS

Models of nursing are the framework of nursing practice and provide a systematic basis for applying the nursing process of assessing, planning, implementing and evaluating nursing care (Gale and Gaylard, 1996). The models indicated below all fit with the interdisciplinary assessment required by the rehabilitative process.

Orem (1985) sees a person as a 'functional, integrated whole with an overall motivation to achieve self care'. Nursing intervention is seen as becoming necessary when the individual or carer is unable to achieve the self care required as a balance between what the individual is able to do and what is the present need for self care. Self-care requirements are measured against three aspects – universal self-care requisites, developmental self-care requisites and health deviation self-care demands (Redfern and Ross, 1999). According to Hoeman (1996), rehabilitation nurses find this model useful when assessing a patient's functional status in order to assist nursing requirements. She also indicates that it may be 'less useful' when the patient has problems of cognition.

Roy's model (1976) focuses on the central rehabilitation concept of adaptation. It is concerned with the ability of the individual to adapt to influences arising from within the individual (endogenous) or from without (exogenous). She identified four types of adaptation – physiological needs, self-concept, role function/mastery and inter-dependence. Easton (1999) sees this model as ideal through interventions promoting positive adaptation and coping skills.

The 'activities of daily living' model by Roper *et al.* (1996) is utilised widely in nursing, generally, it is easy to see how this particular model has become popular in rehabilitation settings. O'Connor (1996) reviewed the most common models in use in stroke units and found this to be the most widely used.

Hoeman (1996) considers this 'activities of daily living model' as 'all the things people do in everyday life on a dependence-independence continuum'.

It is therefore useful at any stage of the life cycle from the very young to the very old and allows for fluctuating changes in our abilities to meet or cope with the essentials of life. This model will be used to demonstrate the nursing role and the key themes of rehabilitation in the case study of Susan Hunter, described in Chapter 8. It covers 12 aspects and, for each, an indication of professional nursing goals will be given. It must also be remembered that certain areas of care do not clearly fall into one specific aspect, but straddle others, indeed complicating others (stroke positioning, for example, may affect pressure area care, communication, breathing, eating and drinking). This may affect professional boundaries and good interdisciplinary relationships are essential in preventing conflict. Nurses will have to work closely with many interdisciplinary partners, such as dieticians, speech and language therapists, physiotherapists, occupational therapists, medical staff, as well as Susan Hunter herself and her family when considering care needs.

It should also be remembered that truly to consider the nursing role in Susan Hunter's care would probably require an entire book and therefore only some indicators can be given. The discussions that follow do not necessarily take account of the 'carry on roles' when other interdisciplinary team members are unavailable, as previously described by Waters (1987).

A NEW STYLE OF NURSING

There are many varieties of rehabilitation units around the country, often arising from unique historical consequences. Some may be multi-functional assessment and rehabilitation wards combined, while some may strive to a single purpose, such as stroke or orthopaedic rehabilitation.

Single purpose wards, particularly in relation to stroke, are seen to offer better patient outcomes (Langhorne *et al.*, 1993). However, some studies cited by Young *et al.* (1999) indicate only 4 per cent of the patient's day is taken up with active 'hands on' therapies and this therefore cannot be the reason for better outcomes. He suggests that this is due to 'a differing approach to patient care that includes a different style of nursing, interdisciplinary teamwork, and an increasing emphasis on goal setting', i.e. a different philosophy of care.

So what is this different style of nursing? Is it that the key themes highlighted earlier are becoming more mainstream in the rehabilitation wards and that there is not just 'basic nursing care' on offer? Are nurses working more as part of the interdisciplinary team? Are we realising by helping patients on a level personal to them (the participation of the ICIDH-2) and not only in the functional aspects of care, that this actually is effective evidence based practice that really makes a difference? This is ideally what nurses in rehabilitation settings generally, and those nursing in care of the older adult settings, should be striving for. What greater place therefore to achieve truly holistic nursing practice as a key component of interdisciplinary patient care than in a care of the older adult setting? The RCN (2000) recognises that as all aspects of practice in nursing the older adult are essentially re-enablement, then regardless of where the care occurs, be it hospital or community based, the approach is rehabilitative.

Nursing itself is changing with the development of 'consultant' nurses and specialist nurse practitioners in areas such as gerontological nursing and in rehabilitation. How these roles will develop in the future remains to be seen. The development of nurse specialists in Parkinson's disease or stroke will also impact widely on nursing practice. The danger is that too many 'specialists' occur that blur roles and responsibilities with 'generic' nurses.

ORGANISATION OF NURSING CARE AND THE NAMED NURSE PROCESS

Organisation of nursing care within wards is the responsibility of the ward manager. However, the actual care is generally delegated to the 'named nurse'.

The named nurse national guidelines define a named nurse as 'A registered Nurse, Midwife or Health Visitor who is responsible for assessing, planning, implementing, evaluating and coordinating patient care on an individual basis with a patient or a caseload of patients from admission/transfer to transfer/discharge.'

The named nurse concept enables the key features of rehabilitation nursing to be realised within the interdisciplinary team. Within differing care settings the organisation of nursing care follows a variety of models. These include patient allocation, team nursing, primary nursing, key worker and caseload management. Generally, for the continuity of care required within a rehabilitation setting, some of these models may be more appropriate than others, such as primary or team nursing. This is also dependent on the environment in which it takes place, e.g. hospital or home.

Primary nursing

Gale and Gaylard (1996) highlighted this as a systematic, organisational method of managing nursing. This concept originated from Manthey (1980), who described four principles that remain true in the provision of nursing care today:

- allocation and acceptance of responsibility for decision-making to one individual
- individual assignment of daily care by case method
- direct person-to-person communication
- one person operationally responsible for the quality of care administered to patients on a unit 24 hours a day, seven days a week.

The concepts of primary nursing link strongly to those principles that guided the named nurse initiative. Wright (1993) indicates this as the 'clearest expression' of the approach, even although other approaches are recognised.

Team nursing

The Scottish Office National Guidelines on the named nurse indicates this approach where a registered nurse leads a team of nurses, planning, implementing and evaluating care, liasing and delegating care appropriately to others involved in the process of nursing.

CASE STUDY NURSING SUSAN HUNTER

Following admission on to the ward, immediate post stroke goals will be the maintenance of vital bodily functions such as breathing and in the prevention of secondary problems. This is potentially a very frightening time for both Susan Hunter and her family, and fears can often be allayed by adequate communication from the outset. It is essential that the nurse should discuss with the patient/or relatives how Susan Hunter would like to be known. Many older people still like to be called by their title and surname, and this should be respected. The role of the named nurse, and details of how to contact them (or their associate), should be clearly explained.

This case study will use the 12 activities of living described by Hoeman (1996).

1. Communicating

Communication is more than speech. It also covers other areas such as vision, hearing, reading, writing, body language, body image and advocacy. It is also more than a one-way process and this must be remembered when developing care plans.

Dependent on local procedure, nurses may be involved along with the speech and language therapist, dentist, audiologist and optometrist and in the assessment and recording of patients' premorbid and presenting communication abilities.

Consideration should also be given to Susan Hunter's position in bed and to her location in the ward generally to utilise available sight. This will also assist orientation and prevent feelings of isolation.

Advising Susan Hunter of nursing care activities before carrying them out will help prevent distress. Explanations of the nurse call systems and emergency call systems should be given to Susan Hunter as soon as possible, checking her understanding and ability to use them. If she is unable to use them, then other forms of 'calling' or frequent checking by nursing staff may have to be considered.

Pain assessment is crucial in ensuring Susan Hunter is as pain free as possible. It is, after all, *her* pain and she must play a pivotal role in its assessment and management. Failing to do this may make her begin to decline involvement in rehabilitative processes, e.g. mobilisation. Validated tools should be used for assessing pain to facilitate discussion with team members who will be involved in pain management. Despite many older people having potentially painful conditions they have been found to under-report pain (Klinger and Spaulding, 1998), and the authors recommend that assessment of pain should be undertaken routinely during clinical examination.

The role of the named nurse in liasing and communicating with Susan Hunter, her family and the interdisciplinary team is central to provision of individualised care, as has been previously described.

This will also prove vital in picking up any signs of detachment and isolation that may present, assisting in the early referral of Susan Hunter to a clinical psychologist (see Chapter 9).

On admission, Susan Hunter's fluctuating conscious level may prevent her from involvement in decisions regarding immediate care. Nursing staff will be heavily involved in any decisions, which will also involve the rest of the team including the family.

Sutor (1993) considers Fowler's four-model framework in the nursing role in advocacy (see also Chapter 4):

- guardian of patient's rights
- preserver of patient's values
- champion of social justice in relation to health provision
- protector of the patient's best interests.

As the professional providing 24-hour care, the nurse has a key role in ensuring that the patient's advocacy needs are met through the appropriate service. The Scottish Health Advisory Service (1991) document on 'Advocacy, A Guide to Good Practice' indicates key roles in two areas – advocacy alongside or on behalf of someone and advocacy by a person or group for themselves. As her condition stabilises and improves, Susan Hunter will be actively encouraged to make informed decisions in her own right.

The importance of listening skills cannot be overly stressed. Time made to listen to Susan Hunter's fears and worries, her concerns for her own and her family's future, and her hopes and aspirations is certainly time well spent (see also Chapter 17). This can often guide professionals not only in the goal setting process but also in early detection of emotional or other problems.

As she approaches discharge Susan Hunter may be anxious about the future and what it holds for her. Adequate discharge planning with the involvement of Susan Hunter, her family, and both hospital and primary care teams is vital for a successful discharge and the prevention of a possible unnecessary readmission.

2. Maintaining a safe environment

As we age, we often face a decreasing ability to carry out the roles and functions that we once performed independently. In maintaining a safe environment, consideration may have to be given to our increasing dependence on carers or to the use of aids. Acceptance of that help, or reliance on others, often depends on our personality prior to the 'event'. Other considerations such as finance may affect a safe environment.

Immediate goals include orientation of Susan Hunter to time and place. Instigation of neurological or stroke specific observation tools, as per current hospital procedures, will assist in the assessment of her fluctuating conscious level and warn of any impending problems. Early identification of Susan Hunter herself is essential in ensuring the correct patient receives the correct treatment. This is usually by nameband or photograph. If the patient was of ethnic origin then special care would be required in how names are recorded (and used) or where photography may be offensive (see Chapters 3 and 20c for pharmaceutical considerations).

The prevention of pressure damage is a primary feature in maintaining a safe environment. If pressure damage occurs, this will cause Susan Hunter undue pain and distress, as well as delaying the rehabilitation process by many weeks or months. Assessment of the risk of pressure damage should be undertaken within one hour of admission using a recognised tool such as a Waterlow or Braden Score. At the very least an appropriate pressure-relieving mattress should be available immediately from stock. The preferred option would be to have it in place awaiting Susan Hunter's admission following communication from the GP/primary care team or the transferring unit such as A&E regarding her physical and mental state. A plan of pressure damage prevention should be commenced, including positioning and turning utilising the 30-degree tilt (Preston, 1988).

Dependent on the unit's policy, consideration may be given to the use of bedrails to prevent falls from the bed, particularly during the period of disorientation. If a no bedrail policy is in operation then local arrangements for continuous supervision will be required. As Susan Hunter's condition becomes more stable the continued use of pressure relieving devices, bedrails or continuous supervision will be discussed with her and her family and relevant members of the team. Instruction in the use of nursing call systems and emergency call systems is essential at the earliest opportunity to both Susan Hunter and her family.

Medicine administration will be vital to Susan Hunter's continued progress. Nurses play a major part in this. A major concern for Susan Hunter's future care is in the taking of medicines where the consequences of the 'thought it/did it' discrepancy can be profound (see Chapter 9). It is important to emphasise that normal age changes in memory will be exaggerated by illness, distress or other difficulties. Interestingly, adherence with medication has been found not to be related to health status but to self-efficacy and the confidence in ability to successfully remember to take the medication. This confidence can be facilitated by health-care professionals, particularly nursing staff with responsibility for medication administration, through positive feedback to reinforce correct regimens. This will be considered more fully in Chapter 20C.

3. Breathing

Breathing is affected by many factors, such as physical activity, mood, emotion and also the body's reaction to illness. For the case study, the main problems in relation to breathing concern Susan Hunter's immediate post stroke management. Correct positioning in bed will assist the normal body breathing mechanisms, possibly augmented by the use of oxygen therapy. Close working with physiotherapy staff is required to maintain adequate air/oxygen intake to prevent secondary complications such as respiratory infection or postural problems. Health promotion strategies may be required if Susan Hunter was a smoker.

4. Eating and drinking

On admission, the maintenance of nutrition and fluid balance is essential. Failure to do this can cause delay in rehabilitative processes through dehydration or weakness due to malnourishment. Utilisation of a nutritional assessment chart will be paramount in this. Fluid intake will probably be maintained by intravenous access or, increasingly, by hypodermoclysis. Nutritional intake may involve nasogastric feeding until swallowing assessment can be made when Susan Hunter's conscious level and visuospatial disturbances settle.

Nursing involvement in swallowing assessment varies unit by unit. It may be a simple water test to a fuller defined swallowing assessment in conjunction with the speech and language therapist. This is covered in Chapter 16. The family can also be asked about Susan Hunter's likes and dislikes in relation to food and drink to assist feeding if required, until she is able to decide for herself. Dietetic input into ensuring effective nutritional intake is covered in Chapter 20A. Nutritional assessment tools and regular weighing will assist the development of a nutritional care plan. Proper care of teeth and dental plates is also essential in aiding eating and drinking (see also Chapter 20B). Consideration of previous weight loss and poor appetite will also have to be made. This will involve liaison with the primary care team.

Care must also be taken in relation to her hemianopia. Staff and family must be aware from admission of the importance of correct placement of food and drinks to ensure they are within Susan Hunter's visual range and reach. Awareness of whether she is right or left-handed will obviously be necessary, as this may also affect her ability to feed herself (see also Chapter 3 for issues for some minority groups on this). Explaining to Susan Hunter the problems she is encountering and re-enforcing the advice given by specialist members of the team will assist in her re-enablement. Liaison with the occupational therapist will particularly help to identify problems and solutions.

5. Eliminating

Details of continence assessment and incontinence management programmes are discussed in Chapter 20D. Urinary and faecal incontinence play a major role in the development of pressure sores and adequate measures must be in place to prevent this. Recognition of the prognostic indicator of continence for stroke patients and its importance in the final rehabilitative outcome, will ensure that this is a high priority area for appropriate nurse management.

6. Personal cleansing and dressing

Premorbid assessment of Susan Hunter's abilities and preferences in maintaining her personal hygiene should be undertaken as soon as possible. Nursing staff will assist with this function until Susan Hunter is able, or until a personal cleansing and dressing assessment is made by the occupational therapists. Dependent on local arrangements, responsibility for personal cleansing re-enablement may be a nursing role while dressing practice could be an occupational therapy function. Ensuring that enabled skills are maintained at every opportunity during the 24 hours would generally fall to nursing staff.

7. Controlling body temperature

In the older adult the control of body temperature may be influenced by differing factors. These can include the time of day, nutritional intake, exercise or lack of it, clothing, environmental issues such as open windows, the ability to pay for heating, or dependence on others to be aware of requirements in preventing hypothermia. Disease processes also require active consideration.

Accurate recording of Susan Hunter's temperature on admission and at designated intervals thereafter may be an indicator in the stroke disease process and in the early detection of any infections that may occur. It also assists nursing staff in ensuring her comfort by checking she is neither too hot nor too cold. As hypothyroidism can make the patient feel cold, nursing staff need to be aware of this and ensure Susan Hunter takes any prescribed medication. As her condition stabilises, Susan Hunter will be able to communicate her own preferences in relation to temperature and clothing.

Nursing input later on would include health promotion issues in relation to prevention of hypothermia.

8. Mobilising

Mobilising affects not only our ability to walk or move around but also influences other areas such as personal cleansing, eliminating, working and playing, and eating and drinking.

Nursing interventions here, guided by specialist physiotherapy and occupational therapy assessment, include proper positioning in appropriate bed and chairs. Special care will need to be taken with the co-morbidity problems of osteoarthritis in her right leg, her old right total hip replacement and changing tone patterns on her left side. Proper support will help prevent drop foot, assist in acquiring a sitting balance, prevent accidents such as falling over and provide security and comfort to Susan Hunter when she feels safe.

Local policies have to be incorporated into manual handling assessments and care plans. These policies, and in fact the Manual Handling Regulations themselves, can often seem to conflict with mobilising/transferring patients. Some Trusts have a strict no manual handling policy. This results in lifting and transferring aids being used at all times and often prevents nursing staff taking part in the 'carry on' role. It is also very dependent on the required aids being available and the need to have staff trained to use them properly. Improper assessment, use of aids or bad practice may cause damage to Susan Hunter, for example, a subluxation of her shoulder on the affected side.

Her previous medical history, including hypothyroidism and osteoarthritis, as well as pain developing in her right knee, requires to be featured in care plans. Pain assessment has already been described under 'communication'. Further discussion of mobilisation issues can be found in Chapter 15.

9. Working and playing

Much of Susan Hunter's life pre stroke centred on caring for her terminally ill husband. Carer support offered her the opportunity to keep up with local church groups and bowling. With the stroke, her lifestyle and abilities, functionally, mentally and socially, have dramatically changed.

Nurses play a vital role in the adaptation process, not just for Susan Hunter, but also for her family. Close nursing observation will indicate her mood and coping mechanisms. These may be used in deciding if early referral to a clinical psychologist (see Chapter 9) is required, not just for issues around the stroke event but also grieving for her recently deceased husband. She may first need to express her grief to someone with listening skills. Involving Susan Hunter's local clergy may be appropriate. This can be discussed with her and her family. Nursing observation will also provide information on family responses to the stroke; interactions and involvement in her care and assist in any referrals for them.

10. Expressing sexuality

This is not just about the sexual act but also about who we are as males or females and how we express that. Altered body image invariably affects the image we have of someone or indeed ourselves. Feelings of, or the fear of, rejection may ensue due to disturbed body image resulting from the stroke and if this were problematic to Susan Hunter or her family then suggest that psychology input should be requested urgently (see also Chapter 9).

11. Sleeping

The importance of sleep is still not properly understood. One theory considered by Roper *et al.* (1996) is that it is a restorative process, where sleep promotes the repair of damaged tissues. How many of us when we are feeling unwell say 'I'm going to bed, I'll feel better in the morning'?

Assessment of Susan Hunter's normal sleep pattern will assist in the individualisation of care plans and assist nursing staff in making decisions for her until she is able to do so for herself. Nursing considerations for Susan Hunter in this aspect may include hunger, thirst, pain or temperature, noise and light. Anxiety can be a major issue. Patients may worry that if they go to sleep they may not wake up again. Sleep disturbances may also act as an indicator of depression, and variances in sleep routines should be recorded and reported on.

12. Dying

Death for us all is inevitable. The circumstances of how we die with the exception of suicide is outside our control, although many nurses would tell of instances where people just 'gave up'.

Apart from grieving for her husband, Susan Hunter will probably be considering her own future, greatly dependent on her current and possible abilities. Maintaining independence of mind, body and spirit as far as possible is essential in dealing with life and death. Influences in her life such as her family, friends and church will play a great part in how she comes to terms with the death of her husband and her own mortality.

Nurses can act as sounding boards for fears and worries and in dealing with feelings of loss. They must be very aware, however, of the potential for serious psychological problems that could result from the stroke, its consequences, and also the death of her husband, and must be aware of their own limitations in this field.

SUMMARY

The central nursing role of rehabilitation nursing practice is in re-enablement, regardless of where the nursing care is practised. Using appropriate frameworks and models for practice assists in clarification of that role. The 'named nurse' process is vital in the communication and coordination of care functions, not just to other nursing staff, but also to the patient, families and carers and the interdisciplinary team.

REFERENCES

Association of Rehabilitation Nurses (1996) *The Appropriate Inclusion of Rehabilitation Nurses Wherever Rehabilitation is Provided,* Policy Statement of the ARN, London.

British Geriatrics Society and Royal College of Nursing (BGS and RCN) (1975) *Improving Geriatric Care in Hospital.* Report of a working party of the British Geriatrics Society and Royal College of Nursing of the United Kingdom.

Department of Health (2000) *The NHS Plan – A plan for investment, A plan for reform,* The Stationery Office, London.

Easton, K.L. (1999) *Gerontological Rehabilitation Nursing,* Royal College of Nursing, London; W.B. Saunders Company, Philadelphia, PA.

Evers, H.K. (1991) Care of the elderly sick in the UK. In: *New Directions in Rehabilitation: Exploring the nursing contribution,* (eds Nolan, M., Booth, A. and Nolan, J.), English National Board for Nursing, London.

Gale, A. and Gaylard, J. (1996) The role of the nurse in rehabilitation of older people. In: *Rehabilitation of Older People,* 2nd edn (ed. Squires, A.), Chapman & Hall, London.

Henderson, V. (1969) *Basic Principles of Nursing Care,* International Council of Nurses, Geneva.

Hoeman, S. (1996) Conceptual bases for rehabilitation nursing. In: *Rehabilitation Nursing: Process and application,* 2nd edn (ed. Hoeman, S.), Mosby, St Louis.

The King's Fund (1998) *Trends in Rehabilitation Policy: a review of the literature,* The King's Fund and the Audit Commission, London.

Langhorne, P., Williams, B.O., Gilchrist, W. and Howie, K. (1993) Do stroke units save lives? *Lancet,* **342,** 395–398.

Manthey, M. (1980) A theoretical framework for primary nursing. *Journal of Nursing Administration,* **10**(6), 54–56.

Nolan, M., Booth, A. and Nolan, J. (1997) *New Directions in Rehabilitation: Exploring the nursing contribution.* Researching Professional Education – research reports series No. 6, English National Board for Nursing, Midwifery and Health Visiting, London.

O'Connor, S. (1996) Stroke units: centres of nursing innovation. *British Journal of Nursing,* **5,** 105–109.

Orem, D. (1985) Nursing – *Concepts of Practice,* 2nd edn, McGraw Hill, New York.

Preston, K.W. (1988) Positioning for comfort and pressure relief – the 30° alternative. *Care Science and Practice,* **6**(4), 116–119.

Royal College of Nursing [RCN] (1994) Rehabilitation Nursing Forum Philosophy. In: *Standards of Care for Rehabilitation Nursing*, Royal College of Nursing, London.

RCN (1997) *What a Difference a Nurse Makes*. An RCN report on the benefits of expert nursing to clinical outcomes in the continuing care of older people. Royal College of Nursing, London.

RCN (2000) *Rehabilitating Older People. The role of the nurse*, RCN Forum for Nurses Working with Older People, London.

Redfern, S.J. and Ross, F.M. (1999) *Nursing Older People*, Churchill Livingstone, Edinburgh.

Roper, N., Logan, W. and Tierney, A. (1996) *The Elements of Nursing. A model for nursing based on a model of living*, 4th edn, Churchill Livingstone, Edinburgh.

Roy, C. (1976) *Introduction to Nursing: An Adaption Model*, Prentice Hall, NJ.

Scottish Health Advisory Service (1991) *Advocacy, A Guide to Good Practice*, The Scottish Office, Edinburgh.

Smith, M. (ed.) (1999) *Rehabilitation in Adult Nursing Practice*, Churchill Livingstone, Edinburgh.

Sutor, J. (1993) Can nurses be effective advocates? *Nursing Standard*, 7(22), 30–32.

Wade, S. (2000) Nursing older people: the keys to success. *Nursing Times*, **96**(2).

Waters, K.R. (1987) The role of nursing in rehabilitation. *CARE – Science and Practice*, 5(3).

Waters, K.R. (1996) Rehabilitation. In: *A Textbook of Gerontological Nursing. Perspectives on practice* (eds Wade, L. and Waters, K. R.), Baillière Tindall, London.

Williams, J. (1993) Rehabilitation challenge. *Nursing Times*, 89(31).

World Health Organisation (1999) *International Classification of Impairment, Disability and Handicap*, WCC WHO Collaborating Centre, The Netherlands.

Wright, S. (ed.) (1993) *The Named Nurse, Midwife and Health Visitor*, Department of Health, London.

Young, J., Brown, A., Forster, A. and Clare, J. (1999) An overview of rehabilitation for older people. *Reviews in Clinical Gerontology*, **9**, 183–196.

15 THE ROLE OF THE PHYSIOTHERAPIST

Suzanne Hogg

AIMS OF THE CHAPTER

This chapter describes the contribution of the physiotherapist to the inter-disciplinary team. Older people are referred to physiotherapy across a broad range of both hospital and increasingly community based health and social care settings and make up the largest group of service users. Input may be at any stage along, and frequently throughout, the continuum of rehabilitation, particularly where problem solving following accurate measurement and analysis of movement, posture and function is required. Physiotherapists and occupational therapists share skills in managing problems of function, and this chapter emphasises the need for these two disciplines to work closely together to ensure that treatment approaches are consistent, complementing and reinforcing each other and enhancing the overall therapeutic benefit to the patient without unnecessary duplication.

INTRODUCTION

The prime purpose of physiotherapy is to restore activity and independence and prevent injury and illness Chartered Society of Physiotherapists [CSP] (1999a). Physiotherapists provide a holistic multi-faceted approach to the management of a wide range of conditions. Chartered physiotherapists work primarily in the NHS, but also in occupational health, education, research and the private, independent and voluntary sectors, practising both autonomously and in collaboration with others. The emphasis of the profession is on the use of a range of physical approaches in the assessment and management of neuromuscular, musculoskeletal, cardiovascular and respiratory conditions (CSP, 1999b).

The Chartered Society of Physiotherapy (CSP) is the recognised professional and educational body for physiotherapists working in the UK and is responsible for setting professional standards of practice and defining the curriculum framework for undergraduate education. It has a strategic function in overseeing the development of the profession, particularly in response to changes within the health economy, providing, for example, a clinical effectiveness strategy that works to develop and disseminate the evidence base underpinning physiotherapy intervention. Special interest groups, such as that for working with older people (AGILE), work with the CSP to facilitate development, communication, support and research.

All chartered physiotherapists must be registered with the Council for the Profession Supplementary to Medicine (CPSM) (to be replaced by the Health Professions Council by April 2002) in order to practise in the UK NHS. According to the latest government data, there are 19,000 physiotherapists employed in the NHS across all specialities in both hospital and community services (Department of Health [DoH], 2000). Physiotherapists can take direct referrals for assessment from any member of the team, although in practice this depends on local service agreements that in the future are likely to be based upon evidence based integrated care pathways for the management of specific conditions.

PHYSIOTHERAPY SERVICES FOR OLDER PEOPLE

Physiotherapy services for older people are provided across a range of primary, secondary and, increasingly, intermediate care settings, the organisation of which will vary according to local commissioning arrangements. Simpson *et al.* (1999) refer to the fact that the percentage of initial physiotherapy contacts made by people aged 65 years or more, at almost 38 per cent, is higher than for any other age group. While much of this activity is generated within designated services for older people, the age-related incidence of falls in the elderly and conditions such as stroke, cardio-respiratory disease and fractured neck or femur, means that older people are referred to physiotherapy across a broad range of both hospital and community based health and social care settings.

For older people admitted to hospital, rehabilitation starts as part of their acute care and may continue in a specialist rehabilitation unit or within an intermediate care setting (Audit Commission, 2000), and within each of those settings physiotherapists are core members of the interdisciplinary team. While physiotherapy services are largely provided on a limited five-day basis it should be emphasised that rehabilitation is best supported by a twenty-four-hour team approach (see Chapters 7 and 14). It is a stated ambition of the NHS Plan (DoH, 2000) to increase the number of physiotherapists; in the interim efficiencies can be achieved by effective use of team goal setting and care planning following assessment.

In the community, physiotherapists work in patients' own homes, nursing homes and residential care, in day hospital and in other day care settings. Historically, funding for and availability of therapy services, given the additional costs of providing a community based service (see also Chapter 10), made this a scarce resource, the use of which has not always been equitable. For example, a survey carried out by the CSP found inequality of access and under-resourcing of physiotherapy provision to older people who were resident in nursing homes, despite the benefits that physiotherapists can achieve in minimising levels of dependency and preventing hospital admission for nursing home populations (Johnstone *et al.*, 1993). In addition the Clinical Standards Advisory Group report (CSAG, 1998) identified 'patchy provision' of rehabilitation including community physiotherapy, a view supported by Dickinson and Sinclair (1998) and the Audit Commission (1997).

In 'The Way to Go Home' (2000) the Audit Commission concluded that investment in preventative and rehabilitation services, including physiotherapy, could reduce the number of unplanned admissions and inappropriate admission into long-term residential care. These findings, together with pressure to reduce the length of acute hospital stay, have already been drivers for the increasing provision of intermediate care and community based rehabilitation services based upon innovative models of integrated service delivery, in which physiotherapy plays a significant part.

Guidance for the further development of intermediate care issued by the DoH (2001) has been built upon in the National Service Framework for Older People (see Chapter 6) and both documents support the delivery of rehabilitation services within a range of community based health and social care environments that should complement specialist provision within secondary care.

PHYSIOTHERAPY WITHIN THE REHABILITATION PROCESS

Rehabilitation must be viewed along a continuum, from prevention; early stage (impairment) management; to the ongoing continuing management of patients with chronic, residual disability (Edwards, 1996). There is evidence to support the role of the physiotherapist within an interdisciplinary team for the assessment and rehabilitation of older people (Dickinson and Sinclair, 1998) and physiotherapy intervention may be indicated at any point along that continuum.

Young and Dinan (1994) describe the relationship between physical function and disability in terms of a critical threshold beyond which independence is compromised. If the key aim of rehabilitation is to enable the individual concerned to regain, as far as is possible, independence that has been lost as a result of illness or injury (Robinson and Turnock, 1998), then the management of physical function is central to that process. Edwards (1996) and Ward and McIntosh (1993) suggest that management of disordered movement and function is a key physiotherapy skill, based on problem solving, is goal directed and reliant on the accurate measurement and analysis of movement, posture and function. The ability of the physiotherapist as problem solver in this context is dependent upon an accurate and extensive knowledge of movement.

INDICATORS FOR PHYSIOTHERAPY INTERVENTION

Physiotherapists are the movement specialists within the rehabilitation team, their key role being to identify and address impairments responsible for disorders in movement and balance and to manage the consequences of residual impairments, in order to increase activity and participation (ICIDH–2, 1999). This involves the use of strategies aimed at prevention, restoration and maintenance.

Physiotherapy may be indicated in the following situations:

- assessment as part of an interdisciplinary diagnostic process to determine rehabilitation and/or long-term care needs in both health and social care settings
- prevention of unnecessary hospital admission and support of early discharge where movement impairment has resulted following acute medical problems
- rehabilitation of conditions that directly impact on mobility, for example stroke

- primary and secondary prevention of falls
- management of dependency in older people with progressive conditions or residual disability.

Where there is a defined need for rehabilitation then the need for a physiotherapy contribution may be clear; however referral patterns may reflect the experiences and perceptions of other members of the interdisciplinary team, as well as patients and carers themselves (Partridge *et al.*, 1991, Age Concern, 1999) (see also Chapters 5 and 7). A key role of the physiotherapist is to be aware of the evidence base that supports the effectiveness of intervention and to use that evidence base to inform the commissioning of, access to and provision of physiotherapy services.

Referral processes are determined at service level and will be defined by clinical setting. Many inpatient teams working in acute or rehabilitation services work to a collective system screening all new admissions for assessment, highlighted as best practice in the NHS Plan (DoH, 2000). The implementation of a single assessment process for older people (DoH, 2001) will necessitate robust triggers to be agreed for specialist assessments including community based physiotherapy services. Given the functions of intermediate care in preventing inappropriate hospital admission and supporting early discharge, the model of physiotherapy provision within acute environments must increasingly focus on assessment as part of an inter-disciplinary diagnostic care and transfer of care planning process. Within this process, rehabilitation needs are identified and recommendations made as to how/where those needs might best be met.

Standards for response to referral will also reflect the clinical setting and in particular are dependent on length of stay. The average length of stay in hospital (acute) fell from 12.7 to 7.8 days for people aged 65–74 and from 17.4 to 10.2 days for the over 75s in the period 1983–1998 (CSAG, 1998). Outside of emergency weekend work (typically for acute respiratory cases only), most physiotherapy services are funded for provision over a five-day week, thus necessitating prioritisation of resources to enable timely assessment and intervention of other acute admissions.

PHYSIOTHERAPY ASSESSMENT

As movement specialists, physiotherapists have particular skills in analysing the impact of impairments within the neurological and musculoskeletal systems, in particular on movement function. Given the complex needs of the older patient, physiotherapy assessment is guided by other physical, social, psychological and environmental factors, and in particular by the subjective history from the patient.

As part of the assessment process the following questions are addressed:

- How has the patient been moving up until now?
- What was the problem that prompted referral?

- What factors will influence goal setting and the subsequent outcome for the patient?
- What are the patient's and carer's expectations of treatment?

In order to answer those questions the following information about the patient is obtained from the patient, the patient's main carers and the patient's clinical record:

- previous level of physical, cognitive and psycho-social function
- social history including environment, information about formal and informal support networks, how adequate that level of support was and whether it is sustainable
- medical history, including diagnosis, medical stability and past history
- medication history
- cognitive function
- communication skills and special senses (see also Chapter 6).

Information sharing between professionals and health and social care agencies is facilitated by the use of a single multi-professional record, thus reducing duplication in those domains common to several members of the team.

Physiotherapists have a key role to play in the assessment of handling risk; where other members of the health-care team have commenced this process, then this information must be accessed prior to examining the patient. Other risk assessments, e.g. skin integrity, may influence treatment planning including, for example, the provision of special seating or resolving problems with footwear (see also Chapter 18).

Assessing physical function

The relationship between physical performance and functional ability is well documented (Young and Dinan, 1994; Gill *et al.*, 1996; Spirduso, 1996). Assessment of physical function aims to quantify the inter-relationship between ageing, disease processes and problems relating to function: physiotherapy assessment of movement must therefore incorporate measures both of impairment and activity. Handford and Jones (1993) suggest a framework for physiotherapy assessment in Parkinson's disease (see Figure 15.1) that describes how this relationship informs the treatment plan:

Assessment of physical function encompasses all aspects of motor control; central to the physiotherapy assessment process are postural stability and movement including the musculoskeletal system, such as posture, joint ranges and soft tissue extensibility, muscle strength and coordination.

The musculoskeletal system is one of the major systems contributing to postural stability and muscle weakness is recognised as a factor contributing to physical decline and falls risk in the elderly (Tinetti *et al.*, 1988; Simpson and Forster, 1993; Fiatarone *et al.*, 1994). Assessment will be guided by subjective history and should include objective measures of joint range and muscle strength.

The ability of an individual to balance underlies the performance of most physical activities (Berg *et al.*, 1989). Hu and Woolacott (1996) describe balance as 'maintaining the centre of gravity over the base of support in response to changing tasks and environmental conditions'. The following is an overview of some of the objective measures of balance thought to be relevant, particularly in the assessment of older people who have fallen (CSP, 2001).

* **Timed unsupported stand:** described by Simpson and Worsfold (1996), this is a test that is easy to carry out, and accommodates levels of frailty associated with acute illness and long-term disability. The authors report that the ability to stand unsupported is a prerequisite for the satisfactory performance of many functional activities, citing Studenski *et al.* (1994) in describing the link between the inability to stand unsupported and increased fall risk. In establishing parameters for the test it was concluded that it was only necessary to time for one minute, as those subjects able to stand for one minute could do so for three minutes or longer.

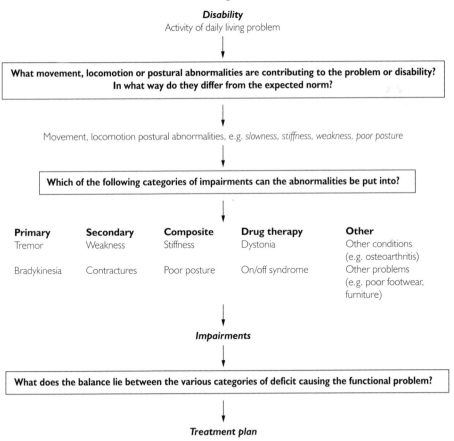

Figure 15.1 The assessment of Parkinson's patients
(Parkinson's Disease Society, 1997)

- **Functional reach:** functional reach (FR) represents the maximal distance an individual can reach forward beyond arms' length while maintaining a fixed base of support in the standing position (Duncan *et al.*, 1990). It has reported predictive value for fall risk (Duncan *et al.*, 1992) and sensitivity to change over time (Weiner *et al.*, 1992). It is easy to perform and accommodates a wide range of physical performance, although it presupposes an ability to stand. Weiner *et al.* (1992) also describe FR as a marker of physical frailty.
- **Timed gait:** the relationship between walking speed and balance has been well documented (Simpson and Worsfold, 1996; Willems and Vandervoort, 1996). Gait speed of less than 0.45 to 0.53m/sec has been reported to be predictive of falls risk (Willems and Vandervoort, 1996), although the same authors caution the use of timed gait as a substitute for other balance measures.
- **Get up and go:** while not in itself predictive of fall risk, this measure is an indicator of the need to complete further investigation of postural instability (Mathias *et al.*, 1986). The subject is instructed to get up from a standard height chair without arms, walk a distance of 3 m, turn around and return to sit in the chair. Observation of difficulty or unsteadiness suggests the need to carry out additional assessment.
- **Berg Balance Scale:** this is an ordinal scale, which rates the ability of the individual to balance while performing 14 movements required in everyday activities (Berg *et al.*, 1989). This is a well-validated tool, reported to have a strong association with gait speed (Willems and Vandervoort, 1996) and, in combination with self-report history of imbalance, to be predictive of fall risk (Shumway-Cook *et al.*, 1997).
- **Performance Orientated Assessment of Mobility:** an assessment of balance (static, dynamic, functional and in response to external displacement) and gait (Tinetti, 1986). The balance subscale is again predictive of falls risk in community dwelling elderly (Arnadottir and Mercer, 1999), although the same authors report a ceiling effect when the complete tool is used with that population.

Functional mobility

While assessment of general function is not the sole domain of the physiotherapist, the physiotherapist has particular skills in analysing disorders of movement and contributing to the identification of probable causes of general functional disability.

Within rehabilitation settings there are probably three key but different purposes to recording functional ability:

- as a baseline of performance in the activities of daily living against which outcome can be measured
- to analyse the impairments underlying physical disability
- as a determinant of long-term care needs.

The physiotherapist's concern with movement necessitates an emphasis on motor skills, and functional assessment of such should include balance, ability to transfer and mobility. The aim is to record both an objective and qualitative assessment of mobility based upon a combination of observation, measurement and the use of handling skills.

Functional ability in the frail elderly is strongly influenced by environment, and assessment within hospital or other clinical settings can be misleading. An obvious example is the patient with a combination of visual and balance difficulties who may mobilise more safely within the familiarity of his or her home. Where mobility needs are complex and/or compromised by other functional disorders, a home visit in conjunction with the occupational therapist may be necessary; routinely, however, effective communication between therapists regarding any particular handling or mobility needs will inform a single discipline home assessment process for individual patients.

Evaluating outcome

Assessment scales provide a record of baseline performance against which change over time can be detected and may demonstrate predictive value in outcome and risk relating to functional ability. There is consensus (Massie, 1993; Simpson and Forster, 1993) that the use of relevant validated tools is preferable to the development of local measures.

The Elderly Mobility Scale (EMS) (Table 15.1 overleaf) is a standardised validated measure of locomotion, balance and the key position changes, which are prerequisites to more complex activities of daily living (Smith, 1994). It was further validated by Posser and Canby (1997) and found to be sensitive to change but not predictive of either falls or discharge destination. Both studies demonstrated significant correlation between the EMS and Barthel Index (see also Chapter 8).

The Barthel Index is the measure of physical function recommended for use in elderly medicine by the Royal College of Physicians and the British Geriatrics Society (1992). While widely validated and easy to use, physiotherapists remain unconvinced by its ability to detect change that might be attributable to physiotherapy intervention (Smith, 1994) and thus assist audit. In a further comparative study, Wright et al. (1998) concluded that the Rivermead Mobility Index (RMI) (Collen et al., 1991) is more responsive to change in patients receiving rehabilitation than the Barthel Index, although it was acknowledged that the RMI had a floor effect for frail hospitalised patients. The use of the Barthel Index within team settings should not preclude the use of measures believed to be more valid to physiotherapy intervention.

GOAL SETTING

Physiotherapists use a problem-solving approach to the management of disability, and both the subjective problems identified by the patient (and his or her carer), together with the objective outcome of assessment, should inform the goal setting process (see also Chapter 8). Bradley et al. (1999), in proposing a theory of goal setting in the care of patients with dementia, describe modifying factors as those relating to the individual and those relating to the disease. There is conflicting evidence about the efficacy of treatment goals in physiotherapy (Bassett and Petrie, 1999), but studies supporting the motivational effects of goals conclude that they should be set collaboratively with patients (and carers where appropriate) (Reid and Chesson, 1998). Goals should be challenging, achievable, specific, measurable, meaningful and predict a time for evaluation

Table 15.1 Elderly Mobility Scale

Key for scoring:	
Lying to sitting	*Sitting to lying*
2 Independent	2 Independent
1 Needs help of one person	1 Needs help of one person
0 Needs help of two+ people	0 Needs help of two+ people
(Maximum score 2)	(Maximum score 2)
Sit to stand	
3 Independent in under 3 seconds	
2 Independent in over 3 seconds	
1 Needs help of one person (verbal or physical)	
0 Needs help of two+ people	
(Maximum score 3)	
Stand	
3 Stands without support[a] and able to reach	
2 Stands without support[a] but needs support to reach	
1 Stands but needs support	
0 Stands only with physical support[a]	
(i.e. help of another person)	
[a]Support means needs to use upper limbs to steady self.	
Gait	
3 Independent (including use of sticks)	
2 Independent with frame	
1 Mobile with walking aid but erratic/unsafe turning	
0 Needs physical help to walk or constant supervision	
(Maximum score 3)	
Timed walk (6 m)	*Functional reach*
3 Under 15 seconds	4 Over 16 cm
2 16–30 seconds	2 8–16 cm
1 Over 30 seconds	0 Under 8 cm or unable
0 Unable to cover 6 m	

(Smith, 1994)

(Bassett and Petrie, 1999).

The goal setting process will determine the physiotherapy treatment plan. Team goal setting facilitates agreement and clarification of individual and shared professional roles. Physiotherapists and occupational therapists share skills in managing problems of function, and on a local level need to work closely together to ensure that treatment approaches are consistent, complementing and reinforcing each other and enhancing the overall therapeutic benefit to the patient without unnecessary duplication.

INTERVENTION: THE EVIDENCE BASE FOR PRACTICE

Following assessment and in discussion with the patient, the physiotherapist will select an appropriate treatment plan that will enable agreed goals to be achieved. Clinical governance (Chapter 1) is now a statutory requirement for all staff within the UK NHS, and in demonstrating clinical effectiveness, physiotherapists must make decisions about intervention that are based on the best available evidence. While the term 'best evidence' primarily refers to scientific research, it also encompasses the consensus of clinical experts and patient preferences (Bury and Mead, 1998).

Physiotherapists work as advisers and educators, as well as practitioners, and intervention may comprise a range of strategies reflecting these varied roles:

- manual therapy techniques including soft tissue and joint mobilisation to reduce pain and stiffness in joints
- exercise approaches, including home exercise programmes, to improve muscle strength and power and to retrain posture and balance
- neurophysiological, cognitive and educational approaches where activity is compromised by neurological deficit
- assessment for mobility aids, assistive devices such as splints (and more recently hip protectors) and footwear (see also Chapter 18)
- functional retraining of transfers and mobility
- recommendations for seating and wheelchairs in conjunction with the occupational therapist (see also Chapter 16)
- advice and education for patients and carers promoting optimal levels of physical activity
- advice and education for carers and other professionals in the management of physical dependency.

The growing evidence base supporting the efficacy of physiotherapy intervention for older people is reflected in clinical guidelines for the management of certain conditions, for example osteoporosis (Mitchell *et al.*, 1999) and stroke (see Case study below) (Intercollegiate Working Party for Stroke, 2000). Clinical Guidelines for the Collaborative Rehabilitative Management of Elderly People Who Have Fallen (Simpson *et al.*, 1998) have been developed and subjected to national audit (CSP/College of Occupational Therapists [COT], 2000), and literature reviews have informed recommendations on best practice for the management of Parkinson's disease (Handford and Jones, 1997).

Key to much of the evidence is the use of exercise by physiotherapists to improve muscle strength and balance. Muscle weakness as a consequence of the ageing process is linked with physical frailty and functional decline (Fiatarone *et al.*, 1994) and activity can be compromised by illness that pushes muscle strength below safety margins. Immobility in older people further weakens muscle strength by 3 per cent a day (Payton and Poland, 1983). Studies have demonstrated the benefits of strength training in both healthy community dwelling and frail institutionalised subjects (Fiatarone *et al.*, 1994; Porter *et al.*, 1995; Skelton and McLaughlin, 1996). Most studies favour the use of moderate to high intensity progressive resistance programmes and task specificity would appear to be necessary in order to transfer strength gains into functional improvements (Porter *et al.*, 1995; Skelton and McLaughlin, 1996). More recently the importance of muscle power and the relationship between decreased muscle power and falls has been described by Skelton (Health Education Authority [HEA], 2000), who reports that older people who fall may have 30–40 per cent less power than those who do not fall. Falls are the most common type of home accident experienced by people aged 65+ and the principal cause of injury (particularly hip fracture) leading to death or hospital admission for that group (HEA, 2000). Non-injurious falls may result in reduced confidence and independence for older people (Salked *et al.*, 2000), leading to increased levels of dependency and accounting for 30–40 per cent of nursing home admissions.

Accidents have been highlighted as one of four key target areas outlined in *Our Healthier Nation* (DoH, 1999), and this, together with the emerging evidence demonstrating the effectiveness of multi-factorial fall prevention programmes (Gillespie *et al.*, 2000), has led to the development of services aimed at both primary and secondary prevention of falls.

The use of exercise aimed at improving muscle strength, balance and functional mobility when used alongside other interventions in fall prevention is supported by the Cochrane review (Gillespie *et al.*, 2000). Other studies have demonstrated the benefits of exercise alone in reducing falls risk in both primary (Campbell *et al.*, 1997) and secondary prevention (Shumway-Cook, 1997). Increasing importance is being attached to the psychological consequences of falls (Cumming *et al.*, 2000).

Behavioural modifications including self-imposed restriction of mobility can lead to inactivity and disuse, resulting in a further decline in mobility and increased fall risk. Physiotherapists have a role to play in helping to improve the older person's confidence in their ability to mobilise safely within their home environment, helping patients and carers balance the risk of falls and inactivity on quality of life, and promoting safe physical activity. Benefits of promoting physical activity may also include a reduction in the rate of bone demineralisation and protection against hip fracture (CSP, 1999a, b). Although high impact exercise is of more benefit to younger people, appropriately tailored exercise can improve or maintain bone mineral density later in life (HEA, 2000).

FALL PREVENTION STRATEGIES

Physiotherapists clearly have a key role to play in the development of services aimed at fall and fracture prevention, and are already working alongside occupational therapists within accident and emergency departments and in specialist 'Falls Clinics', identifying those at risk and providing specifically tailored interventions aimed at secondary prevention.

Those interventions include:

- effective history taking, possibly supported by the use of a 'Falls Diary' to identify frequency, causes and patterns of falls, and to ensure the older person's ability to get up or summon help
- rehabilitation programmes to address impairments in balance and muscle strength in order to reduce postural instability
- assessment of environmental (including clothing and footwear) risk factors and advice on modification of home – alternative layout, equipment and adaptations
- promoting physical activity at all levels of ability
- behaviour modification, including the use of hip protectors where fall and fracture risk is high
- running 'Falls Groups' to provide education and support to those at risk of falling and their carers.

Standard Six of the National Service Framework for Older People advocates a 'whole systems' approach to fall prevention and management strategies, central to which are the key themes of the 'Falls Guideline' (Simpson *et al.*, 1998). As movement specialists within the rehabilitation team, physiotherapists are in a key position to influence the development of local strategies aimed at both primary and secondary prevention across the spectrum of health and social care.

WORKING WITHIN AN INTER-AGENCY TEAM

Successful rehabilitation usually involves a mixture of clinical, therapeutic, social and environmental interventions that are not the preserve of any one agency (Robinson and Turnock, 1998), and the benefits of collaborative team working have been discussed elsewhere in this book (see Chapter 7). The specialist contribution of the physiotherapist within a multi-agency team can be defined as assessing and analysing movement disorders, and supporting the processes of diagnosis, prognosis and risk management, in addition to the role outlined here.

As already stated in Chapter 7, an interdisciplinary approach should facilitate negotiation and agreement of treatment strategies aimed at achieving longer term as well as short-term goals, particularly when the use of early compensation may compromise the restoration and maintenance of physical function in the longer term. Pressure to discharge patients from hospital may result in the provision of equipment and care to support dependency without provision being made for reassessment of longer term needs or the opportunity for rehabilitation potential to be realised (Audit Commission, 1997). Unnecessary admissions to residential care and nursing homes as a result are acknowledged to place an unsustainable demand on social services and other resources that could be aimed at primary prevention (Audit Commission, 1997).

CASE STUDY   SUSAN HUNTER'S PHYSIOTHERAPY

The overall aim of physiotherapy intervention in stroke is to maximise movement ability by:

- assessing the level of neurological deficit and consequent movement disability within the context of the individual's previous lifestyle and co-morbidity
- goal setting within the interdisciplinary team
- implementing preventive strategies to minimise the onset of secondary complications
- reducing neurological deficit
- reducing the level of disability by the use of alternative movement strategies and the provision of mobility equipment where required
- symptomatic treatment of secondary complications
- facilitating discharge following hospital admission
- supporting both patient and carers in maintaining optimal levels of mobility at home.

For the purposes of this case study, physiotherapy intervention will be considered over three stages: early (up to discharge from hospital); intermediate; and long term.

Assessment

Initial assessment: given that Susan Hunter remained neurologically unstable during the first 48 hours, a full physiotherapy assessment was neither indicated nor appropriate. However, in view of the combination of fluctuating consciousness and impaired swallowing, a review of respiratory function was indicated, and agreement would be reached with nursing and speech and language therapy colleagues regarding optimal positioning to:

- minimise the risk of aspiration and promote optimum resting lung function
- prevent the retention of secretions
- minimise the onset of high tone without compromising cerebral circulation.

When medically stable: prior to examination a full history would be obtained from the medical, nursing and other records where possible including:

- confirmation of neurological and cardiovascular stability
- overview of present condition including neurological impairment and resulting functional disability (classification of lesion, continence, swallowing, nutritional status, communication and language skills, cognitive function, visual field deficit, handling needs)

- pre-morbid function including the effects of co-morbidity affecting movement ability, especially arthritis of the hip and knee (baseline pain and function)
- stability of diabetes and hypothyroidism (and whether the integrity of the skin has been compromised by diabetic neuropathy, which may have affected sensation distally in the lower limbs)

- the results of investigations into weight loss prior to admission
- drug history, with particular attention to pain control and treatment for arthritis
- social history – what might be the family's involvement in supporting Susan Hunter after discharge
- patient and carer understanding of the condition and perceptions regarding recovery.

Objective assessment: assessment of physical function enabled identification of problems relating to neurological impairment resultant from Susan Hunter's stroke. The components of assessment included observation and detailed examination of joint and soft tissue range, abnormal tone and associated reactions, postural control, including balance and righting reactions, sensation, voluntary movement and function.

Initially Susan Hunter presented with altered tone affecting her left side (predominantly low but with evidence of effort related associated reactions in her upper limb) and was unable to tolerate sitting out for long periods. Following assessment by the speech and language therapist and dietician, a care plan would now be in place for the management of residual swallowing deficit and therefore the risk of aspiration would be reduced.

The nursing team had completed risk assessments indicating the need for pressure relieving equipment and hoisting for all transfers.

Problems identified following assessment:

1 Left-sided weakness with altered muscle tone and subsequent inability to move in bed without assistance, to achieve or sustain normal sitting posture, to transfer/mobilise.
2 Loss of functional use of left arm.
3 Inattention to left side.
4 Risk of hemiplegic shoulder pain secondary to altered tone and inattention to left side.
5 Compensatory overactivity on right side.
6 Unrealistic goals – lacking insight into extent of disability.
7 Osteoarthritis of right knee and previous right total hip replacement.

Findings following physiotherapy assessment would be discussed with the team to maximise the opportunities for interdisciplinary problem planning and goal setting, and to avoid unnecessary duplication.

Management in the early stages: key aims

1 Keep the patient and family informed
Once Susan Hunter became fully conscious, and in line with the overall team approach for consistency and simplicity, the role of physiotherapy would be explained and an outline of the assessment findings provided. With Susan Hunter's

consent, contact would be actively sought with the family to provide them with the same information and to agree lines of communication. While all the family appear supportive it is clear even at this stage that each had other responsibilities that were likely to make it difficult for them to assume full-time caring roles in the long term.

2 Goal setting within the interdisciplinary team

There is reasonable evidence to support the use of team goal setting in rehabilitation (ICSWP, 2000). The patient must be central to the process and, where appropriate, the needs of any carers should be considered. Goal setting would be used as a tool to manage the unrealistic expectations Susan Hunter had regarding her recovery and her physiotherapy treatment in particular. Susan Hunter's main goals were to walk and to get home; after discussion walking would probably become a long-term goal and its prerequisites – the ability to get out of bed and to move from sitting into standing – would be incorporated into short-term goals. Other mobility related goals would include the ability to achieve and sustain a more normal sitting posture, and to tolerate sitting for longer periods – Susan Hunter would probably enjoy visits from her family and friends, and want to be out of bed when they arrived.

3 Prevention of secondary complications, including hemiplegic shoulder pain

The use of therapeutic positioning handling as a strategy to minimise the onset of spasticity is supported by the evidence underpinning the National Guidelines for Stroke (Intercollegiate Working Party for Stroke, 2000). Shoulder pain occurs in up to 30 per cent of all patients after stroke. It is commonly associated with poor motor recovery and there is believed to be a correlation between poor handling and the incidence of hemiplegic shoulder pain, although this area is one requiring further study (Intercollegiate Working Party for Stroke, 2000).

Sharing of assessment findings with the team would result in a care plan being agreed, which addresses problems and risks associated with residual swallowing deficit, abnormal tone and skin integrity. The most important feature of such a plan is that it is implemented consistently by *whichever staff are in contact* with Susan Hunter throughout the 24 hours (see also Chapter 14).

The care plan outlined would probably resemble the following:

- optimal positions in lying and sitting, together with recommendations regarding seating needs and protection of the hemiplegic upper limb
- recommended handling techniques
- a daily programme for Susan Hunter that enabled time spent in sitting to be gradually increased as her ability to maintain a more normal sitting posture improved, and which coincided with mealtimes once she became able to tolerate food and fluids orally
- awareness of affects of decreased mobility and functional use of right knee and hip with the need to maintain muscle strength in right leg.

Team agreed consistent information and advice would be provided for the family to make them aware of ways in which they could help reinforce optimal positioning and how to handle Susan Hunter's left arm. Again, consistent demonstration by all members of staff will reinforce the advice; failure to do so will confuse patient and carers.

Weekly team meetings enable feedback of changes in functional ability to influence the care planning process, monitor change and review goals.

4 Restoration of movement

There is evidence that, following a lesion of the central nervous system, functional improvement can occur. To date that evidence base appears to favour approaches to the management of disability with no evidence to support the superiority of one approach over another. Such approaches focus on the teaching of adaptive strategies to compensate for neurological impairment and for some patients this may be appropriate. Kwakkel et al. (1997) support the view that treatment should be directed at the level of impairment.

In practice, physiotherapy approaches to the restoration of function following stroke are based on theories of motor control, which recognise the contribution of specific peripheral, spinal, supraspinal and environmental mechanisms (Stokes, 1998). Edwards (1996) describes normal movement as a basis for the treatment of neurologically damaged patients, and in a survey of UK-based physiotherapists, Davidson and Waters (2000) reported that 88 per cent use approaches based on Bobath principles in the belief that the resultant quality of movement optimises functional outcome.

The Bobath concept is 'a problem solving approach to the assessment and treatment of individuals with disturbances of tone, movement and function due to a lesion of the central nervous system. The goal of treatment is to optimise function through the facilitation of improved postural control and selective movement' (IBITAH, 1995). In Susan Hunter's case it might be decided to adopt a treatment approach, which was based on normal movement but that accommodated Susan Hunter's personal goals. While the emphasis would be on eliciting active functional responses and minimising the onset of abnormal tone and movement, in some instances compensatory use of the unaffected side of the body might be accepted as long as its effects were monitored. The inefficiency of the movement produced may cause spasticity, which over time may limit functional recovery and cause muscle and soft tissue contracture.

Progress at three months would be likely to be as follows:

Goals relating to getting out of bed, sitting balance and sit to stand are all progressing. By now Susan Hunter is able to get out of bed with minimal assistance, to sit unsupported and to manage reaching activities. When standing from sitting there is some evidence of compensatory overuse of the right side, but Susan Hunter is able to stand unsupported for ten seconds. Mobility milestones are sitting unsupported; standing unsupported; stepping; walking ten steps; walking 10 m (Warlow et al., 1994).

Susan Hunter is able to walk 5 m; however effort associated with walking in particular might appear to increase tone in the upper limb, requiring review of general levels of activity, positioning and advice to patient and family. Agreed with Susan Hunter that we should try to increase activity in lower limb in preparation for walking. An ankle foot orthosis might be an option, although if provided too early may increase spasticity, but the left foot and ankle are swollen, and discrepancy picked up on formal sensory testing would reinforce concerns regarding integrity of skin. An aircast splint may provide sufficient stability to access dorsiflexor activity in the left foot, thus making it easier to 'step through' and reduce some of the effort of walking. Footwear will need to be wide enough to accommodate both splint and swelling (see also Chapter 18).

It has been observed that Susan Hunter's mood has deteriorated and she appears less interested in treatment sessions. On questioning Susan Hunter might report pain in her right knee on standing, due to combination of compensation and insufficient analgesia for arthritis – an explanation would be given and the doctor asked to review medication. At the regular team meeting the noticeable change in Susan Hunter's mood would be raised and the effects on her progress discussed. Agreement would be reached on the need to screen for depression so that treatment options could be discussed with her.

Awareness is maintained of Susan Hunter's continuing urinary incontinence and support of nursing staff in helping to manage the problem by assessment of pelvic muscular control and appropriate intervention. It may be necessary to refer Susan Hunter to the specialist continence physiotherapist or named adviser.

5 Discharge planning

Team goals that would enable this to be achieved would be agreed, and those relating to physiotherapy involve improving ability to transfer, ability to stand unsupported and to be able to reach in standing for functional tasks. The risk of falls and falls management would be discussed. The key carers within the family would be identified and encouraged to begin to spend more time on the ward, familiarising themselves with Susan Hunter's personal care needs. Special handling needs would be identified and practised within the ward and home environments.

Walking ability would be progressing slowly and the family would be shown how to facilitate the optimal gait pattern for Susan Hunter. The use of a self-propelled wheelchair would be assessed with occupational therapy colleagues, but because of residual visuospatial difficulties and increased tone in the left arm it would probably be agreed that this was not an option. However, an attendant-propelled chair for social outings could be obtained. Rehabilitation needs would be identified and it would be agreed that a referral to the community based rehabilitation team would enable the success of the discharge to be monitored along with progression of goals relating to the following:

- safe independent gait within the home environment
- ability to balance in stand for over one minute
- ongoing prevention of secondary complications including falls.

Community rehabilitation

The physiotherapist working as part of the community rehabilitation team will review Susan Hunter's treatment plan and goals with her following discharge. Family and carers may be involved in those discussions. Changes may be necessary should new problems arise and as progress occurs. As Susan Hunter's social needs change new mobility challenges, including physical access outside her own home, other buildings and transport will need to be met.

When recovery plateaus with no evidence of objective change a decision will be reached with Susan Hunter to discontinue treatment; however, a home maintenance programme will by then have been established and advice will be provided about what action to take if new problems arise. A review appointment will be arranged at an agreed period after discharge from treatment to determine whether change has occurred in the interim and to agree what further follow-up is required.

SUMMARY

The growing recognition of the long-term benefits of rehabilitation in restoring and preserving independence in older people and the planned increase in intermediate care places outlined in the National Service Framework for Older People (DoH, 2001) offer significant challenges to the physiotherapy profession. Changes in working patterns, including a move away from traditional bases on acute hospital sites into a range of community based multi-agency teams, offer the opportunity to extend the scope of traditional clinical practitioner roles. Key to this will be the ability of the undergraduate curriculum to respond and the ongoing development of the evidence base that underpins physiotherapy intervention.

REFERENCES

Age Concern (1999) *Turning Your Back on Us: Older people and the NHS*, Age Concern England, London.
Arnadottir, S. and Mercer, V.S. (1999) Functional assessment in geriatric physical therapy. *Issues on Ageing*, **22**(2), 3–12.
Audit Commission (1997) *Coming of Age*, Audit Commission, London.
Audit Commission (2000) *The Way to Go Home*, Audit Commission, London.
Bassett, S.F. and Petrie, K.J. (1999) The effect of treatment goals on patient compliance with physiotherapy exercise programmes. *Physiotherapy*, **85**(3), 130–137.

Berg, K., Wood-Dauphinee, S.L., Williams, J.I. and Gayton, D. (1989) Measuring balance in the elderly: preliminary development of an instrument. *Physiotherapy Canada*, 41(5), 240–246.

Bradley, E.H., Bogardus, S.T., Tinetti, M.E. and Inouye, S.K. (1999) Goal setting in clinical medicine. *Social Science and Medicine*, 49(2), 267–278.

Bury, T. and Mead, J. (1998) *Evidence-based Healthcare: A practical guide for therapists*, Butterworth Heinemann, Oxford.

Campbell, A.J., Robertson, M.C., Gardner, M.M., Norton, R.N., Tilyard, M.W. and Buchner, D.M. (1997) Randomised controlled trial of a general practice programme of home based exercise to prevent falls in elderly women. *British Medical Journal*, 315, 1065–1069.

Chartered Society of Physiotherapy [CSP] (1999a) *The Difference is Physiotherapy, Here's the evidence . . .* For Healthcare Commissioners No. 1.

CSP (1999b) Services for older people. *Physiotherapy Effectiveness Bulletin*, 1(2).

CSP/College of Occupational Therapists [COT] (2000) *The National Collaborative Audit for the Rehabilitative Management of Elderly People who Have Fallen – Final Report*, CSP/COT, London.

CSP (2001) *Falls Audit Tool* (in press).

Collen, F.M., Wade, D.T., Robb, G.F. and Bradshaw, C.M. (1991) Rivermead Mobility Index: A further development of the Rivermead Motor Assessement. *International Disability Studies*, 13, 50–54.

Clinical Standards Advisory Group (CSAG) (1998) *Community Health Care for Elderly People*, CSAG, London.

Cumming, R.G., Salked, G., Thomas, M. and Szonyi, G. (2000) Prospective study of the impact of falling on activities of daily living, SF-36 scores and nursing home admission. *Journal of Gerontology, Series A, Biological Sciences and Medical Sciences*, 55(5), M299–305.

Davidson, I. and Waters, K. (2000) Physiotherapists working with stroke patients: A national survey. *Physiotherapy*, 86(2), 69–80.

Department of Health [DoH], Executive Letter EL(97)62, *Better Services for Vulnerable People*, October 1997.

DoH (1999) *Saving Lives: Our healthier nation* (white paper) and *Reducing Health Inequalities: An action report*, HSC 1999/152: LAC(99)26, DoH, London.

DoH (2000) The NHS Plan – *A plan for investment, A plan for reform*, The Stationery Press, London.

DoH (2001) *The National Service Framework for Older People*, The Stationery Office, London www.doh.gov.uk/nsf/olderpeople.htm

Dickinson, E. and Sinclair, A. (1998) *Effective Practice in Rehabilitation – reviewing the evidence*, The King's Fund, London.

Duncan, P.W., Weiner, D.K., Chandler, J. and Studenski, S. (1990) Functional reach: a new clinical measure of balance. *Journal of Gerontology*, 45(6), 192–197.

Duncan, P.W., Studenski, S., Chandler, J. and Prescott, B. (1992) Functional reach: predictive validity in a sample of elderly male veterans. *Journal of Gerontology*, 47(3), M53–63.

Edwards, S. (1996) *Neurological Physiotherapy. A Problem-solving Approach*, Churchill Livingstone, Edinburgh.

Fiatarone, M.A., O'Neill, E.F., Doyle Ryan, N., Clements, M.N., Solares, G.R., Nelson, M.E. *et al.* (1994) Exercise training and nutritional supplementation for physical frailty in very elderly people. *New England Journal of Medicine*, 330(25), 1769–1775.

Gill, T.M., Williams, C.S., Richardson, E.D. and Tinetti, M.E. (1996) Impairments in physical performance and cognitive status in predisposing factors for functional dependence among nondisabled older persons. *Journal of Gerontology, Series A, Biological Sciences and Medical Sciences*, 51A(6), M283–288.

Gillespie, L.D., Gillespie, W.J., Cumming, R., Lamb, S.E. and Rowe, B.H. (2000) Interventions for preventing falls in the elderly. *Cochrane Database of Systematic Reviews*, Issue 2.

Handford, F. (1993) Towards a rational basis for physiotherapy in Parkinson's Disease. *Ballières Clinical Neurology*, 2, 141–158.

Handford, F. and Jones, D. (1997) *Parkinson's and the Physiotherapist*, Parkinson's Disease Society, London.

Health Education Authority (2000) *Physical Activity and the Prevention and Management of Falls and Accidents Among Older People – A Framework for Practice*, Health Education Authority, London.

Hu, M. and Woollacott, M.H. (1996) Balance evaluation, training and rehabilitation of frail fallers. *Reviews in Clinical Gerontology*, 6, 85–99.

IBITAH (1995) BBTA Adult Hemiplegia Course Neurophysiology (course notes).

ICIDH–2 (1999) *International Classification of Functioning and Disability*, World Health Organisation, Geneva. (Beta-2 draft) www.who.int/icidh

Intercollegiate Working Party for Stroke (2000) *National Guidelines for Stroke*, Intercollegiate Working Party for Stroke, Royal College of Physicians, London.

Johnstone, J., Judd, M., Langley, J., Stephenson, J., Tutton, J., Underhill, J. *et al.* (1993) Can older people resident in private nursing homes receive NHS physiotherapy? *Physiotherapy*, 79(6), 403–405.

Kwakkel, G., Wagenaar, R.C., Koelman, T.W., Lankhorst, G.J. and Koetsier, J.C. (1997) Effects of intensity of stroke rehabilitation. A research synthesis. *Stroke*, 28, 1550–1556.

Massie, S. (1993) Multi-professional measures of outcome for care of the elderly. *Physiotherapy*, 79(12), 844.

Mathias, S., Nayak, U.S.L. and Issacs, B. (1986) Balance in elderly patients: the 'Get up and Go' test. *Archive of Physical Medicine and Rehabilitation*, 67, 387–389.

Mitchell, S.L., Creed, G., Throw, M., Hunter, A. and Chapman, J. (1999) *Physiotherapy Guidelines for the Management of Osteoporosis*, Chartered Society of Physiotherapy, London.

Partridge, C.J., Johnstone, M. and Morris, L. (1991) *Disability and Health Services: Perceptions, beliefs and experiences of elderly people*, Centre for Physiotherapy Research, King's College, London.

Payton, O.D. and Poland, J.L. (1983) Ageing process – implications for clinical practice. *Physical Therapy*, 63(1), 41–48.

Porter, M.M., Vandervoort, A.A. and Lexell, J. (1995) Ageing of human muscle: structure, function and adaptability. *Scandinavian Journal of Medical Science and Sports*, 5, 129–142.

Posser, L. and Canby, A. (1997) Further validation of the Elderly Mobility Scale for measurement of mobility of hospitalized elderly people. *Clinical Rehabilitation*, 11(4), 338–343.

Reid, A. and Chesson, R. (1998) Goal Attainment Scaling: Is it appropriate for stroke patients and their physiotherapists? *Physiotherapy*, 84(3), 136–144.

Robinson, J. and Turnock, S. (1998) *Investing in Rehabilitation*, The King's Fund, London.

Royal College of Physicians and British Geriatrics Society [RCP and BGS] (1992) *Standardised Assessment Scales for Elderly People*, RCP and BGS, London.

Salked, G., Cameron, I.D., Cumming, R.G., Easter, S., Seymour, J., Kurrle, S.E. *et al.* (2000) Quality of life related to fear of falling and hip fracture in older women: a time trade off study. *British Medical Journal*, 320(7231), 341–346.

Shumway-Cook, A., Gruber, W., Baldwin, M. and Liao, S. (1997) The effect of multidimensional exercises on balance, mobility and fall risk in community-dwelling older adults. *Physical Therapy*, 77, 46–57.

Simpson, J.M. and Forster, A. (1993) Assessing elderly people. Should we all use the same scales? *Physiotherapy*, 79(12), 836–838.

Simpson, J.M. and Worsfold, C.M. (1996) *Assessments of Balance and Function*, Division of Geriatric Medicine, St George's Hospital Medical School, London.

Simpson, J.M., Harrington, R. and Marsh, N. (1998) Guidelines for managing falls among elderly people. *Physiotherapy*, 84(4), 173–177.

Simpson, J.M., Waterman, C. and Zouhar, K. (1999) Raising awareness of older people in undergraduate education. *Physiotherapy*, 85(11), 587–592.

Skelton, D.A. and McLaughlin, A.W. (1996) Training functional ability in old age. *Physiotherapy*, 82(3), 159–167.

Smith, R. (1994) Validation and reliability of the Elderly Mobility Scale. *Physiotherapy*, 80(11), 744–747.

Spirduso, W. W. (1996) *Physical Dimensions of Ageing*, Human Kinetics, Champaign, IL.

Stokes, M. (1998) *Neurological Physiotherapy*, Mosby, London.

Studenski, S., Duncan, P.W. and Chandler, J. (1994) Predicting falls:the role of mobility and nonphysical factors. *Journal of the American Geriatric Society*, 42, 297–302.

Tinetti, M.E. (1986) Performance-orientated assessment of mobility problems in elderly patients. *Journal of the American Geriatrics Society*, 34, 119–126.

Tinetti, M.E., Speechley, M. and Ginter, S.F. (1998) Risk factors for falls among elderly people living in the community. *New England Journal of Medicine*, 319, 1701–1707.

Tinetti, M.E. and Williams, C.S. (1998) The effect of falls and fall related injuries on functioning in community dwelling older persons. *Journal of Gerontology*, Series A, *Biological Sciences and Medical Sciences*, 53A(2), M112–119.

Ward, C. and McIntosh, S. (1993) The rehabilitation process: a neurological perspective. In: *Neurological Rehabilitation* (eds Greenwood, R., Barnes, M. and McMillan, T.), Churchill Livingstone, Edinburgh.

Warlow, C.P., Dennis, M.S., Van Gijn, J., Hankey, G.J., Sandercock, P.A.G., Bamford, J.M. *et al.* (1994) *Stroke – A Practical Guide to Management*, Blackwell, London.

Weiner, D.K., Duncan, P.W., Chandler, J. and Studenski, S.A. (1992) Functional reach: a marker of physical frailty. *Journal of the American Geriatrics Society*, 40, 203–207.

Weiner, D.K., Bongiorni, P.T., Studenski, S.A. Duncan, P.W. and Kochersberger, G.G. (1993) Does functional reach improve with rehabilitation? *Archives of Physical Medicine and Rehabilitation*, 74, 796–800.

Willems, D.A. and Vandervoort, A.A. (1996) Balance as a contributing factor to gait speed in rehabilitation of the elderly. *Physiotherapy Canada*, 48(3), 179–184.

Wright, J., Cross, J. and Lamb, S. (1998) Physiotherapy outcome measures for rehabilitation of elderly people, responsiveness to change of the Rivermead Mobility Index and Barthel Index. *Physiotherapy*, 84(5), 216–220.

Young, A. and Dinan, S. (1994) Fitness for older people. *British Medical Journal*, **309**, 331–334.

16 THE OCCUPATIONAL THERAPY CONTRIBUTION

Jennifer Wenborn

AIMS OF THE CHAPTER

This chapter considers the contribution that occupational therapy offers to health and social care interdisciplinary teams. The author notes that older people comprise the biggest user group across both health and social service departments, and that partnership is crucial for seamless provision. Explanation is provided for the specialist focus of occupational therapy intervention being occupational performance and its restoration, development and improvement through the use of selected occupation. Intervention is described as being influenced by the clients' physical and social environment, and agreed in partnership with them and their carers. The author notes that occupational therapists and physiotherapists share skills in managing problems of function, and emphasises the need for these two disciplines to work closely together to ensure that treatment approaches are consistent, complementing and reinforcing each other to enhance the overall therapeutic benefit for clients without unnecessary duplication.

INTRODUCTION

'Occupational therapists assess and treat people using purposeful activity to prevent disability and develop independent function' (College of Occupational Therapists [COT], 1994). According to the latest government data (Department of Health [DoH], 2000), there are 15,000 occupational therapists employed in the NHS across all specialities in both hospital and community services, in addition to 2,129 employed by Social Services (COT, 2000a). Staffing levels can be patchy, even non-existent, with resulting service delays and pressure on existing staff. The College of Occupational Therapists (COT) is committed to raising the profession's profile and the need to increase its numbers – through more training places and posts (COT, 2000b) and this is reinforced in the NHS Plan (DoH, 2000). Occupational therapists also work independently, under contract or as consultants for the NHS, local authorities and within the voluntary, charitable and private sectors.

Local authority social services departments originally employed occupational therapists to fulfil their responsibilities under the Chronically Sick and Disabled Persons Act 1970. They concentrated primarily on the provision of equipment and adaptations within the home, to enable people with permanent and substantial disability to achieve independence and this still constitutes the greater proportion of the workload. Access is by self-referral or via another person – either a professional or informal carer.

NHS and local authority services have remained separate until now. The need to work in partnership is resulting in jointly commissioned and integrated occupational therapy services (DoH, 1997a, b, 1998a, b, 2000). Hopefully this will break down the traditional divide, enabling all practitioners to utilise their full range of occupational therapy skills to the benefit of clients as 'the needs of vulnerable older people do not respect the health/social care divide and frequently cross over it' (COT, 1998). Occupational therapists need to adapt to the new styles of service delivery within health and social care, for example 'out of hours' initiatives.

As older people comprise the biggest user group of health and social services, it is not surprising that most occupational therapists deal primarily with this client group – not just those who work within specialist units or teams (COT, 1996). Occupational therapists work closely with support staff, including assistants, technical instructors and community care workers. The supervising occupational therapist is responsible for ensuring that whoever work is delegated to is competent to carry it out (COT, 2000c).

OCCUPATION

The concept of occupation is central to occupational therapy philosophy, based on the key assumptions that:

- the need to engage in occupation is a basic human need and is essential for survival
- occupation has the potential to restore and maintain health and well-being.

Occupation is 'the meaningful use of activities, occupations, skills and life roles which enables people to function purposefully in their daily life' (COT, 1994) and occupations are 'the ordinary and familiar things that people do everyday' (American Occupational Therapy Association, 1995). It has been shown that participation in valued occupations can enhance life satisfaction of older people (Gregory, 1983). More recently, Iwarsson et al. (1998) demonstrated a relationship between the level of occupation and health in older people. Indeed, the benefits of promoting health and activity are highlighted in the National Service Framework for Older People (NSF) (DoH, 2001a) (see also Chapter 6).

The specialist focus of occupational therapy intervention with older people therefore is on occupational performance and its restoration, development and improvement through the use of selected occupation.

CLIENT-CENTRED PRACTICE

The occupational therapy profession is 'strongly committed to client-centred practice and the involvement of the client as an equal partner in all stages of the therapeutic process' (COT, 2000c). This is in accord with health and social care services' commitment to client empowerment and involvement in service development, provision and quality assurance, and reflects the standard on person-centred care included within the NSF (DoH, 2001a) (see also Chapter 6). Client-centred practice concentrates on what the client sees as the problem, what the client wants to achieve and the client's priorities (see also Chapter 4).

OCCUPATIONAL THERAPY CORE SKILLS

The profession's unique core skills are the:

> *Use of purposeful activity and meaningful occupation as therapeutic tools in the promotion of health and well-being.*
>
> *Ability to enable people to explore, achieve and maintain balance in the daily living tasks and roles of personal and domestic care, leisure and productivity.*
>
> *Ability to assess the effect of, and then to manipulate, physical and psychosocial environments to maximise function and social integration.*
>
> *Ability to analyse, select and apply occupations as specific therapeutic media to treat people who are experiencing dysfunction in daily living tasks, interactions and occupational roles.*

(COT, 1994)

THE OCCUPATIONAL THERAPY PROCESS

Occupational therapists adopt the same basic philosophy and client-centred approach when working with older people, as with any other client group; and often follow the problem solving approach together with other team members (see Chapter 7).

Observation

Non-verbal signs (for example, facial expression, evidence of increased effort and/or pain), physical and cognitive abilities can be observed in several settings, including interview, performing an activity, formal testing and at rest. It is important to acknowledge the effect that observation can have on a person's performance. A client may be embarrassed – particularly if carrying out personal care activities; and anxiety to 'perform' well can influence behaviour – and either enhance or inhibit function. However, as occupation is about doing, then observation of how and what a person does is the most realistic way of assessing occupational performance.

Interview

The initial interview usually provides the first opportunity to observe a client and gather information. It can also be used to explain the role of occupational therapy, to establish rapport and develop a therapist–client relationship. Obviously the following are not exclusive occupational therapy skills, but their combination to focus on occupational performance is. It is important to liaise with other team members to avoid unnecessary duplication, while each obtains the specific information required:

- **Listen** to what the client is saying, while maintaining focus on what is relevant to occupational therapy – the factors that affect occupational performance.
- **Acknowledge** and respect the individual's life experience and biography.

- **Explore** the client's expectations and aspirations and provide adequate time for the client to ask specific or general questions.
- **Remember** that a client-centred approach and the notion of questioning a health professional may be alien to an older person, based on their previous experience of health and social care services (see also Chapter 5).
- **Consider** the presence of sensory and/or cognitive impairments and adapt the approach accordingly (see Chapter 20).
- **Recognise** and respond appropriately to cultural issues and needs, for example, use an interpreter (see also Chapter 3).

Assessment tools

Many specialist assessment tools are available to occupational therapists. The challenge is deciding which to use.

Occupational therapy assessments include:

- Allen's Cognitive Levels (ACL) (Allen *et al.*, 1995; Conroy, 1998)
- Assessment of Motor and Process Skills (AMPS)
- Community Dependency Index (CDI) (Eakin and Baird, 1995)
- Canadian Occupational Performance Measure (COPM) (Law *et al.*, 1994)

The reader is referred to other texts (Creek and Feaver, 1993; Hagedorn, 1996; Kielhofner, 1992) regarding frames of reference and models of practice commonly used by occupational therapists. While using an occupational therapy model can assist in defining professional boundaries, it can also lead to conflict if it is not in accord with the model(s) adopted by other team members (Feaver and Creek, 1993). If specialist assessment tools are used, occupational therapists must be able to explain their rationale, terminology and results to other team members. However, occupational therapists also need to look forward to their involvement in developing the single assessment process outlined within the NSF for Older People (DoH, 2001a) that aims to provide equitable access and quality service provision, while ensuring the effective use of resources and specialist skills.

When to assess?

Assessment should not be undertaken while a client is medically or psychologically unstable, but equally it should be in sufficient time to allow future planning. The time of day should be realistic to the activity and the client's normal routine, for example, carrying out personal care tasks in the morning (if that is when the client usually washes and dresses). Remember that performance can fluctuate – perhaps caused by medication, or by diurnal variation of the condition, for example, depression or arthritis.

Where to assess?

A patient in hospital may initially be assessed in a ward or occupational therapy department. Home assessments are often conducted to ascertain the feasibility of a 'safe discharge'. Indeed, over recent years, many occupational therapists have found themselves cast increasingly in the role of 'discharge technician' in response to the pressure to increase hospital throughput. The effectiveness of such a 'short term fix', which may prevent the opportunity for rehabilitation to improve function, has been questioned (Clark *et al.*, 1996) due to the potential source of anxiety for clients who may feel judged as having 'passed' or 'failed' – in their *own* home. Imagine the physical and mental stress involved in:

- preparation regarding keys and outdoor clothing
- leaving the ward
- getting in/out of transport
- travelling to and fro
- returning home for the first time following the traumatic event that necessitated admission, for example, a fall or bereavement
- carrying out a range of daily living activities in an unrealistically short space of time
- 'performing' in front of several professionals and relatives – all with different expectations.

The effect of any combination of these factors must not be underestimated. A systematic review (Tullis and Nicol, 1999) highlighted the need to undertake further evaluation into this area of practice with older people who have dementia. It has been noted (Mountain and Moore, 1995) that such short-term assessments and interventions primarily provide professionals with information, but can induce anxiety on the part of clients and carers. In contrast, longer term occupational therapy intervention with older people who have a complex mix of mental and physical health needs, provided in a community setting, is seen as a positive experience.

Within NHS and local authority community services, clients' homes are usually the venue for assessment and intervention, and as such are more realistic. Home is a familiar environment where the client will perform the necessary occupations. Equipment can be installed; its use demonstrated and practised; and relevant safety aspects emphasised in situ. The potential effects of any proposed layout changes, equipment and/or adaptations can be discussed with other household members, for example, would installation of bathing equipment affect access for others?

Carers can be involved in the assessment and subsequent intervention – although there may be occasions when carers involvement can be tricky to deal with, for example, if carers are over-protective or have unrealistic expectations, either negative or positive, or hold expectations at odds with the client (see also Chapter 12). It may be difficult to carry out validated assessments within a non-standard environment and the occupational therapist may need to carry test materials and equipment – a practical consideration, especially for those relying on public transport. Above all, occupational therapists must always remember that they are visitors in the client's home, and avoid making subjective assumptions or comments about the environment based on personal values.

All clients and homes differ, and there are many reasons for carrying out an assessment. However, the following list attempts to highlight the areas most commonly considered when assessing an older person. The information obtained forms part of the holistic assessment made in conjunction with other team members. Again it is important to work together effectively to use resources, avoid duplication and provide a consistent approach with clients. Core areas of assessment for occupational therapy include the following:

- **orientation** – time, place and person
- **cognition** – short-term and long-term memory, sequencing, problem solving
- **mood**
- **mobility** inside and outdoors, using stairs, use of mobility aids
- **transfers** – bed, chair, toilet, bath/shower; note height, type, layout of furniture
- **personal care tasks** – eating and drinking, washing, dressing, grooming
- **domestic activities** – cooking, cleaning, shopping, laundry
- **occupation and usual routine** – completion of a daily/weekly timetable highlights 'gaps' in service provision, occupational opportunities and social interaction
- **environment** – accommodation, access, layout, facilities, lighting, flooring, heating, communication – standard and emergency
- **potential hazards** and safety issues
- **equipment** already provided – by whom and when? is it used? (Wielandt and Strong, 2000)
- **other household members** and pets
- **support and social networks**.

With the client's permission, carers are often present at assessment and can be a valuable source of additional information.

Goal setting and intervention

Following assessment, goals need to be agreed by the team and client/carer and subsequent interventions implemented, audited and reviewed.

Intervention depends on the client's active participation, and the occupational therapist's skill lies in engaging and motivating the client using occupation as the medium.

An endless list of activities can be used. The skill lies in selecting relevant activities valued by the client, and presenting them (adapted if necessary) such that they meet the client's current abilities, while encouraging the desired outcome. Everyday activities are often used, for example cooking; while leisure activities, such as gardening and crafts, can provide either familiar or new experiences. These improve occupational performance through the development of motor and process skills such as balance, strength, reaching and sequencing. Advances in technology provide opportunities to use computers and the Internet, where access to certain databases may increase the confidence of the user to understand their circumstances better, and communicate with professionals from a more informed position (see also Chapter 5). However, the use of such everyday tasks can influence the way in which occupational therapy intervention is perceived – both by clients and other team members. It may not be seen as 'proper' treatment, partly because of the everyday nature of the activities used and partly because of the need for the client's active participation.

Intervention can happen on a one-to-one basis, or within a group setting, and/or in conjunction with other relevant disciplines; often provoking enjoyment and fun, which can be a great motivator. Activities of daily living may be practised using compensatory techniques, and/or equipment. However, the provision of equipment should not compromise the rehabilitation agenda by encouraging compensation too early on. Collaboration with other professions ensures a consistent approach, for example, liaison with physiotherapists regarding mobility and transfers (see Chapter 15); and nursing staff regarding personal care tasks (see Chapter 14).

Practical intervention within the home environment can include the following:

- removal of safety hazards, for example, loose mats, trailing wires
- enhancing client and carer's safety awareness
- altering furniture height and/or layout, for example, moving bed downstairs
- providing and training in use of equipment
- providing minor (for example, grab rails, ramps) and/or major (for example, stairlift) adaptations.

As these can impact on the appearance and function of the client's home, full involvement of the client/carer is essential from initial assessment to implementation and evaluation. The eligibility criteria and timescale for major adaptations may necessitate making the 'best fit' within the circumstances – even as a temporary measure.

The long waiting times for older people to be assessed and provided with equipment are well known (DoH, 1992; Age Concern, 1996; Audit Commission, 2000). The NHS Plan (DoH, 2000) outlined major investment in community equipment services and more detail was included in the Intermediate Care Guidance (DoH, 2001b). The subsequent Guide to Integrating Community Equipment Services (DoH, 2001c) outlined the timetable to achieve full integration and 50% increase in service users by March 2004.

Community equipment includes (but is not limited to):

- home nursing equipment usually provided by the NHS, such as pressure relief mattresses and commodes
- 'equipment for daily living' usually provided by local authorities, such as raised toilet seats and teapot tippers
- minor adaptations, such as grab rails, lever taps, improved domestic lighting
- ancillary equipment for people with sensory impairment, such as flashing doorbells, low vision optical aids

- equipment for short-term loan, including wheelchairs (but not those for permanent use)
- telecare equipment such as fall alarms, gas escape alarms.

The proposed developments are good news; not only for the staff who have previously spent far too long trying to access equipment on clients' behalf; but primarily for clients and their carers who will be enabled to remain more independent within their own homes for longer. Of course, the occupational therapy profession faces the challenge, along with other colleagues and services, of implementing these radical plans, but can look forward to the advantages that will result.

Evaluation

Evaluation occurs throughout the occupational therapy process. It informs the review of progress made and modification of the subsequent intervention and grading of activities towards the corporate goal. Validated reassessments can be used as outcome measures to demonstrate the effectiveness of individual intervention as well as service effectiveness. For example, the Canadian Occupational Performance Measure (COPM) can be used both to guide an initial (semi-structured) interview, and as a comparative outcome measure within the context of client-centred practice (Law et al., 1994). The Community Dependency Index (Eakin and Baird, 1995) is designed as an initial assessment tool and to measure outcome of occupational therapy intervention.

AREAS OF SERVICE PROVISION

The shift away from the traditional hospital rehabilitation unit offers enormous potential for future development of occupational therapy services. Specialist areas of service provision include the following.

Accident and Emergency (A&E) Departments

Many A&E departments employ occupational therapists and physiotherapists (see Chapter 15), although the level and scope of cover varies. Intervention can avoid unnecessary admission, facilitate safe discharge with appropriate support/equipment and follow up those who are admitted. Occupational therapists can:

- assess a client's suitability for discharge taking into account functional and cognitive abilities, social and home circumstances
- provide equipment (using fast-track technical support) and liaise with necessary agencies to facilitate discharge
- follow up at home to provide further equipment and a rehabilitation programme
- provide the above for clients admitted to A&E/observation wards.

Falls

Many of the clients seen by therapists in A&E departments, hospital wards or in the community have fallen. The inclusion of a 'Falls' standard within the NSF for Older People (DoH, 2001a) highlights its significance. Older people need to be enabled to return home quickly, to regain their independence and confidence within their own environment, and occupational therapists and physiotherapists have a key role in achieving this. It is an area of practice that requires collaboration between the two professions, each providing specialist but complementary expertise (Chartered Society of Physiotherapy [CSP]/College of Occupational Therapists, 2000). Therefore, for simplicity and economy of space, this topic is covered in detail within Chapter 15.

Wheelchair provision and assessment

Another area of practice where occupational therapists and physiotherapists work closely is that of wheelchair assessment and provision. For the sake of simplicity and economy of space, this area of practice is covered in this chapter.

Wheelchair provision

In 1991 the wheelchair service was devolved to each health authority (and subsequently to Primary Care Groups [PCGs] and Primary Care Trusts [PCTs]) to commission wheelchair services to meet local needs. While local services can respond more appropriately to the needs of local users, there has been variation of eligibility criteria and inequitable provision (Audit Commission, 2000).

Wheelchairs are available through the NHS for those who have a permanent disability that affects their mobility. Short-term loan is usually provided through voluntary organisations, such as the Red Cross, although some wheelchair services offer this additional service. Wheelchairs for short-term loan are to be included within the proposed Integrated Community Equipment Services, but those for permanent use are not (DoH, 2001c). Some services do not provide wheelchairs to nursing home residents unless they are able to self-propel, or have a named person who regularly takes them out and who will take responsibility for the wheelchair; others provide a 'pool' of transit wheelchairs.

The local wheelchair service team usually comprises a manager, administration staff, wheelchair therapist(s) (occupational therapist and/or physiotherapist), and rehabilitation engineer. Most local services can access a specialist (regional) team that deals with more complex cases. This team includes a consultant in rehabilitation medicine and sometimes a clinical engineer and/or orthotist. Contract engineers provide repair and maintenance support to every registered NHS wheelchair user, free at the point of delivery. Referral systems are agreed locally, but referrals are usually accepted from other health professionals with a GP or consultant referral for new clients. Details of the client's local provider can be obtained through their GP or Social Services office.

The main categories of wheelchairs are:

- manual
  self-propelling
  attendant propelled/transit

- powered
  indoor (EPIC)
  indoor/outdoor (EPIOC).

Two schemes were introduced in 1996. The first was the provision of powered indoor/outdoor wheelchairs for severely disabled people (NHS Executive, 1996a). Eligibility criteria for provision of EPIOCs vary from service to service, but in general are available to anyone unable to walk or self-propel indoors. Secondly, the Voucher Scheme (NHS Executive, 1996b) gives users the choice of three options following assessment:

- **NHS provision** – wheelchair prescribed and provided, using contract repairer maintenance, i.e. the status quo.
- **Independent option** – user contributes to the cost of a more expensive wheelchair of own choice. The user owns the wheelchair and is responsible for maintenance.
- **Partnership option** – user contributes to the cost of more expensive wheelchair from a range suggested by the wheelchair service. The service owns the wheelchair and is responsible for maintenance.

Take up of the scheme has been variable across the UK but is increasing (Sanderson *et al.*, 2000). The evaluation report recommended that funding for EPIOC provision should continue and be ring-fenced. However, although the government has agreed to continue funding, it will not be ring-fenced.

Wheelchair assessment

Many occupational therapists and physiotherapists working with older people carry out routine wheelchair and seating assessments. Clients with more complex needs are usually assessed by a specialist wheelchair therapist either in a clinic or at home, often with other health professionals, for example, community nurse, and/or carers involved.

Assessment for a wheelchair takes into account aspects of the client's needs including diagnosis, height, weight, physical ability such as postural competence and skin condition; environmental issues; mode of transport; attitude, motivation and lifestyle (PMG, 1997; Baxendale and Kelsall, 1998a, b, c; Ham *et al.*, 1998). If a carer will be pushing or handling the wheelchair, their ability and needs are also considered.

The prescription specifies the type of wheelchair, special cushion and any accessories required that are essential for the client's posture and/or independence and that the client can use unaided. All provision should be accompanied by training for client and carer in wheelchair handling and safety issues, day-to-day maintenance, an information handbook for the model provided, plus information on how to access the contract repair service.

Ongoing intervention includes:

- monitoring suitability of equipment
- regular review for clients with changing needs
- information on accessing wider mobility opportunities for wheelchair users, for example, Shopmobility, public transport and local disability groups.

Community rehabilitation

Occupational therapists – often within community rehabilitation or primary care teams – also work with clients in their own homes. Following assessment, intervention may include:

- advice on alternative strategies and methods of carrying out activities
- provision of cues to aid memory and orientation
- adaptation of environment
- provision of equipment, including education and practice for client and carer
- use of selected activities to restore, develop and maintain occupational skills.

Evidence exists to support the effectiveness of community based rehabilitation. For example, Walker *et al.* (1999) demonstrated that occupational therapy intervention provided to people with stroke not admitted to hospital significantly reduced disability and handicap.

Intermediate care

The range of intermediate care services is increasing as a result of the NHS Plan (DoH, 2000) and the NSF for Older People (DoH, 2001a) (see also Chapter 6). The occupational therapist's contribution addresses the transition from dependence to independence, from the care environment back to the client's own home. The occupational therapist can:

- assess a client's occupational performance
- plan, implement, review and modify a rehabilitation programme – often in conjunction with other professionals
- carry out a series of visits with the client to their home, in order to practise daily living activities and enhance self-confidence
- provide appropriate equipment
- set up the necessary care package
- train care staff in the skills required for the implementation of rehabilitation programmes and to change their role from one of 'care' to 'cure'.

Residential and nursing homes

Occupational therapists have an important role to play within care homes – and not just in the context of providing short-term rehabilitation through intermediate care schemes.

The recently published *National Minimum Standards* (DoH, 2001d) *for Care Homes for Older People* require 'the routines of daily living and activities made available' to be 'flexible and varied to suit users' expectations, preferences and capacities'. Residents' interests should be recorded, and social, leisure and recreational activities offered that suit their needs, preferences and capacities.

Occupational therapists can advise on occupational opportunities to enhance residents' quality of life (Green and Acheson Cooper, 2000), and select, educate and supervise 'activity' staff (Hurtley and Wenborn, 2000).

Long-term care insurance

Long-term care insurance policies pay benefits when the policyholder 'fails' either two or three activities of daily living (ADLs) or shows evidence of cognitive impairment – depending on the policy, which may include 'assistive devices' (equipment) benefits. Occupational therapists can:

- assess eligibility for benefits at the point of claim – ADLs/cognitive impairment
- advise on equipment
- identify the potential for rehabilitation packages.

Insurance companies are interested in cost-effective solutions and recognise the potential for rehabilitation and provision of equipment to enable policy-holders to regain and maintain independence. This results in older people remaining at home for longer and reduced costs for insurance companies (Swiss Re Life and Health, 1999).

Prevention of disease and promotion of health

Rehabilitation services traditionally responded to clients who had experienced a crisis, but recognition of the need to adopt preventive strategies and provide support for older people has grown (DoH/Social Services Inspectorate, 1999) and its inclusion within the NSF for Older People (DoH, 2001a) confirms its importance.

There are two aspects:

- services that prevent or delay ill health or disability – and thereby the need for more costly (often institutional) services
- services that enhance quality of life and engagement within the community.

Occupational therapy intervention can:

- identify risk factors within the home and suggest modifications to lifestyle and environment that may enhance safety and prevent falls (Close *et al.*, 1999; Sevigny, 2000)
- develop programmes that offer older people the opportunity to participate in personally selected, meaningful occupation to enhance health and well-being (Jackson *et al.*, 1998).

THE FUTURE FOR OCCUPATIONAL THERAPY WITH OLDER PEOPLE?

The older population is growing, and becoming more culturally diverse. This presents the occupational therapy profession with many opportunities to further develop practice, while also facing the challenges of providing flexible and responsive services, improving recruitment and retention of staff, and developing evidence based practice.

Evidence of effectiveness

The occupational therapy profession needs evidence of its effectiveness to increase well-being, health and independence through the use of occupation, in order to improve cost-effectiveness – be it hospital admission, community services or long-term care. It is important that each occupational therapist provides continuously reviewed evidence based practice and can articulate the rationale underlying his or her intervention.

While the importance of working in teams is acknowledged, occupational therapists must utilise their specialist skills, to ensure the most appropriate and cost-effective use of scarce resources. Occupational therapists need to develop their skills and role as educators, advisers and facilitators, both with clients, carers and other professional groups. The advent of consultant therapist posts acknowledges the specialist contribution that occupational therapy can offer within interdisciplinary teams in health and social care, as well as other sectors such as education and insurance.

CASE STUDY SUSAN HUNTER – OCCUPATIONAL THERAPY

The many impacts of the stroke (physical, cognitive, perceptual, emotional) are superimposed on Susan Hunter's recent bereavement. This results in her loss of roles as wife, carer, homemaker, plus loss of her own occupational performance and routine. Her family is also experiencing their own losses. These aspects must be taken into account throughout assessment and intervention.

Working within the interdisciplinary team requires effective communication, joint assessment and intervention sessions to ensure consistency of approach. This includes Susan Hunter and her family as team members. There is also the need to use outcome measures to demonstrate progress and effectiveness.

The NSF (Department of Health, 2001a) promises that people who have experienced a stroke will be treated by a specialist stroke service and be able to participate in a multidisciplinary rehabilitation programme. This is good news for people such as Susan Hunter, although it will obviously take time to implement.

Admission phase

Data gathering
Collate information from documentation wherever possible; discuss further with team members, family regarding social networks, home environment, previous routine and occupational performance.

Observation
Observe Susan Hunter on ward and throughout interview and assessment procedures. At interview:

- establish relationship
- gather and document information about home environment – accommodation, support, previous occupational performance and routine

- discuss Susan Hunter's priorities and wishes
- agree initial goals and plan of action together with Susan Hunter, her family and the rest of the team.

Assessment

Contribute to multidisciplinary assessment:

- physical – tone, range of movement, balance
- cognitive – initial screen followed by formal testing, for example, Rivermead Perceptual Assessment Battery (RPAB) (Whiting et al., 1985), Behavioural Inattention Test (BIT) (Wilson et al., 1987) (see Resources)
- Activities of Daily Living (ADL)
- emotional – effect of bereavement, level of motivation, insight.

Rehabilitation phase

Reassessment and review of goals, together with Susan Hunter, her family and the rest of team will be required throughout the rehabilitation phase.
A rehabilitation programme will be designed to enhance occupational skills, using:

- bilateral activities with facilitation to normalise tone, promote normal movement patterns and enhance perceptual incorporation of upper limb into task; for example, rolling pastry, baking, ADL
- creative activities to encourage expression of feelings, for example, art and music
- ADL – start with eating and drinking, personal care tasks – progress to kitchen tasks later on. Needs to be a graded process, starting with just parts of an activity and using backward chaining. Emphasise energy conservation and effects of effort. Liaise with nursing staff regarding continuation and consistency on the ward over 24-hour period. Joint sessions with physiotherapist regarding positioning and normal movement. Take into account pain in right knee
- groupwork to provide social interaction, increase confidence, as well as 1:1 intervention to ensure that specific physical needs are addressed. May be done in conjunction with other team members, for example, physiotherapist.

The rehabilitation programme should provide positive experiences and an element of fun.

Provide attendant propelled wheelchair (if part of agreed plan) to enable Susan Hunter to get out and about with her family and to maintain community contacts. Involve family in assessment and choice between NHS provision or voucher options. Ensure wheelchair provides appropriate support and positioning. Later on, could consider indoor powered wheelchair – depending on mobility, cognitive and perceptual abilities, and environment.

Discuss with family strategies for their involvement, and include in activities that they can enjoy together with Susan Hunter (consider life biography).

Discharge planning

- Consider whether current environment is suitable, and discuss with Susan Hunter whether she wishes to return to it.
- Carry out preliminary visit to check access, together with family member and other team members as appropriate, for example social worker.
- Carry out home assessment with Susan Hunter, together with other team members as appropriate, for example physiotherapist if there are specific mobility issues.
- Introduce compensatory methods and assess for equipment needed for safety – beware of providing equipment too early on as it can inhibit rehabilitation by increasing tone and associated reactions – discuss with team colleagues, for example physiotherapist.
- Serial home visits, gradually increasing time spent at home, practising activities, in order to increase confidence.

Community follow up

- Continue rehabilitation programme on discharge, to further improve independence, using valued occupations, for example getting out to bowls club and church group.
- Introduce new interests and occupations.
- Review equipment needs and provide ongoing education and practice if necessary.
- Refer to other agencies, for example Stroke Club and day centre.

SUMMARY

This chapter has considered the specialist contribution of occupational therapy to rehabilitation with older people. Occupational therapists need to work as effective team members, while using their specialist skills to best advantage. Many opportunities exist to further develop practice with this fast-growing population. The fact that many older clients have a range of needs, plus the current emphasis on services working together in partnership enables occupational therapists to be creative in utilising their full range of skills.

There will probably never be a better opportunity for the profession to establish the need for, and the effectiveness of, occupational therapy intervention with this client group, as the NSF for Older People (Department of Health, 2001a) paves the way to develop and implement innovative practice. However, the challenge facing the profession is the need to produce evidence of its effectiveness and focus accordingly. This must be addressed, not just by the professional body, but also by each and every occupational therapist in day-to-day practice.

ACKNOWLEDGEMENTS

The author thanks her occupational therapy colleagues for their assistance in reading the draft text: Patsy Aldersea, Patricia Eyres, Fiona Douglas, Susan Moore, Jo Pereira and Beryl Steeden. And, as always, many thanks to the COT Library staff for their help.

REFERENCES

Age Concern (1996) *Stuck on the Waiting List: Older people and equipment for independent living*, Age Concern, London.

Allen, C.K., Earhart, C.A. and Blue, T. (1995) *Understanding Cognitive Performance Modes*, Allen Conferences, FL.

American Occupational Therapy Association (1995) Position paper: occupation. *American Journal of Occupational Therapy*, **49**(10), 1015–1018.

Audit Commission (2000) *Fully Equipped: The provision of equipment to older or disabled people by the NHS and social services in England and Wales*, Audit Commission, London.

Baxendale, K. and Kelsall, A. (eds) (1998a) *Manual Wheelchairs: A practical guide*, Disability Information Trust, Oxford.

Baxendale, K. and Kelsall, A. (eds) (1998b) *Powered Wheelchairs and Scooters: A practical guide*, Disability Information Trust, Oxford.

Baxendale, K. and Kelsall, A. (eds) (1998c) *Wheelchair Accessories: A practical guide*, Disability Information Trust, Oxford.

Chartered Society of Physiotherapy/College of Occupational Therapists [CSP/COT] (2000) *The National Collaborative Audit for the Rehabilitative Management of Elderly People who have Fallen – Final Report*, CSP/COT, London.

Clark, H., Dyer, S. and Hartman, L. (1996) *Going Home: Older people leaving hospital*, University of Bristol, The Policy Press in association with the Joseph Rowntree Foundation and Community Care magazine.

Close, J., Ellis, M., Hooper, R., Glucksman, E., Jackson, S. and Swift, C. (1999) Prevention of falls in the elderly trial (PROFET): a randomised controlled trial. *The Lancet*, **353**, 9th January, 93–97.

COT (1994) *Core Skills and a Conceptual Framework for Practice: A position statement*, COT, London.

COT (1996) *Membership Survey*, COT London.

COT (1998) *Rehabilitation of Vulnerable Older People Nature of the Evidence Base and implications for Occupational Therapists*, COT, London, p. 5.

COT (2000a) *Occupational Therapy in Social Services Departments: A review of the literature*, COT, London.

COT (2000b) 38,000 sign petition. *Occupational Therapy News*, 8/2, February, p. 1.

COT (2000c) *Code of Ethics and Professional Conduct for Occupational Therapists*, COT, London.

Conroy, M.C. (1998) Allen's Cognitive Levels with people who are dementing. *British Journal of Therapy and Rehabilitation*, **5**(1), 21–26.

Creek, J. and Feaver, S. (1993) Models for practice in occupational therapy: Part 1, Defining terms. *British Journal of Occupational Therapy*, **56**(1), 4–6.

Department of Health [DoH] (1992) *Equipped for Independence? Meeting the Needs of Disabled People*, DoH, Wetherby.

DoH (1997a) *The New NHS: Modern, Dependable: A National Framework for Assessing Performance*, HMSO, London.

DoH (1997b) *Better Services for Vulnerable People*, DoH EL(97)62/CI(97)24, Wetherby.

DoH (1998a) *Modernising Social Services: Promoting independence, improving protection, raising standards*, HMSO, London.

DoH (1998b) *Partnership in Action (New Opportunities for Joint Working Between Health and Social Services): A discussion document*, DoH, Wetherby.

DoH/Social Services Inspectorate (1999) *Promoting Independence Preventative Strategies and Support for Older People: Report of the SSI Study*, DoH, Wetherby.

DoH (2000) *The NHS Plan – A plan for investment, a plan for reform*, The Stationery Office, London.

DoH (2001a) *The National Service Framework for Older People*, DoH, London.

DoH (2001b) *Intermediate Care Guidance*, HSC 2001/01: LAC(2001)1, DoH, London.

DoH (2001c) *Guide to Integrating Community Equipment Services*, DoH, London.

DoH (2001d) *Care Homes for Older People: National minimum standards*, HMSO, London.

Eakin, P. and Baird, H. (1995) The Community Dependency Index: a standardised assessment of needs and measure of outcome for community occupational therapy. *British Journal of Occupational Therapy*, 58(1), 17–22.

Feaver, S. and Creek, J. (1993) Models for practice in occupational therapy: Part 2, What use are they? *British Journal of Occupational Therapy*, 56(2), 59–62.

Green, S. and Acheson Cooper, B. (2000) Occupation as a quality of life constituent: a nursing home perspective. *British Journal of Occupational Therapy*, 63(1), pp. 17–24.

Gregory, M.D. (1983) Occupational behavior and life satisfaction among retirees. *American Journal of Occupational Therapy*, 37(8), 548–553.

Hagedorn, R. (1996) *Foundations for Practice in Occupational Therapy*, 2nd edn, Churchill Livingstone, Edinburgh.

Ham, R., Aldersea, P. and Porter, D. (1998) *Wheelchair Users and Postural Seating*, Churchill Livingstone, Edinburgh.

Hurtley, R. and Wenborn, J. (2000) *The Successful Activity Coordinator: Making the best use of resources to provide activities and leisure opportunities to older people in care homes*, Age Concern England, London.

Intercollegiate Working Party for Stroke (2002) A multidisciplinary stroke audit (2nd edition), London: Royal College of Physicians.

Iwarsson, S., Isacsson, A., Persson, D. and Schersten, B. (1998) Occupation and survival: a 25 year follow-up study of an aging population. *American Journal of Occupational Therapy*, 52(1), 65–70.

Jackson, J., Carlson, M., Mandel, D., Zemke, R. and Clark, F. (1998) Occupation in lifestyle redesign: the Well Elderly Study Occupational Therapy Program. *American Journal of Occupational Therapy*, 52(5), 326–336.

Kielhofner, K. (1992) *Conceptual Foundations of Occupational Therapy*, F.A. Davis, Philadephia, PA, pp. 74–74.

Law, M., Baptiste, S., Carswell, A., McColl, M.A., Polatajko, H.and Pollock, N. (1994) *Canadian Occupational Performance Measure*, 2nd edn, Canadian Association of Occupational Therapists, Toronto. Available from COT, London.

Mountain, G. and Moore, J. (1995) *What Do Occupational Therapists Working with Older People Do?* Report of a Seminar to Present Research Findings held during September 1995. University of Leeds, Community Care Division, Nuffield Institute for Health, Leeds.

NHS Executive (1996a) Health Service Guidelines (96) 34 *Powered Indoor/Outdoor Wheelchairs for Severely Disabled People*, DoH, Wetherby.

NHS Executive (1996b) Health Service Guidelines (96) 53 *The Wheelchair Voucher Scheme*, DoH, Wetherby.

PMG (Posture and Mobility Group) (1997) *Guidelines for Wheelchair Services: Provision of wheelchair mobility and postural assistance services. A reference resource for commissioners and providers*, PMG King's Healthcare, London.

Sanderson, D., Place, M. and Wright, D. (2000) *Evaluation of the Powered Wheelchair and Voucher Scheme Initiative*, York Health Economics Consortium, York.

Sevigny, J. (2000) *The Value of OT in Home Safety*, American Occupational Therapy Association, OT Practice, pp. 10–13.

Swiss Re Life and Health Ltd (1999) *Long Term Care Data Pack*, Swiss Re, London.

Tullis, A. and Nicol, M. (1999) A systematic review of the evidence for the value of functional assessment of older people with dementia. *British Journal of Occupational Therapy*, **62**(12), pp. 554–563.

Walker, M., Gladman, J., Lincoln, N., Siemonsma, P. and Whiteley, T. (1999) Occupational therapy for stroke patients not admitted to hospital: a randomised controlled trial. *The Lancet*, **354**, 24 July, 278–280.

Whiting, S., Lincoln, N., Bhavnani, G. and Cockburn, J. (1985) *Rivermead Perceptual Assessment Battery (RPAB)*, NFER-NELSON, Windsor.

Wielandt, T. and Strong, J. (2000) Compliance with prescribed adaptive equipment: a literature review. *British Journal of Occupational Therapy*, **63**(2), pp. 65–75.

Wilson, B., Cockburn, J. and Halligan, P. (1987) *Behavioural Inattention Test (BIT)*, Thames Valley Test Company, Bury St Edmunds.

ADDITIONAL RESOURCES

Assessment of Motor and Process Skills – AMPS
Assessors must be trained and calibrated – for information about training courses
    contact:
AMPS UK Coordinator
PO Box 2338, Bradford on Avon, Wiltshire BA15 1ZN
Tel: 01225 864847
Fax: 01225 868721
Email: info@amps-uk.com
www.amps-uk.com

Occupational Therapy for Older People – OTOP (The College of Occupational
    Therapists' specialist section for those working with older people.) Contact details
    available from:
The College of Occupational Therapists
106–114 Borough High Street, South Walk, London SE1 1LB
Tel: 020 7357 6480
www.cot.co.uk

17 COMMUNICATION PROBLEMS OF OLDER PEOPLE

Kirsten Beining, Jayne Whitaker and Jane Maxim

AIMS OF THE CHAPTER

This chapter describes the contribution of speech and language therapists (SALTs) to heath and education interdisciplinary teams, frequently on a sessional rather than team member basis, relying on full team members for appropriate referral and inclusion. Approximately 20 per cent of SALTs work with adult clients who have communication problems or swallowing disorders of neurological origin. The authors emphasise the importance of both of these functions to comprehensive rehabilitation through the nutritional and intellectual ability to contribute to active treatment. The authors note that assessment and treatment is frequently in conjunction with nursing, dietitian, occupational therapy, dental, audiology and orthoptist colleagues.

INTRODUCTION

Speech and language therapists are employed in the NHS across all specialities in both hospital and community services. Although the majority of SALTs work with children who have developmental speech and language disorders, approximately 20 per cent work with adult clients who have communication problems or swallowing disorders of neurological origin.

Most SALTs who work with older people want to work as part of an interdisciplinary team (IDT) but, because of the small numbers of SALTs employed in this speciality, they are often only contracted to work on a sessional basis with this client group. If there is a full-time SALT, this is a rare occurrence. In a recent survey, only 67 per cent of speech and language therapy departments provided any service at all to older people with mental health problems (including the dementias) and only 43 per cent of SALTs were working as part of the IDT. Most SALTs in this field will be part-time team members, having to allocate their time between working with older people and other specialities. The ward team need to find out how much time the SALT has to provide the service and to plan jointly what the SALT can realistically contribute to the IDT and the people in their care. If the time allocated is inadequate, then careful collection of statistical evidence of need and a dialogue with senior managers may lead to increased contracted time. The ward team may find that the SALT is only contracted to provide a service to patients who are at risk because of possible swallowing disorders. While this may be the remit, when working with older people, it is vital that a swallowing assessment is carried out in conjunction with a communication assessment, which will provide essential information on the patient's ability to understand and communicate their nutritional needs and problems with eating and drinking. Unless both areas of the assessment are completed, the ward team will not be able to plan management effectively. It may be possible for the SALTs to alter their pattern of work in a way that has been found to be effective (Rainbow *et al.*, 1996). Whereas most SALTs respond to referrals for individual patients, Rainbow *et al.* used a system of block visits to wards of up to four weeks, which allowed time for all staff to work and learn together. While this model of working will probably not be practical in acute settings because patients are on the ward for a short time, when older people remain on wards for a longer period of time, this pattern of service provision can be very effective.

The primary goal of all speech language therapy intervention for communication disorders is to identify the impairment and to maximise activity and participation in communicative interaction. Why is communication important for older people? In their everyday lives, communication fulfils a number of functions; social interaction, communicating needs, expressing emotion. When older people need health care, good communication facilitates team work for holistic rehabilitation, assists the transition back into the community and improves the chances of a successful and sustained return home.

Access to speech and language therapy provision for older people is variable within the NHS. The National Service Framework for Older People (Department of Health, 2001), along with initiatives such as the National Clinical Guidelines for Stroke (Intercollegiate Working Party for Stroke, 2000) have the potential for reducing this variability and in improving access to evidence based services.

Communicating Quality 2 (Royal College of Speech and Language Therapists [RCSLT], 1996) is the primary source of standards and guidelines for speech and language therapists. The guidelines on management of older people with communication problems set out the following as key features of service delivery:

- provision of assessment and intervention for communication and swallowing disorders
- delivery of services with and through other health professionals and carers within the client's environment, as well as to the client
- working within a multidisciplinary framework, sharing goals of intervention with other health professionals and carers
- enabling carers and other health professionals to understand clearly the communication strengths and needs of each client and providing the opportunity for those concerned to develop the appropriate skills in facilitating the client's communication.

NORMAL COMMUNICATION

Speech and language therapists working with clients of any age are required to use their knowledge of normal communication processes. Communication describes a diverse set of skills that allow human beings to exchange information and express emotion. These skills demand the synergy of voice, speech, language and cognition (Maxim and Bryan, 1994) and the ability to convey messages through written text and gesture.

What is involved in communication? Language and cognitive skills (memory, attention) are used together for verbal communication in most contexts. Voice and speech are produced by transforming respiration into sound and by shaping sounds through articulation to produce speech. The language processing system transforms thought into spoken or written words and understands what is heard or read. Cognition is the process whereby knowledge is acquired and includes perception, intuition, memory and reasoning. The term 'communication' incorporates all these skills. In addition, the pragmatic use of language describes the uses of any of these skills within a particular social context (Davis and Wilcox, 1985). An example of the successful synergy of speech, language, cognition, gesture and pragmatics can be observed in everyday communication situations.

NORMAL COMMUNICATION CHANGES IN OLDER PEOPLE

Communication skills in older people may change because of the normal biological ageing process or because of a pathology; an abnormal change. It is necessary to differentiate between these two forms of change when evaluating the need for intervention. However, despite the need to determine cause and effect, a completely accurate differential diagnosis may be difficult to make because of the confounding influences of institutionalisation and social isolation. Biological ageing includes changes to neuro-cognitive abilities, sensory motor and musculo-skeletal systems as follows:

- Verbal and language mediated tasks do not greatly change with age (Craik and Salthouse, 1992; Kemper and O'Hanlon, 2000).
- Some aspects of cognition that support language change with increasing age (Rabbitt, 1965; Clarke, 1980).
- Deficits in cognition contribute to the decline in the understanding and use of language (Maccobby, 1971; Rabbitt, 1979).
- Attention deficits may be caused by changes in both visual, perceptual and auditory processing (Ball et al., 1988; Schonfield et al., 1982).
- The understanding of complex syntax, ambiguous sentences, inferences and word or clause order shows some decline with age (Kemper and O'Hanlon, 2000).

LANGUAGE PROCESSING

Comparative research on language use across the age range is limited due to methodological constraints. The important variables of education, cultural differences, dialect, change in language use and code switching in speaking styles are difficult to control. However, older adults show psychomotor slowing in language processing and an increase in performance errors when speaking that may be attributed to retrieval difficulties; older people need a longer period of time to process and organise language output, fill in this processing time by increasing the frequency of pauses and interjections, and may use sentence repair (changing what is said either to clarify or to correct an error) more frequently.

VOICE CHANGES

There are well-recognised voice changes during the normal ageing process. Frequency, loudness and rhythm are prone to biological change. Voice change in ageing is most often considered to be secondary to normal biological change. These changes are due to:

- irregular patterns of expiration during phonation (Luchsinger and Arnold, 1965)
- changes in the respiratory mechanism and endocrine function (Hollien, 1987)
- inappropriate use of a louder voice that places a strain on the vocal mechanism, secondary to impaired hearing (see also Chapter 20F)
- respiratory problems associated with chronic obstructive airway disease
- changes in natural dentition or badly fitting dentures (see also Chapter 20B).

WHAT FACTORS INFLUENCE COMMUNICATION?

When assessing an older person's communicative competence, it is essential to consider a number of environmental and sensory factors that may have secondary effects on a person's ability to communicate such as:

- environment
- hearing (see also Chapter 20F)
- vision and perceptual difficulties (see also Chapter 20E).

The environment

The environment has a strong influence on communication. 'The improvement of communication skills and opportunities of older individuals in all settings must be considered a right and not a privilege, a priority and not a by-product and a reality not an ideal' (Lubinski, 1991). It is well recognised that a person's ability to communicate is significantly influenced by opportunities to interact, mental and physical stimulation, as well as other people with whom the person may come into contact. Social isolation is commonplace in the older population, whether the person is still living at home or in residential care. The majority of research has been carried out in settings such as hospitals, nursing and rest homes. In many of those settings a 'communication impaired environment' exists (Lubinski, 1991).

Aspects of the environment that are particularly crucial for good communication are the physical and the social environments. The physical environment refers to key features such as the layout of furniture (chairs round the walls is all too commonplace and often done for the best possible reasons, for example safety), lighting, acoustics and privacy. The social environment refers to opportunities to communicate, for instance discussion groups and communication groups, and factors that may limit communication, such as TV and radio as background noise. Ways to change an environment in order to facilitate communication include: through staff training; altering the physical environment (arranging chairs in groups with good access so safety is not compromised); and directly through encouraging setting up of opportunities to interact and communicate, such as giving choices (activities, meals, clothes and outings) and group activities (see Bryan and Maxim (1998) and Orange *et al.* (1995) for reviews of this area).

In a poor communication environment, a communicatively disordered individual's difficulties will often be increased. As a member of the multidisciplinary team, the speech and language therapist has a major role in working with carers and staff on communication disorders in general and specifically with older people who have a communication disorder, to ensure awareness of strategies as well as specific activities to facilitate the communication process.

Older people may use or be helped to use new technology such as a mobile phone, which will reduce possible feelings of isolation and compensate for reduced mobility. Over the next decade, a new generation of older people will need health care who are computer users and have accessed the Internet during their work life or used e-mail to maintain contact with children. This new generation may require support to continue their use of this new technology.

Social networks become increasingly important in old age. The different needs of ethnic minority elders should be considered and contacts maintained with local organisations (see also Chapter 3). If English has not been the first language or most used language for an individual, after a stroke or in Alzheimer's disease the older person may lose the ability to communicate in English, although they may be able to use another language effectively. A speech and language therapy assessment, in conjunction with the family and a trained interpreter, may be necessary to find out the best language for communication. Lack of appropriate social stimulation because of differences in culture or language may also reduce opportunities for communication and increase isolation.

Hearing

Hearing is dependent on the auditory system, which undergoes a number of changes with age in the outer, middle and particularly the inner ear. Hearing loss is an important factor in communication difficulty for a large number of older people. It is vital that members of the interdisciplinary team check on hearing abilities of patients and that they are fully aware of the effects of hearing loss on the individual (Maxim and Bryan, 1994) (see further Chapter 20F). Because hearing loss is seen as part of normal ageing, there is often a delay before advice is sought, which further delays the development of coping strategies (Gravell, 1988). Interaction is often difficult as obviously the listener role is affected, but the patient's own speech may suffer, for example with increased loudness. Non-verbal communication is affected, for instance eye contact is reduced as the listener concentrates on the speaker's mouth. Management should ideally include assessment and provision of appropriate amplification aids as well as training in compensatory techniques (Gravell, 1988) (see also Chapter 20F).

Helpful strategies include:

- reducing background noise
- gaining attention before speaking to the person
- facing the person to allow lip-reading
- ensuring light is on the communication partner's face
- not raising voice loudness, which can distort the speech signal.

The visual system

The visual system also undergoes changes with ageing. The most common disorders include cataracts and glaucoma, often in conjunction with aspects of normal ageing such as changes to long and short sightedness. Neurological disorders (e.g. stroke) may also cause visual and perceptual difficulties, such as neglect, inattention and homonymous hemianopia, all of which need to be considered carefully when assessing a patient. The effects of visual difficulties on communication include direct influences such as reading and writing difficulties, reduced ability in making use of non-verbal communication leading to misunderstandings and indirect influences such as increased isolation. Management includes assessment by the appropriate professional (see Chapter 20e), and the provision of glasses, magnifying glasses, adapted reading material (e.g. large print) and good lighting. In rehabilitation settings, where patients may have visual field or attentional difficulties, it is common for therapists to work from the side that has the visual loss in order to encourage adaptation and visual scanning. For the speech and language therapist, working with a patient who has a communication disorder, this mode of work may only add to the impact of the disorder and make intervention less effective. It is important for the SALT to agree this change of approach with the team, explaining why it may make intervention less effective.

Helpful strategies include:

- using touch to alert the person to the communication focus
- providing extra information to compensate for loss of non-verbal communication
- large print
- taking into account any hearing problems that may be present.

TYPES OF COMMUNICATION PROBLEMS

The main terms used to describe types of acquired communication problems in older people are:

- aphasia
- dysarthria
- dyspraxia.

Aphasia

Aphasia is often used interchangeably with dysphasia; aphasia means a total loss of language, while dysphasia means a partial loss of language. The term 'aphasia' in this chapter is defined by the RCSLT, in *Communicating Quality 2*, as follows: 'A language disorder resulting from localised neurological damage. It may present the patient with difficulties in the perception, recognition, comprehension and expression of language through both the verbal and/or written modalities' (RCSLT, 1996). Using and understanding other symbol systems (gestures, numbers) may also be compromised.

Aphasia is an umbrella term for a number of sub-types of language disorder. These sub-types usually represent as a cluster of symptoms that often occur together. It may be helpful to think of aphasia as having two main forms:

1. **A non-fluent aphasia** is often associated with a right hemiplegia or hemiparesis and right homonymous hemianopia. Broca's aphasia and transcortical motor aphasia are subtypes of fluent aphasia.

Communication is characterised by the following:

- Understanding conversation appears to be better than expression.
- The patient is aware of his or her errors, is often frustrated and attempts to self-correct.
- Spoken output is slow, effortful and consists mainly of content words.
- There are word finding difficulties.
- There is perseveration.
- There is use of non-verbal communication such as gesture, pointing and facial expression to convey information.
- Understanding of written material usually mirrors understanding of spoken language.
- Writing is commonly impaired. There may be a spelling disorder or legibility is often a problem due to paresis of the hand or having to use the left hand in a normally right-handed person.

2. **A fluent aphasia** is not always associated with a hemiplegia or hemiparesis. Sub-types of fluent aphasia are Wernicke's, Anomic, Conduction and Transcortical sensory aphasia.

Communication is characterised by the following:

- Understanding is often impaired, sometimes severely in Wernicke's aphasia.
- There are word finding difficulties – the patient may use non-words in place of real words.
- There is poor awareness of own errors and few attempts at self-correction, consequently the person is often unaware a problem exists with communication. A study investigating people whose fluent aphasia had resolved, found that most people believed that their communication had been either normal or relatively normal (Ross, 1993).
- There is an easy flow of speech, which is often 'empty', lacking in content words and conveys little meaning, though there may be some appropriate language in conjunction with jargon.
- Understanding of written material is also impaired, usually at the same level as understanding of spoken language, though the visual channel may aid understanding in some people.
- Writing is abnormal, often resembling the spoken output by lacking meaning.

Finally, **global dysphasia** presents with a range of accompanying neurological signs representative of severe brain damage. These include visual field defects, hemiplegia and sensory loss. Communication is characterised by severe difficulties in understanding spoken and written language, and in using spoken and written language. People with global aphasia often try to communicate via non-verbal communication such as gestures and facial expression. Relatives and clinicians may mistake such behaviours as an indicator of true understanding of language when it is the context that has been understood rather than language itself. If available, language output is often limited to jargon or repetitive stereotyped utterances that convey little meaning.

Dysarthria

Dysarthria is defined as a 'collective name for a group of related speech disorders that are due to disturbances in muscular control of the speech mechanism resulting from impairment of any of the basic motor processes involved in the execution of speech' (Darley *et al.*, 1975). Anarthria is the most severe form with no speech but vocalisations are still possible.

Traditionally the dysarthrias have been classified in terms of lesion site. However, it may be more helpful to identify the areas of breakdown and undertake a more descriptive analysis of parameters, which enables the speech and language therapist to decide on appropriate management, such as:

- respiration (how well does breathing support voice and speech?)
- phonation (how good is voice production?)
- articulation speech (how clear are speech sounds in words and sentence?)
- resonance (does speech sound nasal?)
- intelligibility (how well can speech be understood?).

Dyspraxia

Dyspraxia of speech is a disorder of voluntary movement for speech. The person may be able to speak or move their orofacial musculature when they are not consciously thinking about doing so, but cannot do the same movements when asked to do so. This leads to reduced intelligibility of spoken output and, for some people with a severe dyspraxia, an alternative form of communication may be needed. It has also been defined by Darly *et al.* (1975) as 'a disorder of motor speech programming manifested primarily by errors in articulation and secondarily by compensatory alterations of prosody. The speaker shows reduced efficiency in accomplishing the oral postures for production of words. The disorder is most commonly associated with aphasia but may also occur in isolation'.

CAUSES OF COMMUNICATION DISORDERS IN OLDER PEOPLE

The most common causes of communication disorders in problems in older people are:

- stroke
- Alzheimer's disease
- multi-infarct dementia
- Parkinson's disease
- pseudo-dementia/depression
- head injury.

Stroke

Stroke (cerebro-vascular accident or CVA) is common in older people and the incidence increases with age. The resulting disability will depend on the area of cerebral tissue that is damaged and the extent of that damage. The communication disorders that may result are aphasia (a disorder of language), dysarthria (a disorder of movement for speech) and dyspraxia (a disorder of voluntary control of speech and orofacial movement). Aphasia and dyspraxia are usually caused by acquired brain damage to the left hemisphere of the brain. For most people, the left hemisphere is dominant for language. That is, most language processing is carried out in the left hemisphere. For people who are left handed, this cerebral dominance is not always so strong and a small minority of left-handed people do most of their language processing in the right hemisphere.

Alzheimer's disease

Alzheimer's disease is the most common form of dementia in the UK and north America. The dementias are a group of diseases that can be defined as: the global disturbance of higher cortical functions including memory; the capacity to solve problems of everyday living; the performance of learned perceptuo-motor skills; the correct use of social skills and control of emotional reactions, in the absence of clouding of consciousness (RCP Committee on Geriatrics, 1981).

In older people, many of the symptoms of a dementia may also appear in other conditions, e.g. confusional states following acute infections, a raised temperature, dehydration or surgery, and also in depressions and anxiety states. In the dementias that damage the cortex, the effect on communication will usually be to make language less easy to understand for the listener, with key information words missing, although language will often be fluently produced and sentences will be well structured.

The language disorders associated with the dementias are often referred to as aphasia/dysphasia, but there are crucial differences between aphasia following stroke and language disorder in the dementias. Bayles *et al.* (1982) identified five key differences between communication problems in aphasia and those secondary to a dementia:

1 Aphasia occurs secondary to a sudden onset (usually stroke), whereas in the dementias, language impairment develops more slowly over time.
2 Deterioration of language in a dementia is progressive, but this is not usually the case in aphasia post stroke where language often makes some recovery in the first few months post stroke.
3 Aphasia is due to focal lesions, whereas a dementia is accompanied by the diffuse brain atrophy.
4 Aphasia usually has a minimal effect on intellect, whereas loss of reasoning and memory abilities are a primary feature of dementing pathologies.
5 Aphasic patients can present with a dissociation between verbal and non-verbal abilities, whereas most patients with a dementia show simultaneous deterioration of both verbal and non-verbal functions.

These differences provide the basis for an accurate diagnosis and appropriate management but, in the clinical environment, this differential diagnosis may be difficult and require an interdisciplinary team assessment. There are often complex communication problems and behaviours: in particular, people with a fluent aphasia post stroke, who may have no other defining neurological symptoms, those in the early stages of Alzheimer's disease or who have multi-infarct dementia (Gravell, 1988), or rare forms of dementia called progressive dysphasia or semantic dementia (Bryan and Maxim, 1996; Snowden and Griffiths, 2000). In a fluent aphasia post stroke, language is produced fluently although the content may be difficult to understand and, because the lesion is posterior to that part of the brain that controls motor function, there is no hemiparesis.

Multi-infarct dementia

Multi-infarct dementia (MID) or vascular dementia, as its name suggests, results from small and often silent multiple infarctions in the cerebral tissue as a consequence of multiple vessel occlusions (Murdoch, 1990). MID is usually marked by an abrupt onset with stepwise deterioration and fluctuating progression (Bryan and Maxim, 1996). MID is likely to arise from occlusion of the carotid and vertebrobasilar artery systems. Signs and symptoms, including speech and language problems, depend on the location of the damage.

Parkinson's disease

Parkinson's disease causes speech problems in at least 50 per cent of cases (Oxtoby, 1982). Speech is notably dysarthric and some of the main features include a monotonous voice, altered and usually fast rate of speech, imprecise articulation and difficulty with initiation, leading to decreased intelligibility (Bryan and Maxim, 1996). There is also some evidence that language changes occur throughout the duration of the disease and it is likely that linguistic behaviour declines in parallel to other cognitive changes (Knight, 1992). Huber *et al.* (1989) identified difficulties arising from a reduced speed in processing information. Other research findings have identified naming difficulties and auditory comprehension difficulties (Matison *et al.*, 1982; Lieberman *et al.*, 1990). In a minority of people with Parkinson's disease, there may also be signs of a dementia.

Parkinson's disease is sometimes listed as a cause of sub-cortical dementia. This form of dementia is often associated with dysarthria. Speech is characterised by monotony, syllabic stress and fading volume, and patients may not exhibit the same level of language problems that are evident in cortical dementia (Murdoch, 1990).

Depressive illness

In depressive illness, language output can be severely limited although linguistic competence is not altered (Bryan and Maxim, 1996). Speech and language symptoms include: poor attention, lack of interaction, repetition of questions, short phrases and sentences, reduced volume, monotonous intonation, frequent pauses and hesitations. Older people have an increased incidence and prevalence of depression, which also puts them at risk of illnesses arising from self-neglect. They may be admitted to hospital or a community programme for assessment of pseudo-dementia, a condition caused by depression, that presents like a dementia but should respond to treatment.

A significant proportion of patients in rehabilitation post stroke suffer from 'low mood' at some point of their treatment (Intercollegiate Working Party for Stroke, 2000). Depression is commonly associated with an affective reaction occurring in patients with a speech-language disorder such as aphasia (Wahrborg, 1991). Speech and language therapists may often identify the signs and symptoms of depression in patients who are attending their clinics. While entry to rehabilitation may help depression, most patients will need referral to a medical specialist for intervention and medication.

Speech and language therapists working with the older patient are often called on to assist with a differential diagnosis of depression and dementia. They must recognise the clinical signs and symptoms that are associated with these disorders, and liaise closely with relatives and other health-care professionals in order to make an accurate diagnosis.

Traumatic head injury

Traumatic head injury has an increased incidence in older people (often due to falls) and can cause communication problems that will vary according to the location of the damage. In older people who have a history of alcohol abuse or who may have undiagnosed cerebrovascular disease, a head injury may lead to a dementia. Head injury may cause a range of communication deficits; speech production difficulties, a specific language disorder or a language disorder caused by cognitive deficits such as poor memory and reasoning.

MANAGEMENT OF COMMUNICATION DIFFICULTIES

Speech and language therapists should become involved at the earliest opportunity in order to advise the team on future management. The emphasis for management will change as the patient moves through the rehabilitation process. In the acute and early rehabilitation phase the emphasis is on identifying the type of impairment, making predictions about the extent of disability that may occur and advising the IDT, the patient and their family on what will assist communication. The ultimate goal in conjunction with the patient/carer is to concentrate on minimising the impact of social disadvantage that may occur as a result of the original impairment and maximising the communicative potential.

Management and treatment options that may be considered include the following:

- face-to-face therapy
- group therapy
- education and advice to other health-care professionals and/or carers
- referral to other agencies.

Initial assessment attempts to establish a differential diagnosis, together with the degree of impairment and handicap (social disadvantage). The speech and language therapist needs to have a clear picture of the following:

- the patient's ability to understand spoken and written language on formal assessment and in a variety of social situations
- the patient's ability to use spoken and written language on formal assessment and in a variety of social situations

- the patient's motor speech function, i.e. how intelligible they are in a variety of social settings
- the patient's use (and potential for use) of communication strategies, facial expression and augmentative methods of communication in order to make their needs known
- the patient's level of cognitive abilities (such as memory, reasoning and orientation to person, place and time), and any sensory deficits (such as hearing loss, or visual or perceptual disturbances).

Following assessment, the therapist will need to discuss future management strategies and options with patients, relatives and other members of the multidisciplinary team. If direct therapy is thought to be of benefit, a designated block of treatment and goals needs to be agreed between therapist and patient. Communication disorders are often complex and it is prudent to outline the experimental nature of some forms of intervention so that therapist, patient and carer do not feel that they have failed if all their goals are not met. Review of goals following a period of treatment is essential in monitoring outcome (Enderby, 1997). It may be that some adjustments will need to be made to goal setting or that an alternative option of management is necessary if primary goals are not being met.

The evidence base for interventions is now strong in some areas of speech and language therapy. Group therapy has shown positive outcomes for patients with Parkinson's disease wishing to improve speech intelligibility (Robertson and Thomson, 1983; Scott and Caird, 1983). This type of group therapy approach is also very popular for enhancing total communication strategies in dysphasic patients and helps reduce social isolation, but evidence of effectiveness in this situation is sparse. The evidence for intensive and specific interventions for aphasia is good for intensive therapy of four to eight weeks (at least daily therapy), for specific language programmes evaluated in small group and single case studies (Intercollegiate Working Party for Stroke, 2000). There is also evidence that assessment and provision of augmentative communication aids is effective (Intercollegiate Working Party for Stroke, 2000) in patients with dysarthria and dyspraxia.

The use of trained assistants, under supervision of a SALT, to help run groups and to act as a communication facilitator for individual patients is an important resource. In the role of facilitator, assistants can accompany patients on shopping trips and aid in successful communication exchanges. This type of support can be compared to providing immobile patients with wheelchairs, which offers them more access opportunities. By providing chronic language impaired patients with communication support, in the form of trained assistants, they have more opportunities to engage in normal communication events outside the home or care setting.

Education and advice to relatives, other carers and the rehabilitation team is essential in ameliorating communication disability. The patient's communication partners need to understand the cause of the difficulty and its manifestations in order to engage in successful communication exchanges and capitalise on the use of compensatory strategies. Where older people are in residential care, a range of activities such as reminiscence groups, life stories, conversation analysis and validation approaches may prove vital in aiding social interaction for patients with a dementia and in improving their quality of life (Bryan and Maxim, 1998; see also Chapter 9).

The speech and language therapist will need to advise members of the multi-disciplinary team on how best to facilitate successful communication between themselves and the language disordered patient. It is therefore essential that SALTs work alongside their colleagues in the therapy, nursing and medical professions, both to understand the SALT's role, in which ways communication can be enhanced and to ensure reciprocity of support. Speech and language therapists are trained to understand the benefits to this reciprocal approach to management and education.

The speech and language therapist may need to refer the patient to other agencies (such as social services), other health-care professionals (when the diagnosis is in doubt) or support groups in the voluntary sector (such as the Stroke Association, Parkinson's Disease Society), which can provide long-term contacts.

Patients need to adjust to the new and often frightening situation in which they find themselves. It is often helpful for those conversing with the patient to use the following strategies:

- Watch the patient's face, maintain eye contact where possible, use appropriate facial expression.
- Keep sentences short and to the point.
- Observe the patient's reaction to gauge if they are listening to you.
- Allow pauses of silence while the patient processes what is being said.
- Be prepared to repeat, rephrase, demonstrate, write or draw your question if necessary (think what it must be like trying to communicate in a foreign country where nobody understands you – What can you do to get the message across?).
- Encourage the patient to respond to you in any way that conveys their meaning
- Use routine situations, such as washing and dressing and mealtimes, to encourage patients to communicate.
- Ask key questions, regarding the lavatory, drink, pain, relatives, etc.

If you completely fail to understand the patient, or they you, admit to the problem and say you will try again later. Do not pretend you have understood the communication attempt if you have not done so.

Managing communication disorders in the acute care setting is often a challenging business. Communication charts or aids may be given or requested by other health professionals with the best intentions, but patients may be unable to use them for a variety of reasons and there is little evidence of their effectiveness, unless they are used in a highly structured context. Patients' difficulties with using communication charts/aids include:

- diminished consciousness level
- impaired concentration/attention
- visual/perceptual impairment
- inability to recognise symbols, letters or words
- lack of knowledge or practice in using communication charts to indicate their needs or convey information.

CASE STUDY A COMMUNICATION PROBLEM

OM, aged 74, was admitted to a non-acute rehabilitation ward four weeks post-onset from an acute unit. The reasons for transfer were severe communication problems, and non-compliance with rehabilitation goals (at this time awaiting appointment of speech-language therapist in acute unit). In the opinion of the admitting consultant, the availability of speech and language therapy was crucial to meeting OM's rehabilitation goals.

Initial assessment showed a moderate dysphasia with difficulty in understanding spoken and written language as well as language production. However, OM made very good use of facial expression and gesture. The initial goals were as follows:

- encourage use of facial expression and gestures by OM, as well as staff and relatives to aid OM's understanding
- encourage automatic speech (e.g. counting) to help regain confidence in speech output
- encourage OM to finish sentences, e.g. wash my face. This was used by the nurses and occupational therapist in activities of daily living.

Understanding improved rapidly but speech returned slowly, leaving OM with dyspraxic type speech, which was often unintelligible to the listener. The following goals were then set:

- continued encouragement of use of gestures and facial expression
- encourage OM to slow down speech
- feedback when speech not understood, in order to encourage OM to monitor and listen to own speech
- encourage activities/games such as Connect Four, Noughts and Crosses, reading newspapers and magazines. Simple cognitive games are useful in engaging patients in social interaction, developing concentration and attention skills and are immediately rewarding in outcome
- writing of own and family names, so able to sign cards
- telling the time to promote independence and orientation.

OM was seen daily and new goals were set on a weekly basis by the interdisciplinary team.

Outcome

Mild difficulties in spoken and written understanding. Moderate difficulties in spoken and written output. Returned home and continued rehabilitation in a local day hospital. Referral to local Stroke Association. OM's future communication needs will be met by the voluntary sector. Needs have been well met by speech-language therapy service, by a combination of direct therapy and close liaison with the relatives who have utilised OM's total communication skills. OM's relatives have been encouraged to contact the speech and language therapist following discharge if the situation alters.

FEEDING AND SWALLOWING PROBLEMS

Older people are more at risk of developing feeding and swallowing problems than younger adults because of the interrelated problems of physical and mental illness and the greater likelihood that they will have multiple pathologies (Nilsson et al., 1996). Age-related physiological changes (such as reduced thirst and increased susceptibility to dehydration), chronic disease and medication (see also Chapter 20c) can influence:

• swallowing function
• behavioural and cognitive function
• ability to self-feed.

These difficulties can lead to additional problems of:

• dehydration
• inadequate nutrient intake (see also Chapter 20A)
• chest infection/aspiration pneumonia.

Swallowing problems are not uncommon in the older population. Steele et al. (1997) found that 68 per cent of residents in nursing homes had a specific dysphagia. The incidence of dysphagia secondary to stroke is reported to be 45 per cent, usually associated with more severe strokes and with worse outcome (Intercollegiate Working Party for Stroke, 2000). Progressive neurological disease and the dementias that are most prevalent in the older population are also well recognised for contributing to dysphagia and feeding disorders. Feinberg et al. (1990) concludes that dysphagia in older people may be due to neuromuscular disease, debilitation, dementia, depression and structural abnormality.

Many older people are prescribed a variety of medications that may have an adverse effect on eating practice and swallowing function (Weiden and Harrigan, 1986; see also Chapter 20C). Some drugs affect nutritional intake by impairing the appetite, causing nausea and altering the sense of taste. Sedative drugs, or those that cause disorientation and confusion, can have a significant influence on swallowing. Medication that has an action or side-effect of diminishing oral secretions can result in drying of the oral and pharyngeal mucosae and adversely influence swallowing in three main ways:

• reduction of saliva to bind food particles to form a bolus
• reduction of saliva to lubricate the oral cavity (this aids oral transit and protects the oral mucosae)
• inhibition of the swallow 'reflex'.

Antipsychotic drugs are known to contribute to dystonia and tardive dyskinesis, movement disorders of the face, jaw and tongue, which interfere with the initiation and control of mastication and swallowing.

Orophayngeal dysphagia (or difficulty with chewing and swallowing) affects both the voluntary and automatic aspects of the oral-pharyngeal swallow function and this may deteriorate or be lost when not practised for even relatively brief periods.

Problems associated with dysphagia

Aspiration is known to occur during sleep in the normal population (Huxley *et al.*, 1978). However, if lung function is impaired then the risk of pneumonia increases with either single or recurrent episodes of aspiration. Aspiration is know to account for 6 per cent of deaths following stroke in ambulant survivors (Elliott, 1988). However, Kidd *et al.* (1995), found that post stroke, while 42 per cent of people were aspirating at 72 hours, only 8 per cent were still aspirating at three months. There is evidence for the effectiveness of assessment using a validated bedside protocol and all patients with a suspected abnormal swallow should be referred to a speech and language therapist (Intercollegiate Working Party for Stroke, 2000).

Dysphagia and severe malnutrition causing admission to hospital carries a 13 per cent risk of mortality regardless of aetiology (Sitzman, 1990). It is known that nutritional state influences both length of stay and eventual outcome in the older patient (Cederholm and Hellstrom, 1992; Unosson *et al.*, 1994). Not only does dysphagia contribute to mortality and morbidity, but also to psycho-social complications such as social isolation and embarrassment, which can be resolved with a team approach to management (Emick-Herring and Wood, 1990).

Management of feeding and swallowing disorders

Dysphagia is now recognised as an important consequence of neurological illness (Whitaker and Romer, 1993). Early identification of swallowing problems is essential in reducing mortality and morbidity, and in minimising psychological sequalae such as fear, embarrassment and social isolation. In some conditions swallowing problems are not evident at the time of the diagnosis of the disease, but as the disease progresses swallowing function can become severely impaired. Some patients exhibit dysphagia as the first and only sign of their disease, while others experience dysphagia in a constellation of other signs and symptoms, which makes it difficult to determine to what extent dysphagia is contributing to morbidity and mortality.

A systematic approach to assessment is essential and should be tailored to individual needs. However, the patient's needs are often complex and management requires a coordinated multidisciplinary approach with both patient and relatives. The keystone of effective multidisciplinary coordination is good communication and liaison.

In acute and community hospitals, the core team members most often called upon for advice are as follows:

- Speech-language therapists, whose main responsibility is often to coordinate the dysphagia rehabilitation programme.
- Dieticians make recommendations regarding nutritional needs, the use of supplements and non-oral feeding methods and regimes. The dietician is the primary resource for ensuring that the patient's nutritional needs are in line with ethnic dietary habits and practice (see also Chapter 20A).
- On the ward, the nursing staff are the key professionals who initially identify swallowing or feeding problems. They have the crucial responsibility for

monitoring the patient's daily nutritional intake, maintaining oral hygiene and supervising eating at mealtimes (see Chapter 14).

- The physiotherapists contribute to assessment of swallowing when patients have a tracheostomy or are ventilated. They provide advice on positioning and deliver chest physiotherapy (see Chapter 15).
- The occupational therapist provides advice on adaptive equipment and may help to promote independent feeding skills in patients who have visual and perceptual impairment (see Chapter 16).
- The patient's physician coordinates specialist investigations from neurologists and the ENT department etc., and contributes to decisions regarding oral/non-oral feeding (see Chapter 13).

Older people often remain in hospital because of an unresolved swallowing disorder and concomitant poor nutritional status. One intervention for older people who are going back home or into residential care is a percutaneous endoscopic gastrostomy (PEG), which allows nutrition via non-oral means. This requires surgery and continuing care of the PEG tube but is much better tolerated than a naso-gastric tube (Intercollegiate Working Party for Stroke, 2000).

CASE STUDY SUSAN HUNTER – A SWALLOWING PROBLEM

Susan Hunter aged 79 years, was referred to speech and language therapy by the nursing team, 24 hours after admission for assessment, and advice regarding her swallowing difficulties. Speech-language therapy assessment and observation identified the following:

- The patient was drowsy but attempted to attend to social contact.
- The chest was clear (according to physiotherapy evaluation).
- At this stage auditory understanding appeared to be severely impaired but situational understanding was apparent.
- Assessment of cranial nerves for swallowing indicated the following level of dysfunction:
    - 7th CN facial nerve; face asymmetrical, affected on left side
    - 9th CN glossopharanyngeal; gag diminished
    - 10th CN vagus; difficult to determine as no speech available, and unable to cough on command
    - 12th CN hypoglossal; tongue asymmetrical on protrusion.

Functional swallow – coughed on thin fluids, managed thickened fluids and puréed food on assessment. However, despite the ability to swallow some food consistencies safely, she was unable to meet her nutritional needs without supplements.

Supplements were provided by the dietician because of severe fatigue during mealtimes, i.e. tended to manage only a few teaspoons. Case discussion between medical, nursing and therapy staff resulted in the following goals being set:

- An adequate oral diet using appropriate food textures and consistency. This consisted of high protein puréed diet, thickened fluids and supplements. All oral intake was monitored on a regular basis to ensure nutritional needs were being met.
- Supervised feeding in the early stages of recovery – was spoon-fed by nursing staff.
- Supervised while self-feeding – equipment provided by occupational therapist to enhance self-feeding skills and independence.
- Weighed weekly.

Outcome

All swallowing problems resolved over the next five to six weeks. Independent with feeding, maintained weight.

Summary

The aim of this chapter has been to describe the range of communication impairments the older person may experience as part of disease or illness, but which may be made worse by the interaction with the normal ageing process. The concept of the 'client' or 'customer' centred approach to rehabilitation is also a key feature. Our definition of rehabilitation is to minimise the impact of communication or swallowing disorders on daily living. Active collaboration with other health-care professionals furthers mutual understanding and drives the need to achieve desired outcomes. Most clinicians will recognise that the focus of 'rehabilitation' often falls to the relatives and carers because it is they who need to understand how best to determine what the issues are, what opportunities the patient has to communicate and what system they can use to indicate their intention to communicate.

Speech and language therapists recognise the need to deliver high quality services that meet the needs of individual patients, their relatives/carers and other health-care professionals. Commissioners need professional advice on how to prioritise services and what form of management they should take. An innovative approach to management is needed if we are to continue supplying speech and language therapy services to a growing older population. The use of assistants and the voluntary sector is often considered to be a cheaper and effective resource, but the evidence for this is lacking. Effective training of volunteers and assistants needs to be researched with carefully targeted patient populations to ensure that an appropriate service is being delivered and that this way of providing a service is cost-effective. Older people with more chronic communication disorders must have access to services that understand their needs to avoid social isolation and retain mental health. Access to group or individual treatment is essential during the patient's lifetime as situations and lifestyles change. We need to consider carefully how to provide this resource from limited means.

The small number of speech and language therapists working with older people in the NHS has required the speech and language therapist to act as a consultant who assesses patients, liaises with primary and secondary health-care teams, and helps design a package of care that fully utilises assistants, the voluntary sector and social services.

This package of care can then be evaluated and changed with input from the team so that the changing needs of the older person are fully taken into account. For this method of service delivery to work, the speech and language therapist has to become an integral member of the interdisciplinary team, with shared knowledge and goals.

REFERENCES

Ball, K.K., Beard, B.L., Roenker, D.L., Miller, R.L. and Griggs, D.S. (1988) Age and visual search: expanding the useful field of view. *Journal of the Optical Society of America*, 5, 2210–2219.

Bayles, K.A., Tomoeda, C.K. and Caffrey, J.T. (1982) Language and dementia producing diseases. *Communicative Disorders*, 7, 131–146.

Bryan, K. and Maxim, J. (eds) (1996) *Communication Disability and the Psychiatry of Old Age*, Whurr, London.

Bryan, K. and Maxim, J. (1998) Enabling care staff to relate to older communication disabled people. *International Journal of Language and Communication Disorders*, 33, 121–125.

Cederholm, T. and Hellstrom, K. (1992) Nutritional status in recently hospitalized and free-living elderly subjects. *Gerontology*, 38, 105–110.

Clarke E.O. (1980) *Semantic and Episodic Memory Impairment in Normal and Cognitively Impaired Elderly Adults*, Language and Communication in the Elderly, DC Heath, Lexington, MA.

Craik, F. and Salthouse, T. (1992) *The Handbook of Ageing and Cognition*, Lawrence Erlbaum, Hillsdale, NJ.

Darley, E., Aronson, A. and Brown, J. (1975) *Motor Speech Disorders*, Lea & Febiger, Philadelphia.

Davis, G.A. and Wilcox, M.I. (1985) *Adult Aphasia Rehabilitation; Applied Pragmatics*, NFER-NELSON, Windsor.

Department of Health (2001) *The National Service Framework for Older People*, Stationery Office, London. www.doh.gov.uk/nsf/olderpeople.htm

Elliott, J.L. (1988) Swallowing disorders in the elderly: a guide to diagnosis and treatment. *Geriatrics*, 43, 95–113.

Emick-Herring, B. and Wood, P. (1990) A team approach to neurologically based swallowing disorders. *Rehabilitation Nursing*, 15.

Enderby, P. (1997) *Therapy Outcome Measures: Speech-language pathology*, Singular, London.

Feinberg, M.J., Knebl, J., Tully, J. and Segall, L. (1990) Aspiration in the elderly. *Dysphagia*, 5, 61–72.

Gravell, R. (1988) *Communication Problems in Elderly People: Practical approaches to management*, Croom Helm, London.

Hollien, H. (1987) Old voices: what do we really know about them? *Journal Voice*, 1(1), 2–17.

Huber, S.J., Shuttleworth, E.C. and Freidenberg, D.L. (1989) Neuropsychological differences between the dementias of Alzheimer's and Parkinson's disease. *Archives of Neurology*, 46, 1287–1291.

Huxley, E.J., Viroslav, J., Gray, W.R. and Pierce, A.K. (1978) Pharyngeal aspiration in normal adults and patients with depressed consciousness. *American Journal of Medicine*, **64**, 564–568.

Intercollegiate Working Party for Stroke (2000) *National Clinical Guidelines for Stroke*, Royal College of Physicians, London.

Kemper, S. and O'Hanlon, L. (2000) Semantic processing problems of older adults. In: *Semantic Processing: Theory and Practice* (eds Best, W., Bryan, K. and Maxim, J.), Whurr, London.

Kidd, D., Lawson, J., Nesbitt, R. and MacMahon, J. (1995) The natural history and clinical consequences of aspiration in acute stroke. *Quarterly Journal of Medicine*, **88**, 409–413.

Knight, R.G. (1992) *The Neuropsychology of Degenerative Brain Diseases*, Lawrence Earlbaum, Hillsdale, NJ.

Lieberman, P., Friedman, J. and Feldman, L.S. (1990) Syntax comprehension in Parkinson's disease. *Journal of Nervous and Mental Disease*, **178**, 360–366.

Lubinski, R. (1991) Language and aging: an environmental approach to intervention. *Topics in Language Disorders*, September, 89–97.

Luchsinger, R. and Amold, G.E. (1965) *Voice, Speech and Language*, Constable, London.

Maccoby, E.E. (1971) Age change in the selective perception of verbal materials. In: *The Perception of Language*, Charles E. Merrill, Columbus, OH.

Matison, R., Mayeux, R., Rosen, J. and Fahn, S. (1982) 'Tip-of-the-tongue' phenomena in Parkinson's disease. *Neurology*, **32**, 567–570.

Maxim, J. and Bryan, K. (1994) *Language of the Elderly: A clinical perspective*, Whurr, London.

Murdoch, B.E. (1990) *Acquired Speech and Language Disorders*, Chapman & Hall, London.

Nillson, H., Ekberg, O., Olsson, R. and Hindfelt, B. (1996) Quantitative aspects of swallowing in an elderly nondysphagic population. *Dysphagia*, **11**, 180–184.

Orange, J.B., Ryan, E.B., Meredith, S.B. and MacLean, M.J. (1995) Applications of a communication enhancement model for long term care residents with Alzheimer's disease. *Topics in Language Disorder*, **15**, 20–35.

Oxtoby, M. (1982) *Parkinson's Disease Patients and their Social Needs*, Parkinson's Disease Society, London.

Rabbitt, P. (1965) An age decrement in the ability to ignore irrelevant information, *Journal of Gerontology*, **20**, 233–238.

Rabbitt, P. (1979) Some experiments and a model for change in attentional selectivity with old age. In: *Brain Function in Old Age*, Springer, New York.

Rainbow, D., Painter, C. and Bryan, K. (1996) Working in the community – care and legislation. In: *Communication Disability and the Psychiatry of Old Age* (eds Bryan, K. and Maxim, J.), Whurr, London.

Robertson, S.J. and Thomson, F. (1983) Speech therapy in Parkinson's disease: a study of the efficacy and long term effects of intensive speech therapy. *British Journal of Disorders of Communication*, **370**, 10–12.

Ross, E.D. (1993) Acute agitation and other behaviours associated with Wernicke aphasia and their possible neurological bases. *Neuropsychiatry, Neuropsychology and Behavioural Neurology*, **6**, 9–18.

Royal College of Physicians Committee on Geriatrics (1981) Organic mental impairment in the elderly. *Journal of the Royal College of Physicians*, **15**, 142–167.

Royal College of Speech and Language Therapists [RCSLT] (1996) *Communicating Quality 2. Professional Standards for Speech and Language Therapists*, RCSLT, London.

Schonfield, D., Truman, V. and Kline, D. (1982) Recognition tests of dichotic listening and the age variable. *Journal of Gerontology*, **27**, 487–493.

Scott, S. and Caird, F.I. (1983) Speech therapy for Parkinson's disease. *Journal of Neurology, Neurosurgery and Psychiatry*, **46**, 104–144.

Sitzman, J.V. Jr (1990) Nutritional support of the dysphagic patient: methods, risks and complications of therapy. *Journal of Parenteral and Enteral Nutrition*, **14**, 60–63.

Steele, C.M., Greenwood, C., Ens, I., Robertson, C. and Seidman-Carlson, R. (1997) Mealtime difficulties in a home for the aged: not just dysphagia. *Dysphagia*, **12**, 43–50.

Snowden, J. and Griffiths, H. (2000) Semantic dementia: assessment and management. In: *Semantic Processing: Theory and practice* (eds Best, W., Bryan, K. and Maxim, J.). Whurr, London.

Unosson, M., Ek, A.C. Bjurulf, P. von Schenck, H. and Larsson, J. (1994) Feeding dependence and nutritional status after acute stroke. *Stroke*, **25**(2), 36–71.

Wahrborg, P. (1991) *Assessment and Management of Emotional and Psychosocial Reactions to Brain Damage and Aphasia*, Far Communications, Leicester.

Weiden, P. and Harrigan, M. (1986) A clinical guide for diagnosing and managing patients with drug induced dysphagia. *Hospital Community Psychiatry*, **37**, 3396–3398.

Whitaker, J. and Romer, J. (1993) The assessment and management of neurogenic swallowing disorders. In: *Neurological Rehabilitation* (eds Greenward, R., Barnes, M.P., MacMillan, T.M. and Ward, C.D.), Churchill Livingstone, Edinburgh.

18 FEET FIT FOR REHABILITATION

Olwen Finlay and Colin J. Fullerton

AIMS OF THE CHAPTER

This chapter describes the podiatrist's contribution to the interdisciplinary team. The authors describe older people as by far the biggest user group through both accumulation of problems over many decades, as well as problems specific to the disorder presented to the team. The importance of the feet and footwear to rehabilitation is emphasised, together with the need for all team members to identify and refer appropriate problems, especially of those at particular risk through circulatory disease and problems of balance. The authors describe the levels of footcare, emphasising the importance of good basic care by patients themselves, carers and care staff. The authors note that assessment and treatment of disordered feet and footwear is enhanced through a partnership between podiatrists and physiotherapists.

INTRODUCTION

Chiropodist is a title no longer used in the rest of the English-speaking world, so the profession in the UK has gradually been adopting the title 'podiatrist' in line with practice elsewhere. Until legislation changes, the term state registered chiropodist and podiatrist are used interchangably.

In older people, mobility, which is vital to the maintenance of many aspects of health, function and independence (Plummer and Stewart, 1996), is often hindered by foot problems, which are not felt to be important enough for the older person (family or formal carers) to seek advice or treatment. They may be embarrassed by the shape of their feet or other pathologies may possibly predominate their mind.

Many people accept foot problems as an inescapable accompaniment of ageing and often do not realise that change has occurred, due to its insidious or long-standing nature (Neale and Boyd, 1989). The most common reasons people seek medical attention for their feet are pain, deformity and instability (Goldman, 1993). Shoes have been noted by many authors as a contributing factor to falls in older people (Finlay, 1986; Nuffield Institute for Health, 1996; Richardson and Ashton-Miller, 1996; Munro and Steele, 1999), yet the effect of footwear on stability is often overlooked (Menz and Lord, 1999). While substitution of a shoe that lessens the risk of tripping may not prevent falls, it may represent an important feasible intervention in a complex situation.

A general assessment of the older person (see Chapter 8) by any team member is incomplete without including the feet and footwear, as many are admitted to hospital with ill-fitting, inappropriate, potentially dangerous or no shoes (Finlay, 1987; Kwok, 1994). It is essential that footcare teams have the skills and knowledge required of what to look for, how to manage it and when to refer (McInnes *et al.*, 1999).

INITIAL ASSESSMENT OF THE FEET

A brief screening assessment of the feet by any team member can quickly determine if referral is required for further management. It is estimated that 50 per cent of older people require foot health services (Clarke, 1969), while others require more basic care. The key is ensuring that needs are met appropriately, and carers' access to appropriate services for advice, training and assessment of the patient where warranted is essential.

Foot health management covers:

- basic footcare
- podiatry
- surgical podiatry.

All levels are complemented by the availability of suitable footwear and a team approach to ensure that feet are fit to facilitate rehabilitation. Although various health-care professionals can provide this service, physiotherapists are in a unique position to assess the patient's total mobility needs, and where this can be done in conjunction with a podiatrist, the outcome can be further enhanced. The philosophy and general remit of physiotherapy is included in Chapter 15.

Podiatry provides a comprehensive foot health service for conditions affecting the foot and lower limbs. For patients who have previously been examined by a state registered podiatrist, footcare assistants provide simple footcare under supervision. There are approximately 4,000 podiatrists employed in the NHS across all relevant specialities in both hospital and community services and a similar number employed in the private sector. While all podiatrists must be registered with the Council for the Profession Supplementary to Medicine (CPSM; replaced by the Health Professions Council in April 2002) in order to practise in the UK NHS, this is not a requirement for the private sector. State registered podiatrists have access to local anaesthetics with vaso-constrictor substances. They also have limited dispensing rights.

Where foot problems cannot be fully met by conservative methods, surgery may be needed. Until recently this would have been undertaken by an orthopaedic surgeon, but a growing number of podiatrists are qualifying as surgical podiatrists, and are able to undertake some of this work (Department of Health, 1994).

Access to podiatry can be by self or team referral against clear evidence based criteria for a service where need always exceeds demand, and podiatry has been identified as the most sought after service after that of the GP.

ACCESS TO THE PODIATRY SERVICE

Historically, those aged 65 and over had access to the podiatry service, widely regarded as an entitlement of pensioners irrespective of need. Recently there has been a trend towards need and not age as an access criteria. Patients who are 'at risk' include older persons with the following conditions:

- diabetes
- arthropathies, e.g. rheumatoid arthritis
- peripheral vascular disease
- neuropathy.

Other categories are terminally ill patients; children; and the general public suffering pain that can be alleviated with skilled podiatry treatment.

BASIC FOOTCARE

Basic footcare is part of personal care. At the most rudimentary level it involves foot washing, drying and nail cutting. These tasks are generally undertaken by individuals or their carer as part of personal care. However, for those patients with pathological foot conditions and/or a systemic disorder such as diabetes or peripheral vascular disease, there may be a requirement for podiatry, in conjunction with ongoing self-care.

Where older people cannot continue with their own uncomplicated self-care, voluntary organisations in some areas provide a nail cutting service. Age Concern England has liaised with the Society of Chiropodists and Podiatrists to produce ethically based guidelines on simple nail cutting for volunteers (Society of Chiropody and Age Concern England, 1995). This includes state registered chiropodist involvement in training of volunteers; initial and annual assessment; and provision of care for 'at risk' patients.

PODIATRY

At the initial consultation between patient and podiatrist, and using the contribution by other team members to the patient's central records as a baseline, a detailed subjective account of the patient's concerns must be recorded. These may range from basic footcare problems to more complex foot pathologies related to systemic disease. A detailed objective examination by the podiatrist should include toenails; skin; the alignment of toes; the patient's medical history to discount systemic disease that indirectly may affect the feet; medication such as steroids, which, like any anti-inflammatory drug, can suppress an inflammatory response and therefore mask preceding ulceration or infection; observation of the patient's gait; examination of the patient's foot for biomechanical imbalances; assessment of the patient's neurological and vascular status; and footwear. The use of further laboratory analysis and imaging techniques may be necessary to obtain an accurate insight into the patient's pathology.

The podiatrist must discuss the proposed treatment plan with the team, patient and/or carer, and this may or may not include podiatry treatment. It is important that the patient or carer be given as much information as relevant about the patient's foot health in the form of verbal and written explanations. Where treatment is indicated, goals and initial duration must be discussed and the outcome evaluated by the podiatrist and patient/carer at the end of the episode of care. As practitioners may not have instant cures for pathologies within the ageing foot, the major aims should be to provide comfort, advice on footwear, prevent complications, encourage walking, reduce pain and improve healing.

The following covers problems commonly seen in the older foot; their causes; management by informal or formal carers; and indications for referral to podiatry.

Toenail disorders

Toenail disorders are common in older people. The common causes of toenail pain are as follows:

- **Ingrown toenails** result in symptoms ranging from mild discomfort to acute pain and can cause infection and abscess formation where referral to the podiatrist is advised for conservative or surgical treatment, and, when appropriate, to the general practitioner for antibiotics.
- **Thickening of the toenail** occurs following some permanent damage to the nail matrix caused by trauma, footwear, fungal infections or systemic conditions such as psoriasis. The nail plate is abnormally thickened and discoloured, causing pain, discomfort and nail cutting difficulty. Using a nail drill, the chiropodist can reduce the thickness of the nail painlessly. As the damage is irreversible, regular treatment by the chiropodist will be necessary (Figures 18.1a and 18.1b).
- **A fungal infection** of the nail plate causes the nail plate to thicken and discolour (Beaven, 1984). Routine care by the podiatrist with nail nippers and a nail drill and/or systemic treatment from the general practitioner will keep these nails reduced in bulk and pain free.
- **Infection of the soft tissues adjacent to the nail plate,** such as Paronychia, can spread to the underlying bone, especially in the presence of diabetes mellitus and vascular insufficiency, and requires immediate treatment with systemic antibiotics and local drainage of the wound with suitable sterile dressings.
- **A bony exostosis** occurs under the nail plate near its distal aspect. Surgery may be used to reduce discomfort.
- **A subungual corn** is located under the nail plate. Management consists of partial removal of the toenail and the underlying corn, with measures to modify footwear to remove pressure from the toe.

Lesser toe deformities

Lesser toe deformities are often described as hammer, claw, retracted or mallet toes, and causes include muscle imbalance due to wasting of the distal intrinsic muscles.

Corns and callouses are a reaction of skin to compressive, shearing and tensile stresses or unyielding footwear. A callus is a diffuse hyperatrophy of the stratum corneum caused by compression and shearing stress. A corn is a circumscribed area of callus that has become increasingly compacted at the point of pressure from the shoe. The deepest portion of the corn impinges on the sensory nerve endings, resulting in pain. As corn and callus are derived from the stratum corneum, this can be removed painlessly without bleeding. Shields can be fabricated out of wool, felt or silicone material to reduce pressure on the affected toe. However, shields can only be comfortably worn if there is adequate accommodation within the shoe.

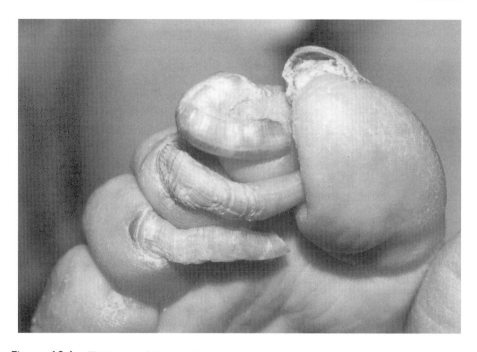

Figure 18.1a Thickening of the toenail

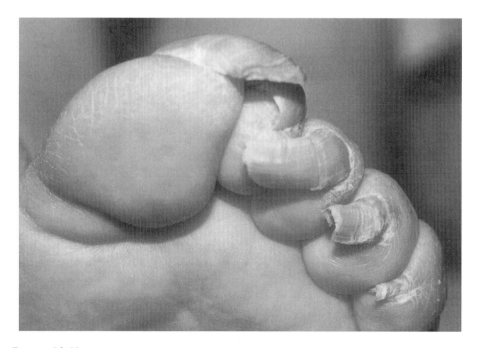

Figure 18.1b Thickening of the toenail

Forefoot disorders

Forefoot disorders are often the end result of primary biomechanical defects such as postural deformities and structural malalignments of the lower limb and foot, which are compounded by contributory factors such as ill-fitting footwear or previous unprotected occupational stresses (Boyd, 1993). These structural defects should be treated at an earlier stage, before the sequel of forefoot deformities become irreversible and chronic in nature. Where appropriate, orthoses can be fabricated to enhance foot function. However, in the aged foot the chronic outcome of biomechanical defects are clinically apparent and include hallux valgus (Figure 18.2) and hallux rigidus and Morton's neuroma – a degenerative condition of the plantar digital nerve exacerbated by metatarsal pressure. Functional orthoses are utilised to functionally correct the biomechanical imbalances of the foot. Softer material, although providing less correction, is better tolerated by the older patient.

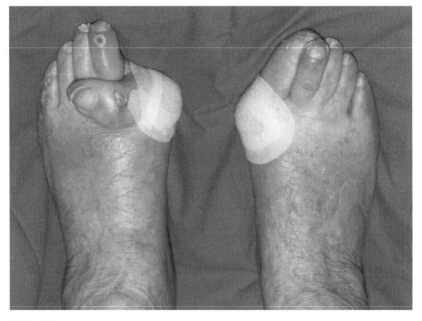

Figure 18.2 Hallux valgus

Mid-foot disorders

The three most common mid-foot disorders are as follows:

• **A ganglion** is a fluid-filled cyst usually derived from a tendon sheath or a joint capsule. The swelling can be readily manipulated from one part of the cyst to another. This, together with the very soft character of the swelling, distinguishes it from a bursa. Ganglia are often asymptomatic and may be left alone.

- **Osteoarthritis** resulting from the wear and tear effects on the mid-foot joints affects foot function. Management of this problem includes modification to footwear to allow greater accommodation for the oesteophytic outgrowths. Alternatively, the osteophytic lipping may be removed surgically.

- **Tenosynovitis** may affect the tendon sheaths anterior to the ankle that stand out from the dorsum of the toe and are liable to be continually irritated by the crease in the upper of the shoe. A small hard corn may first develop, with swelling and pain along the tendon sheath, stiffness and crepitus on movement. Removal may expose a sinus leading to the tendon. Management involves removal of pressure with regular saline soaks if infection occurs. Referral is to the patient's general practitioner for antibiotics if infection is a recurring problem.

Heel disorders

Heel disorders can be difficult to diagnose and treat, the thickness of the heel pad masking the clinical signs of inflammation. The main causes of disorders are as follows:

- **Lipoatrophy** is a reduction in the thickness of the heel pad. The property of shock absorption is reduced and the transmission of pressure is directed on to the underlying heel bone with resulting pain and a tendency to walk by putting as little weight on the heels as possible, risking instability. Heel cushions and soft-soled footwear will help reduce the pain.
- **Plantar fasciitis** is an inflammatory lesion at the junction between the plantar aponeurosis and the calcaneum. This common heel condition may be associated with a heel spur. Localised pain occurs first thing in the morning or after a period of rest. Management includes reducing the tensile stress on this attachment by the use of functional orthoses, physiotherapy to reduce the inflammatory response and finally steroid injection if other measures fail.
- **Posterior calcaneal bursitis** is usually inflammation of subcutaneous bursa overlying the Achilles' tendon insertion. Tenderness will be palpable directly over the calcaneus at the tendon insertion. A noticeable bursal thickening may be present over the bony prominence lateral to the tendon attachment. Footwear with a soft heel counter or soft cushion material adhered to the inside of the heel counter may reduce pressure on the overlying skin.
- **Marginal heel callus** with fissures commonly occur in the elderly population. This is associated with dry skin, obesity and wearing open-heeled footwear and is a particular problem for some minority groups. If the skin is excessively dry, it will split to form fissures as a result of the tensile and shearing forces that occur around the heel margins with the risk of infection. Treatment consists of skin moisturising lotions and advice on footwear such as avoidance of an open-heel shoe.
- **Plantar heel pain** is also caused by systemic pathology such as sero-negative arthropathy. Pain occurs at the attachment of ligaments and tendons to the

underlying bone. A characteristic fluffy heel spur occurs at the junction of the plantar aponeurosis and the calcaneum (Jacoby, 1991).

Whole foot disorders

The incidence of pes cavus (high arched foot) and pes planus (flatfoot) are not linked with the ageing foot. However, the ageing skin predisposes to the formation of corn and callus in areas of excessive pressure. The main disorders are of the skin, systemic disease, swelling, infections and ulceration, and malignancy.

Skin disorders of the foot

Tinea pedis (fungal infection) commonly presents between the toes or in the area of the longitudinal arch. Symptoms include erythema and pruritis. The use of topical anti-fungal agents and footwear that permits ventilation (sandals) is the first line of action. Occlusive footwear made from synthetic substances are to be avoided. For the more acute and resistant fungal infections, referral to the general practitioner for systemic anti-fungal agents is necessary.

The incidence of **verrucae** is relatively low in the elderly population compared to the teenage population (Hefland, 1981), but is very resistant to treatment. One theory about the low incidence of verrucae in the elderly is that their immune system has built up resistance to the particular viral infection throughout their lifetime, whereas it is the opposite with children. If the verruca is giving no pain, the lesion can be left untreated. If painful, proprietary lotions can be used with care.

Foot conditions as residuals of systemic disease

Diabetes mellitus is known to be responsible for multiple foot complications, which may lead to the detection of this disease that increases with age. Foot manifestations often result from the sequel of peripheral neuropathy and vascular pathology (Davidson, 1991).

Foot infection is a serious complication for the older person. It may be related to systemic disease or result from poor self-care of a local foot problem. Residual deformities of earlier conditions, together with the ageing process, provide an excellent medium for the development of foot infections. Foot infections are the most common precipitant of amputation. Common causes of foot infections are:

- any trauma that causes a break in the skin
- ill-fitting footwear and lack of self-care
- dryness of the skin due to the ageing process
- metabolic diseases such as diabetes mellitus combined with peripheral vascular disease.

Management involves removal of exciting cause, saline foot soaks, referral to the general practitioner for systemic antibiotics, and ultimate hospitalisation if systemic disease is uncontrolled.

Gout may produce symptoms in any joint of the foot and should always be suspected where intense pain is present without trauma. The signs and symptoms include chronic painful and stiff joints, soft tissue tophi, deformity and functional impairment. Referral to the general practitioner for investigation is appropriate. If the diagnosis is confirmed, systemic medication is required to control the metabolic imbalance.

Osteoarthritis elsewhere in the body is reflected in the weight-bearing joints of the foot. A reduced range of joint motion, altered foot pressures and the laying down of additional bone surrounding the focus joint is manifested. With altered plantar pressure distribution, corn and callous may occur, and this should be referred to the podiatrist for management.

Peripheral neuropathy consists of one or all three of the components of sensory, autonomic and motor neuropathy, which together have the potential to put the foot at major risk.

Peripheral vascular insufficiency is present to varying degrees in the majority of older people (Hefland, 1981), accompanied by pain, coldness, pallor, paraesthesia, burning, atrophy of soft tissues, dry skin, loss of hair and absent foot pulses. The final result of severe arterial occlusion is gangrene. Referral to the general practitioner for vasodilator medication or referral to a vascular surgeon for assessment is necessary.

Rheumatoid arthritis is accompanied in its later stages by exacerbation of pain, joint swelling, stiffness, muscle wasting and marked deformity of the feet. Management involves basic footcare, skilled management of foot ulceration and pressure dispersion pads for the sole of the foot. Referral for appropriate footwear is essential to alleviate pressure on the forefoot joints (Kinsman, 1980; Harrison, 1984).

Sensory neuropathy makes the patient unaware of minor abrasions to the foot and the risk of pressure related ulceration. With **motor neuropathy**, the most distal muscles of the foot no longer obtain innervation, which results in clawing of the toes, thus increasing the weight-bearing pressures underneath the metatarsal heads. With **autonomic neuropathy**, the controlling innervation to the blood vessel wall is absent or reduced, and the sebaceous and sweat gland secretions are reduced.

Swelling of the foot has many causes, but in the elderly is more likely to be linked with vascular insufficiency. Change may be insidious and feet pushed with increasing difficulty into pre-morbid shoes with the risk of skin damage, infection and ulceration. Medical referral for investigation, together with specialist advice on footwear that will cope safely with variation in swelling is essential.

Ulcerative lesions in the ageing foot are the result of localised pressure due to biomechanical dysfunction and are usually associated with metabolic disease such as diabetes mellitus or peripheral vascular insufficiency. Ulcers in the diabetic patient are usually painless but an ischaemic ulcer is very painful and usually exhibits early local necrosis. Referral to the appropriate clinical department is essential. When healing occurs, all steps must be taken to prevent recurrence.

Vascular pathology associated with diabetes consists of:

- microangiopathy (involving arteriolar vessels of the skin)
- macroangiopathy (involving the medium and large-sized arteries of the lower limb).

Both conditions reduce the lumen of the vessel and therefore a reduced blood flow to the foot. The clinical effects are diminished or absent foot pulses, an increased risk of infection, and possible ulceration and gangrene. Systemic antibiotics are ineffective in these cases as the blood supply is unable to distribute the drug to the target site. Neuropathic ulcers in elderly diabetics can be resistant to treatment. Management involves rest, systemic antibiotics to control infection, removal of dead tissue in ulcerated sites and measures to redistribute weight-bearing pressures. Many patients can be managed by conservative means for long periods of time with an ulcerated lesion. Once the ulcer is healed, prevention of future ulceration is essential. Referral to the diabetic multidisciplinary team is indicated for appropriate management (McInnes, 1994).

As can be seen from the above, suitable footwear complements awareness, prevention and treatment of foot problems.

FOOTWEAR

The importance of assessing foot health and footwear needs, and having an efficient method of responding, is essential if the impact of a proactive and timely rehabilitation programme is to be achieved (Finlay, 1994, 1996). The majority of older people can have their needs met satisfactorily from the commercial market, but the frail elderly may need additional help with supply and fitment. Uncomfortable shoes and painful feet discourage mobility. The footwear needs of older people may be quite simple and basic (Table 18.1), while others may require semi-bespoke or bespoke made-to-measure shoes (Pratts, 1989).

Table 18.1 Objectives of a footcare and footwear scheme

- To identify those people with footwear unsuited to their needs and provide explanation and advice, decreasing the number of older people who are at risk wearing unsafe shoes.
- To facilitate feet fit for rehabilitation.
- To reduce pain and maximise comfort.
- To identify foot risk early and cross-refer to other disciplines.
- To provide sufficient information to help the patient and carer reach an informed decision, thus improving patient satisfaction.
- To assist the elderly (especially the frail elderly) to cope with purchasing a correct product in a complex market place.
- To provide in-house economical, well-fitting shoes suited to individual needs.
- To refer on for specialist provision where needs cannot be met through the commercial market or by adaptation.

Footwear problems likely to be encountered in a rehabilitation programme

Many common foot disorders that are a minor nuisance in young persons become potentially serious in the elderly (Lee and Dedrick, 1995). One of the problems associated with this area of care is the complexity of the variables, such as weight, age, range of joint movement, gender and cadence, and it is often a complex issue to cater for individual need (Finlay, 1995a). Little account may be taken in retail outlets of the differences in foot structure of minority groups. Foot dimension change may be the result of both generation and ethnic origin. For example, mongoloid populations, including the Japanese, have a wider foot compared to the caucasoid and australoid population, and the East Asian population, including the Japanese, have a smaller foot length for height compared to South East Asians and Africans (Kouchi, 1998), yet all those resident in the UK have to be accommodated in a European mould. There are obvious foot health and general safety issues, and poor fitment may lead to loose fitting with a sliding gait to keep the shoe on or 'treading down' of the back of the shoe, with a subsequent effect on mobility and possibly heel traumatisation.

Aims of a footwear scheme

The essential components of good shoes are that they fit well, help the wearer to stand and move in comfort and safety, maximise stability, protect the feet, keep them warm but not overheated, are easy to put on, take off, to fasten and unfasten and suit the individual's lifestyle. Footwear is of real, but often unrecognised psychological importance to the wearer and 'special shoes' may be the first confrontation with a visible symbol of disability (Disabled Living Foundation, 1990).

- Fastenings must be adequate and hold the foot well back in the shoe (Finlay, 1987). Laces provide maximum accommodation (Oxford Health Authority, 1981). Impaired fine finger movements may require Velcro fastenings.
- Fabric should be washable if incontinence is a problem.
- Heels should be non-tapered, low height (<3.6cm) and wide to improve stability (>5.5cm) (Gould, 1982).
- High collar provides better balance than those with low collars (Lord *et al.*, 1999).
- Insole should be well padded (Evanski, 1982), with a smooth lining especially for patients with ischaemic problems or neuropathy.
- Lightweight and supportive (Survana, 1992).
- Soles should be non-slip, except when slippage is required to facilitate movement (e.g. Parkinson's patients).
- Width, length and depth should be correct (Knowles, 1998) with at least 1.2cm between the longest toe and the inside of the shoe to allow the toes to move normally without undue pressure or friction (Finlay, 1987) with increased depth at the toe box.

CASE STUDY FOOTWEAR PROVISION FOR SUSAN HUNTER

Discussion with Susan Hunter's relatives/carers should take place when appropriate and they should be requested to bring (if possible) her regularly worn shoes. Nursing staff can liaise if necessary with the relatives and the nursing records should identify the footwear need. it is also advantageous to provide footwear information leaflets to ensure an informed decision can be reached. If no suitable product is available then assistance should be given regarding supply. If an 'in house' facility for purchase of commercial footwear is available this should enable fast provision, avoiding both the delay and complications associated with high street visits. This service enables the relatives/carers to purchase a suitable product at discount prices.

Footwear examination

The footwear of Susan Hunter should be carefully examined. Remember to examine both the internal and external aspects. Decomposition or wear and tear patterns may be used to confirm any problems in gait prior to admission, as the wear patterns can often support or refute the history provided by the patient or relative.

- Misshapen uppers often indicate the presence of bunions and potential areas of excessive friction (see Figure 18.3).
- If Susan's shoes have pristine soles, then it is probably that these are 'Sunday best' rather than those worn on a daily basis.
- Wear patterns of the product are largely influenced by the shape, size, bone structure and biomechanics of the wearer (Bodziak, 1990). Excessive heel

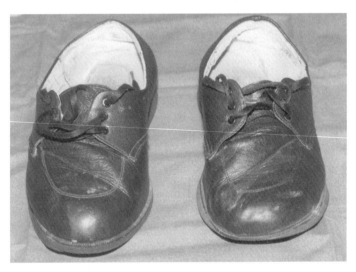

Figure 18.3 Misshapen uppers

wear may indicate long periods of sitting with repetitive heel shuffling. Wear on the anterior sole may indicate foot drop before it is visible to the eye. Excessive wear on either the medial or lateral borders of either sole or heel will reflect uneven alignment of weight or possibly instability. Heels require special attention as this is the common problem found in female shoes.

The importance of obtaining the correct shoes prior to weight bearing and ambulation cannot be over stressed. Should Susan Hunter wear slip-on shoes or slippers then this may increase the tendency to shuffle; shiny or plastic soles may produce a small, fearful step gait; while narrow styles will inhibit normal foot function movement, reducing toe function and preventing normal toe 'push off', thus affecting gait pattern and weight transference. In the case of Susan Hunter, normal low heels will probably satisfy her need (however, in the case of obese patients or if the lower limb swelling is excessive then wedged heel shoes may be more supportive than a 'waisted shoe').

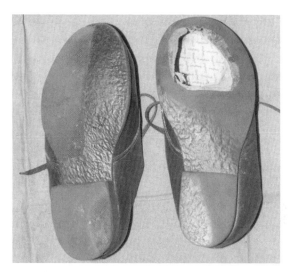

Figure 18.4 Wear patterns

When swelling is present, as with Susan, the toe box shape is of paramount importance. In general, high fashion styles should be avoided, as they often have a triangular toe box that constricts the normal rectangular dimensions of the forefoot (Coughlin, 1998). High heels should also be avoided, as they constitute a needless balance hazard (Lord and Bashford, 1996). Narrow, tapering heels will increase instability and with the swelling the problem will increase, caused by lack of support caused by the tapering. Robbins *et al.* (1992) stated that thick mid-soles will increase the tendancy to falls in older people as these tend to have an 'edge effect', whereby they resist compression less at their edge rather than in the centre, resulting in destabilisation, while increased sole softness probably worsens foot position awareness and impairs stability by reducing afferent feedback to the central nervous system regarding the foot position (Robbins et al., 1995). However, Lord et al. (1999) do not support this theory and state that subjects have better balance wearing shoes with high collars and that sole hardness is not related to balance.

It is difficult to state exactly the make and style of shoe that would be the most useful adjunct in Susan's rehabilitation programme. In footwear supply there are so many variables that one must respond to this on an individual basis. Susan's lifestyle, expectations and medical problems will affect choice; however, this will be further compounded by environmental factors (e.g. the frictional variations between shoes and floor covering must be taken into consideration). It is advantageous to have various styles easily available from an 'in-house' supply, permitting various designs to be tested and when supported by information technology, this provides the most satisfactory approach. In this case study, one would expect that a semi-bespoke product (providing both increased width and depth) from the commercial market to be the most satisfactory. In view of Susan's diabetic history it is imperative that the inside of the shoe should be as smooth as a 'velvet glove'. Some manufacturers will recommend specific products.

Swelling has been identified as a problem; however, the type of 'pitting' should indicate whether this is gravitational or long standing in origin. Depending upon the cause, the need for graduated compression stockings may be identified. Usually below-knee stockings are more easily tolerated by elderly people. Suisan's poor hand function will increase difficulty in application (assistance will probably be required). An advice leaflet on correct application should be provided.

A shoe style that accommodates fluctuating swelling should be recommended to ensure that as swelling alters the footwear can cope with change. Should Susan require an othosis, then this should be supplied before shoe fitment. The unaffected side may require a smaller shoe so the supply of odd sizes may require consideration; however, if the swelling is slight, then a tongue pad may suffice.

The physiotherapist should check whether there is any condition that requires referral to the podatrist (e.g. nail problems, corns or callosities).

Analysing gait problems

The initial assessment of the feet should include history, palpation, measurement, record of circulatory problems, mapping of areas of vulnerable skin, range of movement and gait observation, as well as shoe examination. The hind foot function of the patient should be observed by the therapist standing from behind. Records should include essential information from all concerned disciplines.

When weight bearing commences, gait should be observed, as described above. If underplantar pressure technology is available this can be a very useful method of monitoring gait changes. Underplantar pressure technology (the Musgrave System) is but one type currently in use (see Figure 18.5). Susan would be required to walk over two plates (preferably unassisted or just requiring minimal suport). It is beneficial to let Susan have a trial walk over the plates before recordings are taken.

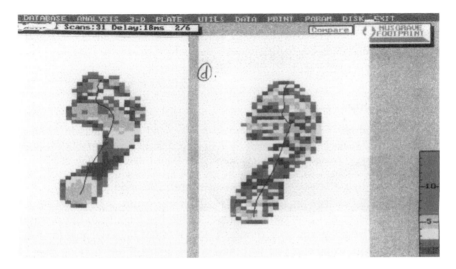

Figure 18.5   Musgrave System

Recordings of Susan walking in bare feet provide the basic gait pattern. Walking in various types of footwear provides information as to the most satisfactory product. The position of the plates should haave been adjusted to suit her stride length.

A total of 2,048 sensors record the underplantar pressure. The footprint data is displayed as coloured squares, each corresponding to the sensor on the plate. The colour of each area represents the pressure against time applied to that sensor, and different colours correspond to different values, with the pressure values being displayed. The pressure is recorded in kg/cm squared. This system also provides colour dynamic footprints that can be obtained in two or three dimensions (Finlay, 1995b, c; Finlay et al., 1999). Heel strike loadings and forefoot function can be clearly identified.

Following the recording being taken and stored on computer, an explanation of the prints can provide a very useful feedback method for Susan, thus increasing her understanding of associated gait problems and increase her motivation in achieving goals. The printouts can also help the decision-making process in shoe selection by providing quantitative data as to why a new product should be purchased.

Modifications

Susan Hunter's shoes may require wedging or floating (widening of the heel) to improve alignment when weight bearing and increase ankle stability. A tongue pad may be essential if there is insufficient room in the toe box by preventing foot slippage within the shoe. Poron insoles will be required if the underplantar pressure technology has identified areas of abnormal high pressure, often found in the diabetic patient whose circulation may be compromised.

If a modification is required and can be completed 'in-house' this is very efficient as it can be completed the same day (Finlay and Fullerton, 1996) and this intervention alone can improve gait (Finlay et al., 1999). 'In-house' modification usually provides a cost-effective measure, as if they do not improve or maximise function or are unacceptable to the patient, then more expensive modifications do not have to be pursued.

Decision making

Susan Hunter and her relatives/carers should be involved in the decision making, thus increasing that unnecessary waste by ensuring that an unacceptable product will not be rejected at the point of delivery.

Evidence shows that efficiency and effectiveness are maximised when a comprehensive rather than an ad hoc footwear service exists. It has been reported that there is a waste of £2 million per annum within the NHS from the provision of unacceptable bespoke footwear (Pratts, 1989). It is not unreasonable for the majority of patients to be supplied with new shoes within three working days of referral (Finlay, 1996), if the hospital operates an 'off the shelf service'; however, if she requires bespoke footwear under national contracts this should be delivered within six weeks (Michaelson, 1989).

Effect of shoe style on gait

Susan Hunter should be advised to wear the footwear supplied on all occasions as unsafe footwear is frequently cited as a contributing factor for instability and falls in older people (Gabel et al., 1985; Finlay, 1986; Edelstein, 1987; Dunne et al., 1993; Chartered Society of Physiotherapy, 1998 and Lord et al., 1999). Examples of poor footwear can be given if necessary, e.g. Wellington boots, heavy boots and slippers with worn soles (Gabel et al., 1985).

Susan should be reminded that footwear may improve balance and gait (Arnadottir and Mercer, 2000), as footwear may be an important factor in affecting balance and stability (Nuffield Institute for Health, 1996).

SUMMARY

Comfortable feet and safe footwear are essential for the mobility and well-being of older people. While basic footcare is normally undertaken by people as part of their personal care, older people may need assistance, thus there is a need for increased awareness education of the public, and formal and informal carers. Due to the general lack of awareness relating to hazards of poor footwear, innovative methods are required to alert the public and carers to the associated problems. More advice in the form of leaflets could be provided in doctors' surgeries, mail order companies, retirement clubs, leisure centres, multinational stores, and on the Internet and in the media.

Hopefully this short description will illustrate the importance of good foot health and the importance of how inter-professional collaboration can help maximise function in older people.

REFERENCES

Arnadottir, S.A. and Mercer, V.S. (2000) Effects of footwear on measurements of balance and gait in women between the ages 65 and 93 years. *Physical Therapy Journal*, 80(1), 17–27.

Beaven, D.W. (1984) Fungal infections and onychomycosis. In: *Colour Atlas of the Nail*, Wolfe Medical Publications, London, pp. 82–89.

Bodziak, W.J. (1990) *Footwear Impression Evidence*, Elsevier, New York, Amsterdam, London, pp. 326–330.

Boyd, P.M. (1993) The adult foot. In: *Neale's Common Foot Disorders*, 4th edn (ed. Lorimer, D.L.), Churchill Livingstone, Edinburgh, p. 51.

Chartered Society of Physiotherapy (1998) *Guideline for the Collaborative Rehabilitative Management of Elderly People Who Have Fallen* (Aim 2), Chartered Society of Physiotherapy, London.

Clarke, M. (1969) *Trouble with Feet*, G. Bell & Sons, London.

Coughlin, M.J. (1998) Foot problems in women, why those shoes aren't made for walking. *Consultant*, 38(10), 2511–2516.

Davidson, M.B. (1991) An overview of diabetes mellitus. In: *The High Risk Foot in Diabetes Mellitus* (ed. Frykberg, R.G.), Churchill Livingstone, New York, pp. 1–22.

Department of Health (1994) *Feet First*, Department of Health, London.

Disabled Living Foundation (1990) *Footwear – A Quality Issue*, Disabled Living Foundation, London.

Dunne, R.G., Bergman, A.B., Rodgers L.W. and Rivara, F.P. (1993) Elderly persons' attitude towards footwear – a factor in preventing falls. *Public Health Reports*, 108(2), 254.

Edelstein, J.E. (1987) If no shoe fits. Footwear consideration for the elderly. Physical and Occupational Therapy Geriatrics, 5, 1–16.

Evanski P.M. (1982) The geriatric foot. In: *Disorders of the Foot and Ankle* (ed. Jahss, J.), W.B. Saunders, Philadelphia, PA, pp. 964–978.

Finlay, O. (1986) Footwear management in the elderly care programme. *Physiotherapy Journal*, 72(4), 172–178.

Finlay, O. (1987) Footwear management in the elderly care programme. *Journal of the Society of Chiropodists*, 42(5), 159–170.

Finlay, O. (1994) *Stay Safe, Stay Steady, Post Malta Conference Report*, World Confederation of Physical Therapists, London.

Finlay, O. (1995a) *Proceedings of the World Confederation of Physical Therapists in Washington*, World Confederation of Physical Therapists, London.

Finlay, O. (1995b) The use of computers to assess problems associated with gait in elderly people. *Information Technology in Nursing*, 7(1), 9–12.

Finlay, O. (1995c) Foot problems and footwear prescriptions. In: *Physiotherapy with Older People* (eds Pickles, P., Compton, A., Cott, C., Simpson, J. and Vandervoort, A.), W.B. Saunders, London, pp. 392–398.

Finlay, O. (1996) Step forward. *Health Service Journal*, 8 February, 31.

Finlay, O. and Fullerton, C. (1996) Feet and footwear. In: *Rehabilitation of Older People* (ed. Squires, A.J.), Chapman & Hall, London, pp. 167–193, (a) p. 187, (b) p. 188.

Finlay, O., van de Meer, D.C. and Beringer, T.R.O. (1999) Use of gait analysis to demonstrate benefits of footwear assessment in elderly people. *Physiotherapy Journal*, 85(8), 451–456.

Gabel, A., Simmons, M. and Nayak, U. (1985) Falls in the healthy elderly; predisposing causes. *Ergonomics*, **28**, 965–1075.

Goldman, F. (1993) *Podiatry for the Non Podiatrist*, Kaiser Permanente Medical Centre, Santa Clara, CA.

Gould, N. (1982) Shoes and modifications. In: *Disorders of the Foot* (ed. Jahss, M.H.), W.B. Saunders, London, pp. 1745–1782.

Harrison, R.A. (1984) A simple pattern for plastazote shoes. *Physiotherapy Journal*, 70(6), 114–115.

Hefland, A.E. (1981) Primary foot care for the elderly. In: *Clinical Podigeriatrics* (ed. Hefland, A.E.), Williams & Wilkins, BA, pp. 1–4.

Jacoby, R.K. (1991) The painful foot in systemic disorders. In: *The Foot and its Disorders* (ed. Klenerman, L.), Blackwell Scientific, London, p. 131.

Kinsman, R. (1980) The do it your self shoe. *Physiotherapy Journal*, **69**(9), 304–305.

Knowles, A. (1998) The role of pressure relief in diabetic foot problems. *The Diabetic Foot*, 1(2).

Kouchi, M. (1998) Foot dimensions and foot shape: differences due to growth, generation and ethnic origin. *Anthropological Science*, **106**, 161–188.

Kwok, T. (1994) A survey of in-patients' footwear. *Care of the Elderly Journal*, March, 118.

Lee, J. and Dedrick, D.K. (1995) Preventing and managing geriatric foot problems. *Journal of Musculoskeletal Medicine*, January, **12**(1), 29–31, 35–36, 39–40.

Lord, S.R. and Bashford, G.M. (1996) Shoe characteristics and balance in older women. *Journal of the American Geriatrics Society*, **44**(4), 429–433.

Lord, S.R., Guy, B.M., Howland, A. and Munroe, B.J. (1999) Effects of shoe collar height and sole hardness on balance in older women. *Journal of the American Geriatrics Society*, 47(6), 681–684.

McInnes, A.D. (1994) The role of the chiropodist. In: *The Foot in Diabetes*, 2nd edn (eds Boulton, A.J.H, Connor, H. and Cavanagh, P.R.), Wiley, Chichester, pp. 77–91.

McInnes, A., Booth, J. and Birch, I. (1999) Multidisciplinary diabetic footcare teams: skills and knowledge. *The Diabetic Foot*, 2(2), Summer, 67–70.

Menz, H.B. and Lord, S.R. (1999) Footwear and postural stability in older people. *Journal of American Podiatric Medical Association*, July, 7, 346–357.

Michaelson, P. (1989) Surgical footwear [letter]. *British Medical Journal*, 299, 1217.

Munro, B.J. and Steele, J.R. (1999) Household-shoe wearing and purchasing habits – a survey of people aged 65 years or over. *Journal of the Americian Podiatric Medical Association*, 89(10), 506–514.

Neale, D. and Boyd, P.M. (1989) In: *Common Foot Disorders*, 3rd edn (eds Neale, D. and Adams I.A.), Churchill Livingstone, Edinburgh.

Nuffield Institute for Health, University of Leeds and NHS Centre for Reviews and Dissemination (1996) *Effective Health Care Bulletin: Preventing Falls and Subsequent Injury in Older People*, 2(4), Churchill Livingtone, Edinburgh.

Oxford Health Authority (1981) *Clothing and Dressing for the Disabled*, Oxford Regional Health Authority, Oxford, p. 2.

Plummer, E.S. and Stewart, G.A. (1996) Focused assessment of foot care in older adults. *Journal of the American Geriatrics Society*, **44**, 310–316.

Pratts, R.G.S. (1989) The NHS boot. *British Medical Journal*, **299**, 932–933.

Richardson, J.K. and Ashton-Miller, J.A. (1996) Periphera; neuropathy – An often-overlooked cause of falls in the elderly. *Postgraduate Medicine*, **99**(6), 161.

Robbins, S., Gouw, G.J. and McClaren, J. (1992) Shoe sole thickness and hardness influence balance in older men. *Journal of the American Geriatrics Society*, **40**, 1089–1094.

Robbins, S., Waked, E. and McClaren, J. (1995) Proprioception and stability: foot position awareness as a function of age and footwear. *Age and Ageing*, **24**, 67–72.

Society of Chiropody and Age Concern (1995) Voluntary nail-cutting guidelines. *Journal of British Podiatric Medicine*, **50**(5), 74.

Survana, R.R. (1992) The ageing foot. In: *Common Foot Disorders*, 3rd edn (eds Neale, D. and Adams, I.M.), Churchill Livingstone, Edinburgh, p. 154.

USEFUL RESOURCES

Musgrave Method:

Musgrave Medical
Musgrave House,
22A Castle Street
Llangollen
Denbighshire
LL20 8NV
Tel: 0870 243 5061
Fax: 0870 243 5062
Email: muslab@aol.com

Useful mail order footwear addresses:
Natureform
Athertonholme Mill
Bacup
Lancashire OL13 0LS
Tel: 01706 873304
E-mail: natureform@bacupshoe.co.uk
Website: www.natureform.co.uk

Cosy Feet
The Tanyard
Leigh Road
Street
Somerset
BA 16 OHR
Tel: 01458 447275
Fax: 01458 445988
Website: www.cosyfeet.co.uk

The British Footwear Association produces a booklet called *Footwear for Special Needs* (£3), available from:
5 Portland Place
London
W1N 3AA

19 THE POTENTIAL OF SOCIAL SERVICES

Jill Manthorpe

AIMS OF THE CHAPTER

In this chapter the potential for Social Services and social workers to contribute to helping older people improve or maintain their quality of life and maximise their independence and citizenship is explored. The focus is on recuperation or rehabilitation after a period in hospital, although many of the ideas and models presented should help to prevent unnecessary admission to hospital or entry to long-term care. Rehabilitation as a term is not yet widely used within social work and so much of the discussion draws on other pertinent debates. A brief overview of Social Services is followed by a discussion of the case study of Susan Hunter. The role of the hospital-based social worker in assessment is discussed, together with the systems of support available through care management. Comment is made on the links with housing and benefits agencies, and concludes with an evaluation of Social Services' practitioners' experience in advocating for service users and their needs.

SOCIAL SERVICES STAFF

With over a million people working in Social Services in the statutory, voluntary and private sector this is a growing and complex workforce. The growth is associated with an ageing population and the shift to community care. The complexity is related to the sheer number of organisations and responsibilities involved, and the range of staff falling under the umbrella of Social Services and social care. A recent study, for example, of five local authority Social Services departments in England found 90 different job titles for staff working as managers and 70 different job titles for those working directly with people (Balloch *et al.*, 1999). In addition, there are several terms used to refer to people who make use of social work and social care services: clients, users or services users, or even consumers in the community and residents in the long-term sector or institutionally based care.

The world of social care is mostly staffed by women. Many of these work part time and relatively few are found at higher levels. Parallels with the health service are evident. These also include the location of work, which can be varied: ranging from an established institutional base within a day centre, for example, to being part of a team that offers a mix of peripatetic or domiciliary based services, such as a support service for carers.

One key distinction in this confusing world is that between a professionally qualified social worker and those who do not hold the qualification (the Diploma in Social Work, Dip SW, the Certificate of Qualification in Social Work, CQSW or Certificate in Social Services). This qualification is not compulsory for many people work in Social Services before qualifying and some never do, but for some parts of Social Services work it is a requirement, particularly work with children and child protection. Many working in residential care or care management will be trained but not qualified. Confusingly, they may be known as social workers, care managers or similar titles.

The world of training and professionalism within Social Services is changing. New policies such as the White Paper *Modernising Social Services* (Department of Health [DoH], 1998) set out the government's commitment to increasing the capacity of Social Services staff. The Care Standards Act 2000 brings these proposals into fruition; setting out:

- a General Social Care Council to act as the regulatory professional body, initially for those with the professional qualification
- a Commission for Care Standards to act as an independent inspectorate for social care (including all nursing home and residential care).

At the same time the body formerly responsible for professional social work education (the Central Council for Education and Training in Social Work) is being reformulated into the national training bodies, in this case the Training Organisation for the Personal Social Services. This broadening of interest into all the workforce looks set to remould a previously pyramid shaped workforce – with small numbers of qualified staff at the top and a mass of semi or unqualified workers at the bottom – into a workforce where training should be expected and enforced for all, and there is step-by-step progress towards qualifications through acceptance of the value of experience.

A final contextual point needs to be made about the organisations or agencies by which Social Services personnel are employed. Currently local authorities in England, Wales and Scotland employ the great majority of Social Services staff. While many run Social Services departments in England and Wales or social work departments in Scotland, a growing number of local authorities have merged parts of their services, for example, Social Services and housing and/or public protection (environmental health) in moves to become more corporate or streamlined. However, the latest proposals (DoH, 2001) see adult Social Services transferring to the NHS, with Care Trusts (perhaps for different client groups) based on the primary care group/Trust model. The director of a combined service that includes Social Services may no longer be a social worker. An understanding of the local geography and organisational structure is constantly complicated by internal and external reorganisations. In Scotland, health, social work and housing are encouraged to pool resources and jointly manage community care services. (Scottish Executive, 2000). For those with NHS backgrounds this sense of upheaval will be familiar. With this changing organisational context in mind, we shall move on to discuss Susan Hunter's engagement with Social Services.

CASE STUDY   MEETING SUSAN HUNTER

The first point of contact with Susan Hunter in hospital came from a telephone call to the social work department, located at another part of the Trust's large site. In this instance the call came from the named nurse and was made because Susan Hunter fitted the criteria for referral – she was elderly, living alone and appeared to need an assessment of her needs. Brief details were passed to a student who was taking telephone calls as part of a shift pattern. The names of Susan Hunter's ward and named nurse were recorded. At an allocation meeting later that week, as it was not assessed as an emergency, Julie Gray was allocated the 'case', since she knew the ward and its staff. One of her colleagues focused mainly on children and another on mental health: Julie and her senior covered other areas.

Julie had been a hospital social worker for six years. She enjoyed her work, particularly contact with patients and nursing staff. She was keen to see hospital discharges handled well: with 'proper' arrangements in place and reliable services ready for people on their return home. In her experience many older people had quite low expectations but occasionally relatives could be quite demanding and confrontational. While her training had placed great value on user and carer empowerment, she appreciated that this could be quite difficult for professionals. She respected many nurses but had a variety of opinions about the doctors, particularly those who referred to 'my beds' on the wards and to patients as 'fractures' or 'bed-blockers'. Her knowledge of the rest of the hospital staff was limited, constant reorganisations in her own department and in the Trust appeared to frustrate exercises such as team building or even social events.

Julie's initial meeting with Susan Hunter took place when her named nurse was off sick. She introduced herself to the ward manager and had a quick discussion with her about whether the time was right to approach Susan Hunter about arrangements for home care. The ward manager considered Susan Hunter was feeling strong enough to talk. As the ward was quiet and Susan Hunter seemed awake and unoccupied, Julie decided to talk to her. She introduced herself and asked Susan Hunter whether she had any general concerns or ideas about what care she might need on discharge from hospital. Julie hoped the nursing staff might have told Susan Hunter of her proposed visit but knew that even if they had, it could well be that this information had been forgotten.

Julie found Susan Hunter spoke slowly, but she seemed very keen to go back home and to do so as soon as possible. Julie learned from her details of Mr Hunter's illness and death, and of her family, friends and church involvement. The case notes were rather limited and Julie knew from experience that such a conversation was a useful way of building a relationship. Susan Hunter described herself as a 'good manager' and someone who coped well – after all, she had nursed her husband 'up to the end'. She had never had any help in the house but her children had helped her financially with the purchase of a replacement washing machine, freezer and central heating. Money was 'tight', however, although she was very economical and did not go in for 'luxuries'.

Julie did not want to tire Susan Hunter on this interview and so returned the next day having had the opportunity to talk to the named nurse, as team communication avenue, about the expected date of discharge. The named nurse was central and fortunately was on duty – Julie knew it could be more difficult if this communication avenue was disrupted by a change of shift or unplanned absence. Julie also met the occupational therapist (OT) working in the ward with Susan Hunter and managed to discuss the assessed needs for the home environment. They also discussed the practicalities in arranging a series of home visits prior to discharge. With Susan Hunter's permission she spoke to her son and daughter about the arrangements for going home and the practicalities of the flat. Julie wanted to identify and clarify a number of points:

- Susan Hunter's wishes and her choices from a range of options
- the family's ability and willingness to help
- Susan Hunter's resources – her determination, priorities and social networks
- Susan Hunter's particular needs to establish a return home and continued physical improvement, or at least maintenance of the progress made in hospital.

To explore these points, Julie used her skills in listening, counselling and risk assessment. She used the Social Services department's community care assessment document as an *aide-memoire*, filling its sections in later in the office to keep her records up to date. Once her assessment was complete, she went back to Susan Hunter to explain what it meant and to ask whether she considered it accurately represented her circumstances and wishes. She found it difficult asking about money in the rather public setting of the ward with no privacy available, but knew this had to be done. Then, Julie spoke on the phone to the OT, who was planning a home visit to collect her impressions of possible problems but also resources. Both considered Susan Hunter's own determination to get home to be a key element of their assessments.

FROM ALMONER TO CARE MANAGER

In many ways social workers such as Julie continue a century-old tradition of hospital social work, which was established in the 1890s as a system of almoners who checked patients' financial entitlements and sought to facilitate their move from hospital to home. The issues of 'bed-blocking' and 'winter pressures' causing problems for hospitals thus predate the NHS hospitals, and Social Services staff continue to make compatible the team objectives of providing a safe and considered return home for patients and assisting their NHS colleagues to make available beds for those in greatest need. At times, of course, these aims may be conflicting (Bradley and Manthorpe, 2000).

Many social workers will practise according to the guidance proffered by the Department of Health's helpful *Hospital Discharge Workbook* (Henwood, 1994). This provides a checklist and a group of performance indicators outlining good practice from admission (or pre-admission), assessment, treatment, discharge and any follow-up. The Department of Health clearly took the view that it would be fruitless to apportion blame for problems with hospital discharge – for any one of a number of staff could practise in such a negative way that discharge could be poorly coordinated, even injurious, upsetting and ineffective (in that patients returned quickly). The DoH was keen on emphasising that while multi-disciplinary or multi-agency approaches were essential, staff had 'complementary responsibilities'. All needed to accept that frequently:

> ... *a discharge from hospital is an admission – or transfer – to community care; and an admission to hospital is a transfer from the community. It is crucial, therefore, to recognise that actions and decisions made at any point in a care episode can have consequences for other parts of the health and social care system.*

> (Henwood, 1994, p.1)

The NHS and Community Care Act 1990 placed certain responsibilities upon local authorities of direct relevance to hospital discharge. In particular, at the level of individuals, it passed responsibility and finance to Social Services departments for the funding of residential and nursing home care for those it considered eligible on grounds of need and resources. Social Services, therefore, have devised their own assessment criteria and 'banding' systems to allocate financial support. Under section 47 of the Act they are empowered to carry out such assessments of need – many of which are informed by contributions from the interdisciplinary team.

For social workers, such as Julie, her assessment may benefit from contributions from the team via Susan Hunter's named or key nurse – particularly if Susan Hunter has confided in her or if her condition is better at certain times than others. The nurse, too, might be able to inform Julie if Susan Hunter's mental capacity is affected – or of certain communication needs. One of the strengths of basing social workers within hospital teams is their ability to appreciate and engage with the hospital perspective and priorities (Manthorpe and Bradley, 2000). From the nurse, or doctor, or therapists, Julie would find both a diagnosis and prognosis helpful – with details, perhaps, of certain anticipated needs. Will Susan Hunter, for example, have medication, and can she take this on her own? Can she get up and dressed? Can she feed and wash herself? Such activities of daily living may be provided to Julie in a report – or more informally. She will be keen to learn if and when any proposed trial visit home has been arranged. In some areas, joint assessment visits between therapists and social workers appear to have significantly improved the quality of assessment

(Cumella and Le Mesurier, 1999). Julie will in turn contribute her assessment to the comprehensive assessment record.

This process of assessment is but one part of the system of care management (see also Chapter 8). It is followed by care planning, care delivery, monitoring and review in a cycle when care or support increases or decreases according to need. The emphasis of the policy document *Caring for People* (Department of Health, 1989) was to turn a resource led system to one that was more flexible or needs led. While this may remain an ideal in many areas, the aim of care management is to respond to individual need as effectively as possible.

RHETORIC AND RESOURCES

The Audit Commission (1997) noted a 'vicious circle', which constituted:

- increasing pressure on hospital beds
- earlier discharge
- insufficient rehabilitation services
- increased admissions to residential or nursing home care
- less money for preventive services
- more admissions to hospital.

Two main effects on Social Services can be observed. Firstly their funding is becoming increasingly 'blocked'. Once a person is eligible for and admitted to residential or nursing home care the cost to the local authority is considerable and largely non-negotiable. Furthermore, even if a high level of community care services can be set in place – the cost is high. The second effect is that much attention becomes focused on patrolling the entry into Social Services care and funding: low level needs may not be met until a crisis develops. Any help is scaled down and may be withdrawn too quickly. Where possible care is charged for and income from service users is maximised.

Commentary on the implementation of the NHS and Community Care Act 1990 has noted the limiting of the process of care management to a narrow focus on assessment as a means of controlling resources. Fewer people now receive domiciliary support, but those who do, receive it at higher levels (Harding, 1999). Such a shift is perhaps best illustrated by the home help service. It has been transformed from a low level domestic service, typically undertaking housework, shopping and pension collection, to a personal care service, which can provide assistance with bathing, toilet needs, meals, dressing and so on – activities that in the past might have been seen (mistakenly or otherwise) as basic nursing care. This process of targeting has been quickly accomplished: in 1992, approximately 58,000 households received six or more visits from home care services per week; by 1996 this number had risen to 123,000 (England only) (Warburton and McCracken, 1999). The numbers of older people in residential care has now stabilised after a period of growth in the 1980s.

It is generally agreed that one factor to improve the level of services for older people is to develop rehabilitation or recuperative services. The Audit

Commission (1997) placed emphasis on local areas 'taking stock' of their current range of services to identify particular needs or shortfalls before rushing to develop a series of new service models. It commented, for example, that few Social Services departments recorded the demand that they faced from hospitals. In other words, most did not know how many cases they might expect that are similar to Susan Hunter. Most did not have a service map from which they could develop information systems: they therefore found it difficult to identify shortfalls systematically.

It is not surprising that when resources are limited each agency seeks to offload or try to pass costs or responsibilities on to others. One illustration of this is the 'blocked bed' where a person stays in hospital, although hospital staff consider the person could and should receive care outside the hospital. The Audit Commission (1997) reported on one local response to such problems: at the start, hospital staff attributed most (65 per cent) of the problems of discharge delays to Social Services. After looking more carefully at the factors involved, they considered that only 12 per cent of the problems were Social Services' responsibility, for it was discovered that other sections of the hospital had been causing delay – or relatives had been resisting discharge (see Chapter 12).

For Social Services staff, a place in hospital for an older person who is in need of a high level of support provides at least a 'holding' station where the person's basic needs are being met, while the urgent (at times) search for a place in a residential home continues or home based care can be assembled and the funding agreed. While a hospital bed may be needed for an emergency or planned admission, Social Services may equally be waiting for a vacancy or agreement from a range of services and agencies about the 'package' of care services. Problems arise when timescales and also power levels differ – a bed is needed now for an emergency but assembling a package takes time. It is possible to see, from Social Services' point of view, that increasingly needs are filtered to their door while they are expected to listen to the views and choices of older people and their carers. Susan Hunter, for example, may insist on going home and may refuse to accept a place in residential care. Her neighbour in the next bed may insist on the opposite.

To respond to issues around 'bed-blocking' and in particular political concerns about hospital waiting lists and distress at times of peak demand (often characterised as 'winter pressures'), the Labour government instituted a series of policy reforms and exhortations. In August 1997, for example, the Minister focused on delays in hospital discharge to prevent winter pressures (DoH, 1997a). By October, the government had issued a government circular, *Better Services for Vulnerable People* (DoH, 1997b), requiring joint investment plans between health and local authorities, emphasising the need to develop multidisciplinary assessment and promoting the development of recuperation and rehabilitation. The later aim has continued to be emphasised in the 1997 White Paper, *The New NHS* (DoH, 1997c), the Social Services White Paper, *Modernising Social Services* (DoH, 1998), and the Report of the Royal Commission on Long-Term

Care, *With Respect to Old Age* (Sutherland, 1999). Despite the latter's focus on funding of long-term care, the Commission took pains to emphasise the potential for rehabilitation to prevent institutional care by aiding recovery. It successfully recommended, for example, that the value of the person's home should be ignored in financial calculations for up to three months to avoid making irreversible decisions.

This emphasis on rehabilitation continued with the White Paper, *The NHS Plan* (DoH, 2000):

> *In future, the NHS and local Social Services should support older people to make a faster recovery from illness, encouraging independence rather than institutional care, and providing reliable, high quality on-going support at home.*

Specifically this White Paper sets out a time frame for many of the measures exhorted in earlier pronouncements. From 2002, there will be a single assessment process for health and social care – starting with the most vulnerable – such as those recently discharged from hospital (para. 15.9). The most vulnerable will also have a 'personal care plan' covering health and social care (para. 15.10). Care Direct will provide a parallel advice and referral service similar to NHS Direct (para. 15.12). Investment and 'beds' will deliver 'active recovery and rehabilitation services' to benefit 150,000 more older people each year (para. 15.14). To prevent unnecessary admission rapid response services will be enhanced (para. 15.14), while to facilitate home care, funds and equipment (ranging from low level to high 'tech') will be augmented. The Royal Commission's recommendation of a 'breathing space' of three months will be in place by 2001 (para. 15.18), while changes to funding formulae are intended to remove the perverse incentives making residential care 'cheaper' for local authorities than some home care packages.

JOINED UP RESPONSES

The policy agenda emphasises joint working, joint delivery and joint financing. For some working in Social Services, there is concern that their particular contribution to the holistic support of older people will be marginalised. Utilising social models of disability in the main and valuing concepts such as choice, independence and autonomy, social workers have been able to offer a certain independence from the hospital and NHS systems. At best they have conceived of themselves as being able to represent older people's point of view in face of a more unified health edifice and to have advocated on their behalf. In particular they have managed difficulties around social relationships, including conflict between family members, service users who are reluctant to engage with services and been able to sustain relationships with those whose mental capacity is frail. Many working in Social Services have accumulated substantial experience in working with complex care 'packages' of home based support involving the independent sector, supporting informal carers and managing risk. This range of skills may be pertinent to what is described as 'active rehabilitation', which may well involve a number of agencies, personnel and funding streams. These can be as relevant to preventing hospital or institutional admissions as much as developing robust discharge arrangements.

One particular contribution from Social Services may lie in their established relationships with local housing agencies. Housing can at times seem the distant relation of community care but it may be central to the whole enterprise of successful rehabilitation. At its most narrow, a focus on housing can be the identification of the right place or location for the individual. Is the right place at home, in residential care, in sheltered housing or with relatives? Such decisions may be made hastily and with little regard to the older person's choices, well-being or principles of ordinary life (Hawtin, 2000). A broader interpretation of housing and home places the individual at the centre of the picture. If their own home is at all practical then there will need to be a considered view of its strengths and weaknesses. Colleagues from Social Services and occupational therapy may work on this together, but may also draw on the wide experience and capacity of housing agencies.

In the case of Susan Hunter, for example, Julie has heard her speak of repairs that should have been sorted out a long time ago. One key local resource in such circumstances for people who are home owners or private/independent sector tenants (in some cases local authority tenants also) is the housing improvement agency, which may work with older people to carry out minor or substantial works and draw in grants or create financial packages to cover costs. Julie's local authority is represented on this agency and she has had previous clients who have been helped in this way. In other areas, community based OTs may have access to such resources.

Susan Hunter's wish to go home may be further assisted by access to resources that will improve her quality of life. As part of the care package Julie may consider forms of assistive technology (see the discussion in Sutherland, 1999), and will discuss these with the therapists and whole family. While there are many devices or systems available, in this case Julie may wish to consider with Susan Hunter whether some aids to daily living may be helpful in helping with domestic matters. It may be of course that this has already been considered by the OT, but if none are available it is likely to be a matter for Social Services. For example, she may find that Susan Hunter has been using a local laundrette because she has no washing machine. Julie may be able to establish whether a washing machine would be acceptable and may be able to propose ways of financing this through the Benefits Agency (Social Fund) or through referral to a local charity. At the very least Julie may pass these ideas on to the Social Services' care manager who will be Susan Hunter's key worker in respect of community care.

At a slightly more sophisticated level, Susan Hunter, her family or any of the professionals in contact with her may consider that an alarm system would be useful. It is presumed – but of course would need checking – that Susan Hunter is one of the 93 per cent of households aged 65 years and over who have a telephone (Sutherland, 1999, p. 84), but if not, a telephone may be an item that it would be helpful to arrange promptly. Julie or her successor care manager should have details of the local systems, some of which will be available through the housing department of the local authority and some of which may be linked to a form of warden service that may provide emergency assistance or reassurance. Most local authorities run such schemes and some have been increasingly integrated with community care services. Finally, housing improvement agencies working with Social Services may play a larger and more sophisticated role in helping the built environment to maximise independence. The development of 'smart houses' that can link into tele-medicine services to monitor individuals' health, to confirm care staff's identity and record their arrival, to control lighting and heating, and so on offers enormous potential for home-based care. Such developments may also be worrying to older people and so the role of a trusted professional in explaining their functions will become increasingly important. Care managers in the future will need to be able both to draw on the expertise of others but also to present the 'human face' of such developments and to support those at the receiving end.

OUT OF HOSPITAL

Hospital discharge, as Henwood and Wistow (1999) observe, has been remarkable for the extent of central mandate behind policy. One further element has been the high level of monitoring of this area and the identification of 'continuing care' as a special case requiring almost unparalleled agreement at local level about the precise level of funding responsibility for individual patients or service users. Continuing health care is a term coined to describe health-care responsibilities at the interface with social care. Patients with high levels of need are included in this area, as long as they are not deemed to be 'acute'. Local agreements have been constructed to clarify responsibility for funding, discrete routes for complaint have been devised and, in many areas, specific groups of staff offer high levels of care to those funded under the system (see Malin, 2000).

It is possible to see these arrangements as presaging new forms of services for larger amounts of people. A 'can do' attitude that concentrates on finding solutions may be one important legacy from the hard-won achievements of continuing care services. As Browning (1999) notes, however, some of the elements of a rehabilitation service need to encompass far more than those associated with social and health services. Delays in housing assessments or problems with provision of adaptations, for example, may make moving back home too difficult. Similarly, while professionals may have some confidence in the value of a short stay in a residential home for rehabilitation, limited as these may be in resources or trained staff, the views of the older person and his or her family will need to be taken into account. One key element of social work research is the importance of establishing that older people's views about their care are variable and highly influential (Stanley, 1999). Their wish to enter residential care, at times, will be a powerful dynamic, influencing all assessments and their contribution to the rehabilitation process.

CASE STUDY SUPPORTING SUSAN HUNTER

We return now to the present to consider Susan Hunter and the arrangements that Julie has made on her behalf. Primarily Julie has tried to support the family in providing a safe return home. She has completed her assessment, which notes Susan Hunter's needs for support at certain times of day, and has found that particular days are likely to be difficult. She suggests that a care worker, from a local private home care agency, visits at lunchtime on Tuesday and Thursday to help Susan Hunter prepare her lunch, to talk with her and to supervise the taking of medication in line with goals identified by the team. Julie proposes this happens for a two-week period and then is reviewed. She explains to Susan Hunter that there will be a charge for this service and how this will be collected. At the same time Julie helps Susan Hunter to apply for Attendance Allowance, which should cover the cost of this care and provide extra income.

Julie explains the arrangements to Susan Hunter and her family – leaving the contact name and number of the care manager who will be taking over Susan Hunter's 'case' once she goes home. In respect of the professionals engaged, she copies such details to the GP and any staff who are likely to be engaged in follow-up work. While such details might be noted in face-to-face meetings, in this case Julie deals with them through letter or memo, noting ruefully that shared electronic systems will be of great assistance. She provides them with a copy of the care plan, pointing out the details of the home care agency. In addition she checks that the family has received details of the local stroke support group.

Such limited activity on behalf of the hospital social worker reflects the demands on their time and their conceptualisation of their role. The demands of the hospital environment place pressure on the social worker to respond quickly to requests for assessment and to make practical arrangements as quickly as possible. From their own agency they receive instructions, at times, that resources are extremely short or that certain services are unavailable. While present on the hospital site and part of the hospital system, their accountability is outside the NHS. To some this represents a strength, while to others it imposes another hurdle to efficient care.

We have outlined the scope of Julie's involvement, but need to stress that her role lies in assessment, communication with Susan Hunter and the family, and initial coordination of the home care 'package'. Much of the day-to-day work with Susan Hunter at home will be the responsibility of a local care manager who will in turn pull together the domiciliary care funded by Social Services, monitor its delivery and liaise with other professionals, as well as Susan

Hunter and her family. Because Susan Hunter may require limited help for a specific period, the home based service may be part of an 'intermediate' service. While there are no precise definitions of this term, it is generally used to describe a service that provides a rapid response, is designed to be flexible and highly responsive, offers a mix of social and health-related care and is oriented to rehabilitation. Other terms commonly used for similar models may be 'intensive home support' or 'hospital at home' schemes (see also Chapter 10).

For some patients the existence of such schemes may be a key in enabling them to leave hospital for home. Their staff may be able to provide regular and frequent assistance and to facilitate action from other agencies – such as 'fast-tracking' loans or equipment. Services may have the advantage to Susan Hunter of being free or charged at a relatively low rate. Many older people have been critical of traditional home care services as being unreliable, inflexible and inconsistent (Sutherland, 1999): intensive schemes may deal with such problems by having the resources to employ and monitor trained staff with smaller case-loads.

Whether such schemes are termed intermediate, intensive or rehabilitative is often a matter of local choice, politics or experience. This movement may reflect the extent to which staff employed in such schemes see themselves as providers of care, doing things for older people, or as agents of change, promoting independence, helping people to regain lost skills and restoring their confidence.

Much, then, will depend on the qualities and abilities of those staff who ultimately may support Susan Hunter at home; providing her with social contact, helping her to choose, prepare and cook her lunch, possibly working alongside her to practise old skills or exercise. Home carers, domiciliary workers or support staff may be their occupational label: it is highly probable that they will be women and at the lower end of pay and qualifications. As Towers and her colleagues (1999, pp. 227–228) also observe:

> *Women and ethnic minorities are heavily over-represented at the lowest levels of home care employment. Despite the emphasis that many local authorities have placed upon training opportunities, this remains a largely formally untrained occupation . . . so many models of integrated care ignore the people who do the bulk of it, the home carers and the informal carers . . . we are seeing Home Carers as the occupational group who are being placed in the impossible position of being the linchpin in the community care health/social care interface, whilst not being accorded the status, influence or remuneration of either their health or social work colleagues.*

While there is increasing attention to the potential of home based rehabilitation, it should not be forgotten that the staff who deliver such a service will need training, advice, support and monitoring. These frontline staff will have a key role in translating the rehabilitation agenda into a reality. Whether employed directly by Social Services, a Care Trust or part of a joint commissioning approach with other agencies, some agreements will be needed about the responsibilities for training, monitoring and service development. While some schemes may be able to develop posts such as rehabilitation assistants (for example, the 'respite' project described by Slack, 2000), it is clear that they too pass much of personal care and support work to home care staff. Slack describes how care plans need to be widely shared among staff 'explaining how much assistance to give and in what areas to encourage independence' (p. 42). At the moment care managers often have little experience on which to build or guidance about their role.

SUMMARY

The new emphasis on rehabilitation will demand some shifts in thinking and practice within Social Services. A recent Social Services Inspectorate report (1999), for example, found many examples of 'separate care plans for the same individuals' (para. 4.23) between Social Services and community nurses. As Hudson notes 'to a large extent, Social Services and primary health care services and staff still run on parallel lines' (2000, p. 247). The potential of Primary Care Trusts to address these issues may be another spur to change at a level closer to practice. The changes proposed by the NHS Plan for Care Trusts may help converge these parallel lines.

The contribution of Social Services staff to the rehabilitation agenda lies both at a strategic level: mapping services, developing new resources and managing the care market; and at the operational level of individuals and the families. New policy developments suggest that some of the major difficulties and perverse incentives are being tackled by joint activities at planning, funding and assessment stages. Nonetheless, the established skills of Social Services staff in communication between agencies (not simply with the NHS), dealing with conflict and empowering service users to make choices, remain highly relevant. Their experiences in working with and sustaining relationships with those who have dementia are also valuable (see also Chapters 9 and 17). New policy developments in relation to decision-making for those who are mentally incapacitated look set to require further skills in assessment, care planning and monitoring (see the proposals of the Lord Chancellor's Department, 1997) for groups whose rehabilitation may involve psycho-social as well as physical contributions. While Susan Hunter's mental capacity appears not to be cause for concern, in many cases Social Services staff will be working with those with dementia or similar disabilities.

The training, value base and practice experience of Social Services staff in the social model of disability offer a perspective that has much to offer older people and their carers, as well as their colleagues in interdisciplinary and multi-agency teams.

Social workers, for example, may be alert to social issues that impact on the whole recuperative process. For example, they are likely (according to research from the Social Services Inspectorate, 1998) to place a high value on ensuring that services to ethnic minority older people are relevant and accessible (see also Chapter 3). While recognising that many resources are ethnocentric they generally appeared to understand the importance of race and culture, and many had been involved in developing a range of innovative services. Similarly, many social workers are sensitive to the impact of poverty on the lives of older people and appear keen to maximise resources available to individuals and to take a sympathetic view regarding charging and ability to pay (Bradley and Manthorpe, 1997). The low incomes and limited resources of many older people, often combined with their dignity in such circumstances, may place serious constraints on the extent to which they have the means to help themselves to maintain a healthy, warm and comfortable home. Many social workers have skills in advocacy and these may be particularly appropriate to the needs of older people who are marginalised.

REFERENCES

Audit Commission (1997) *The Coming of Age: Improving care services for older people*, Audit Commission, London.

Balloch, S., McLean, J. and Fisher, M. (eds) (1999) *Social Services: Working under pressure*, The Policy Press, Bristol.

Bradley, G. and Manthorpe, J. (1997) *Financial assessment: A practitioners' guide*, Venture Press, Birmingham.

Bradley, G. and Manthorpe, J. (eds.) (2000) *Working on the Fault Line*, Venture Press, Birmingham.

Browning, D. (1999) Value for money. In: *With Respect to Old Age* (ed. Sutherland, S.), The Stationery Office, London, Research Volume 3, Chapter 8.

Cumella, S. and Le Mesurier, N. (1999) Re-designing health and social care for older people: multi-skill case teams in primary care. *Managing Community Care*, 7(6), 17–24.

Department of Health [DoH] (1989) *Caring for People: Community Care in the Next Decade and Beyond*, Cm. 849, HMSO, London.

DoH (1997a) *Managing Winter*, 1997/98 MISC(97)62.

DoH (1997b) *Better Services for Vulnerable People*, EL(97)62, CI(97)24.

DoH (1997c) *The New NHS: Modern and dependable*, The Stationery Office, London.

DoH (1998) *Modernising Social Services: Promoting independence, improving protection, raising standards*, The Stationery Office, London.

DoH (2000) *The NHS Plan: A plan for investment, A plan for reform*, Cm. 4818–1, The Stationery Office, London.

DoH (2001) *Care Trust: Emerging framework*, The Stationery Office, London.

Harding, T. (1999) Enabling older people to live in their own homes. In: *With Respect to Old Age* (ed. Sutherland, S.), The Stationery Office, London, Research Volume 3, Chapter 3.

Hawtin, M. (2000) Social care and housing. In: *The Changing Role of Social Care* (ed. Hudson, B.), Jessica Kingsley, London, pp. 123–152.

Henwood, M. (ed.) (1994) *Hospital Discharge Workbook: A manual on hospital discharge practice*, Department of Health, London.

Henwood, M. and Wistow, G. (1999) Clarifying responsibilities and improving accountability? In: *With Respect to Old Age* (ed. Sutherland, S.), The Stationery Office, London, Research Volume 3, Chapter 7.

Hudson, B. (2000) *Social Services and Primary Care Groups. Health and Social Care in the Community*, 8(4), 242–250.

Lord Chancellor's Department (1997) *Who Decides? Making decisions on behalf of mentally incapacitated adults*, Cm. 3803, The Stationery Office, London.

Malin, V. (2000) From continuous to continuing long-term care. In: *Working on the Fault Line* (eds Bradley, G. and Manthorpe, J.), Venture Press, Birmingham, pp. 127–150.

Manthorpe, J. and Bradley, G. (2000) Care management across the threshold. In: *Working on the Fault Line* (eds Bradley, G. and Manthorpe, J.), Venture Press, Birmingham, pp. 71–97.

Scottish Executive (2000) *Community Care: A Joint Future – report of the Joint Future Group*, Scottish Executive Health and Community Care Department, Edinburgh.

Slack, H. (2000) From respite to rehabilitation, Review. *Managing Community Care*, 8(3), 40–43.

Social Services Inspectorate (1998) *They Look After Their Own, Don't They? Inspection of Community Care Services for Black and Ethnic Minority Older People*, Department of Health, London.

Social Services Inspectorate (1999) *Of Primary Importance: Inspection of Social Services Departments' Links with Primary Health Services*, Department of Health, London.

Stanley, N. (1999) User-practitioner: transactions in new culture community care. *British Journal of Social Work*, **29**, 417–435.

Sutherland, S. (ed.) (1999) *With Respect to Old Age: Long term care – rights and responsibilities*, The Stationery Office, London, Royal Commission Research Vol. 2, pp. 81–91.

Towers, B., Smith, P. and Mackintosh, M. (1999) Dimensions of class in the integration of health and social care. *Journal of Interprofessional Care*, 13(3), 219–228.

Warburton, W. and McCracken, J. (1999) An evidence-based perspective from the Department of Health on the impact of the 1993 reforms of the care of frail, elderly people. In: *With Respect to Old Age* (ed. Sutherland, S.), The Stationery Office, London, Research Volume 3, Chapter 2.

20 Other essential services

Aims of the chapter

The generally considered 'core' services for assessment and rehabilitation of older people have been described. There are also a number of other services that play an important role in certain circumstances. An understanding of the criteria for referral and their timely contribution will enable the expanded team to provide a truly comprehensive and effective rehabilitation service. Examples such as nutrition and dietetics, dentistry, pharmacy, continence, optical and hearing services are described, and local developments may offer an even wider range. As will be seen from these and the previous contributions, the linkages and overlaps are considerable – but often overlooked. Good lateral working relationships between all members of the team will do much to facilitate a smooth and timely rehabilitation process. Smaller departments having episodic contact with the core team may feel isolated and excluded from its work and social activities, and opportunities for reciprocal involvement should be actively pursued – and responded to.

PART A: NUTRITION AND DIETETICS IN OLD AGE – KIRAN SHUKLA

INTRODUCTION

Nutrition plays a key role in the health of an older person. Good nutrition for older people is important for both long-term and short-term health. The impact of illness and disability on nutritional status, and the effects of this on the ability to recover from illness are of special concern in this age group. The ageing process affects the majority of the body systems, including the gastrointestinal, cardiovascular, endocrine, renal, neurological, immune, sensory and skeletal systems. Along with these, social and financial circumstances may change. All these changes have a direct or indirect effect on the nutritional status. Good nutrition is not only important for the maintenance of health, but also for recovery from illness. This is particularly important for this age group where, as a consequence of the natural ageing process, ill health is more common.

The nutritional intake of older people relates closely both to physical and mental health. It also reflects on their social well-being, but economic, psychosocial and physical factors also play a very important role in the general nutrition of this age group. It is well known that older people entering residential care are often malnourished. This could be because of long periods of poverty, illness, social isolation, personal and psychological problems. Over the past decade, many changes have taken place in the provision of long-term care for older people.

'Not because they are old' – an independent inquiry into the care of older people on acute wards in general hospital (Health Advisory Service, 2000, 1998) looked at the care given and the factors that might influence the quality of that care. Some of the areas of concern were specific to food, drink, feeding and nutrition.

The important role the dietitian plays in ensuring minimum requirements for older people are adequately met for specific conditions like diabetes, cardiovascular disease and osteoporosis, along with the need to maintain normal weight, preventing the health hazards of being over or underweight, has been addressed by the National Service Framework for Older People (Department of Health [DoH], 2001) (see Chapter 6).

It is very encouraging to note that this mentions dietitians as the core members of the specialist old age multidisciplinary teams. Existing teams that operate without a dietitian will therefore need to review their membership.

ROLE OF THE STATE REGISTERED DIETITIAN AS PART OF THE MULTIDISCIPLINARY TEAM

Only state registered dietitians can practise within the National Health Service. The role of the dietitian is to make sure that older people achieve and maintain optimum nutritional status and have their quality of life enhanced through inter-professional teamwork. The interdisciplinary team works together to achieve the best care for the clients at all times. It is important that the dietitian is a part of this team to work through the stages of the disease and match patients'/clients' therapeutic needs with the changes in the disease status.

DIETETIC INTERVENTION

A dietitian working in a dedicated unit for care of older people or in the community needs a considerable amount of background information before appropriate advice is offered. This information can be as basic as:

- Is the patient living at home or in residential care?
- If at home, who cooks the food?
- Who delivers the food?
- How is the food delivered?
- Who does the shopping?
- What does the meal look like?
- Is the meal culturally/religiously acceptable?
- Is the patient used to this type of food?
- Can the patient handle crockery/cutlery?
- Will the patient get help in feeding?
- Are the meals rushed?
- How long does it take to finish the meal?
- If dentures are used, is the fitting right, are the dentures within the patient's reach?
- What is the nutritional value of the meal?
- How much food is eaten?
- Are likes and dislikes of the patient/client considered?

This information can be obtained by one member of the team and should be available to others as required. This way duplication can be avoided. Other team members likely to be particularly interested in dietary issues are the nurse (Chapter 14), occupational therapist (Chapter 16), speech and language therapist (Chapter 17) and social worker (Chapter 19). The National Service Framework for Older People promotes integration to provide a whole system of care with a single assessment system for health and social care.

REFERRAL TO THE DIETITIAN

Individual dietary advice is available for those referred to the service by a registered medical or dental practitioner. However, general nutrition or dietary advice may be given to groups of clients without the need for such referral. Local procedures for referral to the dietitian can be agreed by the rehabilitation team and dietetic department.

Older adults can be referred to the dietitian if they are:

- diagnosed as needing a special/therapeutic diet
- not eating a full mixed diet, e.g. liquids only
- showing a poor appetite or refusing food
- unable to maintain body weight composition/biochemistry due to poor oral intake
- overweight.

ASSESSMENT

The dietitian assesses nutritional status by considering:

- weight changes
- hydration
- dietary intake
- clinical condition
- social assessment, e.g. home circumstances and mental condition
- drug therapy
- biochemical profile/haematological measurements if available or needed.

After assessment, individual goals are agreed with the patient and/or carer, and the dietitian:

- liaises with appropriate people to ensure that the patient receives the prescribed dietary therapy
- educates the patient/carer on the modified or therapeutic diet and gives written information
- continues to assess the patient and review the therapeutic diet
- evaluates dietary intervention, either directly or by advising others on appropriate monitoring method
- provides information relevant to their needs.

As a member of the interdisciplinary team the dietitian can:

- act as a resource to the health-care team in providing his/her expertise
- devise simple nutritional assessment forms for the care staff to use
- train the care staff in using the assessment tools
- train staff to look out for signs of malnutrition
- provide support, including education, to health professionals and others involved in the care of the older adult
- facilitate an optimum nutritional intake in all older adults
- enable carers to appreciate and act to ensure patients receive nutritionally adequate food
- develop dietetic care pathways from secondary to primary care.

THE ROLE OF THE DIETITIAN IN HELPING WITH SPECIFIC CONDITIONS

Dysphagia

Close working with speech and language therapists and nursing staff is essential. Dietitians can advise on appropriate nutrition in conjunction with the patient following swallowing assessment by the speech and language therapist (Chapter 17). Interdisclipinary dysphagia groups to look at protocols for the treatment of the dysphagia patient can be very useful.

Appropriate thickeners for the food can be recommended by the dietitian. The method of feeding the patient is usually decided by the dietitian in conjunction with nursing staff. If the patient is to be fed enterally, the dietitian advises on the appropriate feed and the regime for the patient, which is regularly reviewed and monitored.

While considering stroke, the standard in the NSF sets out four main components for the development of integrated stroke services:

- prevention
- immediate care, including care from specialist stroke team
- early and continuing rehabilitation
- long-term support, for the patient and their carer.

The need for nutrition and dietetic involvement cannot be ignored at any one of these stages. The proportion of time devoted may vary for different organisations, but when looking at it as a seamless service, dietitians play a key role. This starts with prevention within the community, which might take the form of dealing with hypertension, obesity or general healthy eating. At the second and third stages, the dietitian will be working as a core member of the rehabilitation team. For long-term support, the dietitian may be a key member of contact if the older adult is fed artificially, or if they require nutrition support or texture modification.

Constipation

Constipation is a common complaint particularly in immobile patients. In elderly people, not only is prevalence higher than in the general population but the impact on quality of life is greater (Pettigrew *et al.*, 1997).

Simple constipation can usually be prevented by:

* increasing the intake of dietary fibre of both cereals and vegetable origin
* increasing fluid intake
* increasing activity.

The use of high fibre diets is only effective if there is sufficient liquid to absorb the fibre and soften the stools. Some older adults may be reluctant to increase fibre because of fear of pain or discomfort on defecation. Older people should be advised to gradually increase the fibre in the diet by introducing new sources of fibre slowly over a few weeks. By doing so the body adjusts to the new diet more easily and the feeling of discomfort can be avoided.

Starchy foods like bread, rice, potatoes and fruit and vegetables are a valuable source of vitamins along with the soluble fibre.

Patients fed artificially will be advised on the appropriate feed by the dietitian. The habit of sprinkling 'bran' over food should be discouraged as it impairs the absorption of trace elements and minerals like iron, calcium and zinc, and affects the palatability of the food. Dietitians can advise on the appropriate diet.

Prevention of malnutrition/pressure sores

The prime objective of nutrition policies and practices concerning older people should be directed towards the prevention of malnutrition. Those older people who are relatively inactive require fewer calories because they use less energy. Although the energy requirement of such people may be lower, their requirements for other nutrients will not have changed and may well have increased. Their diet therefore should be one of quality rather than quantity. Wheelchair users or bedridden people are likely to put on weight because of immobility and are at greater risk of pressure sores. It is advisable to consult the dietitian prior to putting patients on the weight reducing diets that may not be nutritionally adequate. Dietitians can be actively involved in developing nutrition screening tools to prevent pressure sores.

APPROPRIATE DIET

Dietitians can advise and ensure that adequate nutrition is not only given to the patient, but also is actually eaten by the patient. The nutritional value of the food not eaten is nil, hence the food served needs to be acceptable, palatable, of correct consistency and presentable to excite the patient's appetite. Over-zealous attempts to apply healthy eating guidelines to older people can result in nutritional problems. If someone has poor appetite and is eating very little, it is very important to give nutrient dense foods that are palatable and look attractive. The overall message should be to keep up an interest in and enjoy the food. If older people could be encouraged to be more physically active, their energy requirements and their appetite would increase. Physical activity would also improve their body fitness and their general health and well-being.

The National Service Framework for Older People recognises the risks that hospital admission can pose for this group. Particular attention is drawn to hydration, nutrition, skin care and continence from arrival at hospital, to discharge. Under Standard 5 on Stroke the National Service Framework addresses actions to reduce the risk factors for stroke in the population. The interventions are broadly the same as those of coronary heart disease, i.e. increasing levels of physical activity, encouraging healthy eating, particularly reducing salt intake and increasing fruit and vegetable consumption.

CASE STUDY	**SUSAN HUNTER – SPEECH AND LANGUAGE ASSESSMENT**

Following the speech and language therapy assessment, the nursing staff reported that Susan Hunter was too tired at mealtimes and was not getting enough nutrition. A case discussion between medical, nursing and therapy staff resulted in the following goals being set:

- An assessment of how much food and drink are consumed daily.
- Identification of her normal weight and how much she has lost.
- Clarification of diabetic control and medication.
- Ensuring an adequate oral diet using appropriate food textures and consistency. This consisted of a high protein puréed diet, thickened fluids and supplements. All oral intake was monitored on a regular basis to ensure nutritional needs were being met.
- Supervised feeding in the early stages of recovery – was spoonfed by nursing staff.
- Supervised while self-feeding – equipment provided by occupational therapist to enhance self-feeding skills and independence.
- Weighed weekly.

Throughout the hospital admission the dietitian would ensure that Susan Hunter's dietary needs were being met and discussion with the occupational therapist about her nutritional needs and cooking abilities made post discharge. Susan Hunter had previously managed her own diabetic control and it was important to teach her carers what her needs were and to liaise with the community team about her nutritional needs on discharge.

Dietitians must be prepared to work with and influence Primary Care Trust colleagues to ensure that the important role of the state registered dietitian is recognised, valued and resourced throughout services for the older adult.

Some older people, especially those with infections (Lehman, 1991; Mobartham and Trumbore, 1991), may require a higher level of protein, but advice should always be sought from the dietitian and/or doctor on the level of protein required.

While advising the carers, dietitians can give ideas of appropriate foods, shopping on a budget for their relative or friend and information on a store cupboard.

Here the dietitian can work very closely with other professionals, particularly occupational therapists (Chapter 16) and carers (Chapter 12) to ensure that their advice is reinforced and is consistent.

THE FUTURE

Dietitians have a crucial role to play in tackling the concerns identified in the latest national diet and nutrition survey of the over 65s (Finch *et al.*, 1998) and national health improvement intentions (DoH, 1998).

Dietitians can help in determining the type of practical dietary advice offered to older people living in the community and the hospitals. The nutritional policies for the institutions providing meals for the older adults should be produced by expert advice from the dietitians.

Dietitians will also be involved in the nutritional health promotion programme in hospitals and will identify areas for active promotion of health to patients/relatives and carers within the hospital or the community. Dietitians have a vital role to play in the education and training of patients' caterers, nursing, social services staff and other members of the primary care team involved in the care of the elderly.

REFERENCES

Department of Health [DoH] (1998) *Our Healthier Nation*, HMSO, London.
DoH (2001) *The National Service Framework for Older People*, The Stationery Office, London.
Finch, S., Doyle, W. and Lowe, C. (1998) *National Diet and Nutrition Survey: People aged 65 years and older, 1: Report of the Diet and Nutrition Survey*, The Stationery Office, London.
Health Advisory Service 2000 (1998) *Not Because They are Old – an independent Inquiry into the Care of Older People on Acute Wards in General Hospitals*, Health Advisory Service, London.
Lehman, A.B. (1991) Nutrition in old age: update and questions for future research, Part 1. *Reviews in Clinical Gerontology*, 1, 135–145.
Mobartham, S. and Trumbore, L.S. (1991) Nutritional problems of the elderly. *Clinics in Geriatric Medicine*, 7(2), 191–214.
Pettigrew, M., Watt, I. and Sheldon, T. (1997) Systematic review of the effectiveness of laxatives in the elderly. *Health Technology Assessment*, 1(13).

FURTHER READING

Caroline Walker Trust (1995) *Eating Well for Older People: Report of an expert working group.*
Department of Health (1993) *The Nutrition of Elderly People*, COMA Report No. 43, HMSO, London.
Nutrition Advisory Group for the Elderly People (1993) *Dietetic Standards of Care for the Older Adult in Hospital*, British Dietetic Publications, Birmingham.

PART B: DENTISTRY IN OLD AGE – JOYCE M. SMITH

ORAL HEALTH AND DISEASE

The last quarter of the twentieth century saw a general improvement in oral health in many Western countries, which has resulted in more people keeping their natural teeth throughout life. In the UK, for example, the proportion of older people with some natural teeth more than tripled during this time, with a resulting 64 per cent of people aged 65–74 and 42 per cent of those aged 75 and over, being dentate in 1998 (Kelly, 2000). Furthermore, the most pessimistic estimate suggests that by the year 2028, only 8 per cent of those aged 65–74, 15 per cent of those aged 75–84 and 31 per cent of those aged 85 and over will have no natural teeth (Kelly et al., 2000). When considering the oral health of older people, therefore, although problems with dentures do still need to be recognised, the prevention and treatment of diseases of the natural dentition are now the main priority. Indeed, the maintenance of extensively restored dentitions in older people is one of the major challenges for dentistry in the new millennium.

Dental caries (decay) and periodontal (gum) diseases are the principal diseases of the oral cavity and they are both prevalent among older people. The majority of dentate older people have been found to suffer from some form of periodontal disease and evidence of a high level of caries experience is found either as active decay, or in the restorations provided as a consequence of past disease (Steele et al., 1998). The 1998 UK Adult Dental Health Survey found that dentate people aged 75 and over had an average of 15 remaining teeth, of which 50 per cent were sound and untreated, one was decayed and the remainder were restored (Kelly et al., 2000). In general, dental caries activity in older adults is different to that in the young, in that secondary, or recurrent, decay tends to predominate over primary lesions and caries of exposed tooth roots, where the gum has receded, is particularly prevalent (Billings et al., 1985).

Ill-fitting dentures are also common among older people and some authors have reported a high prevalence of associated diseases of the oral mucosa (Smith and Sheiham, 1980; Steele et al., 1998). Carcinomas in and around the mouth are another important consideration. These account for between 1 and 4 per cent of all malignant disease in the UK and amount to 1,900 new cases and 950 deaths each year. Eighty-five per cent of cases of oral carcinoma occur in people over 50 years of age (Johnson and Warnakulasuriya, 1993).

All of these oral conditions may affect the quality of a person's life and detract significantly from his or her general and social well-being by causing pain and discomfort, problems with eating and speaking (see also Chapter 17) and suffering from the prejudices associated with a poor appearance (Smith and Sheiham, 1979; Steele et al., 1998). In the National Diet and Nutrition Survey for people aged 65 years and over, Steele et al. (1998) found that a reduction in the number of functional natural teeth and the reduced effectiveness of dentures may result in altered food choices, which in turn can lead to alterations in nutrient intake and nutritional status. They found that some of these effects may even result in levels of nutritional status that are close to deficiency status (see also Chapter 20A). It is important, therefore, that the oral health of older patients should be maintained during rehabilitation, in order that preventable, or treatable, conditions should not become added burdens for those whose health is already compromised.

ORAL SCREENING

Despite the high prevalence of oral disease in older people, there is a reluctance among many in this age group to seek dental care. Indeed, in 1999, only 29 per cent of people aged 75 and over in England and Wales were registered with a National Health Service dentist (Dental Practice Board, 1999). Reasons for this low demand for care include fear, the cost of treatment, lack of mobility and the feeling that 'older people should not trouble the dentist' (Smith and Sheiham, 1980; Lester *et al.*, 1998). The under 75s may be less inhibited (see also Chapter 5).

In many instances, chronic oral problems, which have been ignored by the patient, become acute or obvious and are brought to the attention of carers and members of the rehabilitation team at the time of a generally debilitating illness. In particular, patients may complain of pain, swellings, oral ulceration and loose dentures. It is essential that none of these symptoms should be ignored, but that arrangements should be made for a dentist to examine the patient as soon as possible, either in a practice or through a domiciliary visit. For new patients, carers and members of the rehabilitation team might find it helpful to complete a short checklist on oral symptoms in order to identify those in immediate need of dental care. Such a list might include items from the D-E-N-T-A-L screening form developed by Bush *et al.* (1996):

- Dry mouth
- Eating difficulty
- No recent dental care
- Tooth or mouth pain
- Alteration or change in food selection
- Lesions, sores or lumps in the mouth.

Because of the high level of oral pathology in older people, however, it is important that both those with natural teeth and those without should have regular oral examinations, whether or not they are experiencing symptoms. Oral screening allows for the identification and treatment of disease, and for the implementation of appropriate preventive regimes.

People should be encouraged to attend a general dental practice for routine check-ups, but where this is not possible, the examinations can be carried out on a domiciliary basis. In many districts, oral screening programmes are carried out in residential homes and hospitals. Clinical protocols should also provide for all older people admitted to hospital to receive an oral examination as part of the overall assessment of health.

Prevention of oral disease

During a debilitating illness, a person's eating habits may alter and the ability to carry out adequate mouth care may be compromised. This may result in a poor level of oral hygiene and a marked deterioration in oral health. It is essential that carers and members of the rehabilitation team should be aware of this and help the patient to adopt good oral health practices. Where a patient is unable to maintain adequate oral self-care, occupational therapists may be able to provide adapted products for self-care (Chapter 16), carers should be encouraged to assist with oral hygiene with help from a dental hygienist and provide balanced diets (see also Chapter 20A).

Dental decay occurs when bacterial plaque produces acid as a result of the metabolism of refined carbohydrates, especially sugars. The acid initially causes demineralisation of the enamel surface, but caries and the breakdown of the tooth results if there are frequent acid attacks. Limiting the frequency of consumption of sugary foods and drinks is, therefore, one of the most important ways of preventing dental decay (Levine, 1996). In particular, older people should be warned about sudden changes of diet. Constant 'snacking' on sugary foods and drinks, instead of eating balanced meals, should be discouraged because of the risk of dental decay as well as from the general nutritional point of view.

Many older people suffer from dry mouth, xerostomia, and may be highly susceptible to dental caries, especially if they suck sweets, or take frequent sips of sugar-containing drinks to alleviate the symptoms. The dry mouth is usually due to the ageing process, or the patient's medication (Chapter 20C), but it should always be investigated as it may be caused by an underlying systemic disease such as diabetes. If the dryness persists, 'safe' alternatives such as sipping drinks with no added sugar, sucking sugar-free sweets, or the use of artificial saliva may be suggested. Sugary medicines are another potential cause of dental caries, particularly in people with a dry mouth, and should be replaced by tablets, capsules or sugar-free formulations wherever possible. As well as diet control, regular brushing with a fluoride toothpaste and the use of fluoride rinses are important measures for the prevention of dental decay. The fluoride increases the resistance of the enamel to acid attack and helps arrest early carious lesions (Murray *et al.*, 1991).

Periodontal diseases affect the tissues supporting the teeth. The main cause is dental plaque, which initially produces inflammation, redness and bleeding of the gums. If the disease is not controlled at this stage it will progress to the underlying tissues; recession of the gums may occur and eventually the teeth will become mobile and may be lost. The older dentate patient should be encouraged, therefore, to maintain a level of oral hygiene that is adequate to prevent any further progression of periodontal disease (Jenkins, 1989; Palmer and Floyd, 1995). This may be carried out by regular brushing of the teeth, particularly near the gums, using a small-headed nylon toothbrush. For people who have difficulty holding a thin handle, an occupational therapist should be consulted for advice on toothbrushing aids such as adapting the toothbrush handle to increase its size and allow it to be gripped more easily. Similarly, an electric toothbrush may prove beneficial for a patient with a weak grip. If a patient is suffering from severely bleeding gums, a chlorhexidine gel may be used to brush the teeth and gums until the situation has improved, and then brushing should continue with a regular toothpaste. If gross bleeding persists, the patient should be checked for an underlying medical condition such as leukaemia.

Carers should be encouraged to brush a patient's teeth if the patient is physically unable to do so. The carer should stand behind the patient and support the patient's head under the chin with one hand while brushing the teeth with the other. If co-operation is difficult, extra help may be required and the patient may need a great deal of encouragement and reassurance. Initially it may only be possible to clean one or two front teeth until sufficient confidence is built up to brush all the dentition. The importance of oral hygiene for the older patient cannot be over-emphasised if the deterioration of extensively restored 'surviving' dentitions is to be prevented.

Much of the pathology of the oral mucosa associated with denture wearing may be prevented by the correct care and maintenance of the dentures. Plaque and food debris should be removed regularly by brushing with soap and water and a small nylon brush (Levine, 1996). If this is carried out over a basin of water, breakages may be prevented. Persistent staining and hard deposits may be removed by the careful use of a proprietary cleaner. Dentures should be left out at night to allow the tissues to 'rest' and this, together with good denture hygiene, will help prevent denture stomatitis, a candida infection that may occur under dentures.

Carers should be aware that traumatic ulcers caused by ill-fitting dentures may occur and can be resolved in most cases by leaving the dentures out and by arranging for a dental surgeon to modify the appliance. If necessary, the denture may be relined, or remade, at a later date. An ulcer that does not resolve after two weeks should always be investigated further in case of malignancy (Dimitroulis and Avery, 1998).

Denture marking is another important preventive measure (Harrison, 1986). Many older patients lose their dentures during the initial stages of a debilitating illness, particularly as they move between accommodation and have a series of different carers. This loss of dentures causes further problems at an already distressing time. Some dentures are marked when they are made, but where this has not been done, a denture marking kit may be used, or, as a temporary measure, the patient's name may be written on the smooth surface of the denture with a pencil and the lettering covered with clear nail varnish.

DENTAL TREATMENT

Dental treatment needs to be integrated into the overall plan for rehabilitation and should seek to alleviate any problems that might hinder the process. As many medical conditions may affect dental treatment, it is important for a dental surgeon to liaise closely with other members of the rehabilitation team.

The dentist will need to assess the patient's general and oral health, and propose a realistic treatment plan in conjunction with the wishes of the patient and carers. The aim of the treatment should be to secure a standard of oral health that enables the patient to eat, speak and socialise without active disease, discomfort or embarrassment (DoH, 1994).

Initial treatment must seek to relieve pain and discomfort. For people with natural teeth, this may involve the stabilisation of carious lesions and, in some cases, the extraction of grossly carious, or very mobile teeth, providing the treatment will not compromise the patient. Once this first phase has been completed, preventive care should be implemented as outlined above, together with a thorough scaling to remove gross deposits. Further treatment, including more complex restorative treatment, may be carried out at a later date when the patient is able to cope with longer treatment sessions.

Older people may have worn complete dentures for many years and be very skilled at controlling them. After a debilitating illness, however, the dentures may become loose for a variety of reasons including weight loss, a loss of muscle control following a stroke, or a dry mouth caused by medication. Initially, it is preferable to try and modify the existing dentures as the older patient may not be able to adapt to a new set, and this approach should be explained to avoid perceptions of economy. In many instances the dentures may be adjusted and relined to improve their fit and make them 'tighter'. If this is not successful, new dentures, of a similar design to the old ones, may be made using a copying technique. For a person with a very dry mouth, where there is little retention of the dentures, consideration may be given to the use of artificial saliva. People whose dentures have been lost during their illness should be made new dentures as soon as they are able to cope with treatment. Where possible, photographs of the patient with natural teeth, or their previous dentures, should be consulted to aid in the construction of the new denture. It is crucial, however, that care staff should recognise the importance of keeping patients' dentures safely in order that new appliances do not have to be made at a time when the patient is psychologically frail and least able to adapt to them.

DENTAL SERVICE PROVISION

A number of alternatives exist for the delivery of dental care. Where a person is registered with a general dental practitioner, he or she should be encouraged to seek care from that dentist, either at a surgery, or on a domiciliary basis. Denture work, oral hygiene measures, and some simple fillings and extractions may all be carried out at home, or on a hospital ward. There is no reason, therefore, for the older patient to be unable to obtain treatment simply because he or she is unable to visit a surgery.

The availability of NHS dental care, however, varies markedly between different parts of the UK, with some areas having a multiplicity of NHS dental practices, while others have very few practices that continue to accept patients for care under the NHS. A growing number of dental practitioners are preferring to provide continuing care for their patients through private dental plans, which may be paid for on a monthly basis, rather than remain within the NHS fee per item payment system. For some older people this is an acceptable alternative, particularly for those who already pay significant NHS charges, but for those who receive benefits and are exempt from charges, private treatment may not be a feasible option. In the NHS Plan (DoH, 2000), however, the government does make a commitment to making high quality NHS dentistry available to all who want it by September 2001. It is envisaged that NHS Direct will be able to provide the necessary information to enable a person to locate an NHS dentist and it is proposed that a number of new dental access centres will be developed to provide easier access to dental care.

If a person is still unable to obtain treatment from a general dental practitioner, care may be provided by members of the Community Dental Service who have a remit to provide care for people with special needs, including those with disabilities and older housebound people. Community dental officers provide dental care from health centres, hospitals, mobile clinics and on a domiciliary basis. Community dental staff are particularly well placed to work closely with community nurses and other members of the primary health-care team in order to provide appropriate dental care as part of a client's total care plan.

On occasions, the rehabilitation team might need to arrange for a patient to be treated by a hospital maxillo-facial surgeon. This would be the case if the patient had a potentially malignant oral lesion, or if they required an extraction while being on anti-coagulants.

At the end of a course of treatment, wherever it is provided, it is important to ensure that arrangements are made for future check-ups to monitor and help maintain the patient's oral health. Ongoing surveillance and prevention are keys to ensuring that older people are not burdened by poor oral health.

CASE STUDY   SUSAN HUNTER – DENTAL GOALS AND INTERVENTIONS

Aim

To enable Susan Hunter to maintain/achieve a level of oral health that does not detract from her quality of life.

Interventions

As soon after admission as practical, nursing staff should:

- establish daily oral hygiene procedures
- ensure that any dentures are marked and, if they are not able to be worn initially, that they are kept in a container of water in a safe place
- administer checklist to establish if Susan Hunter is experiencing any oral pain or eating problems etc.
- refer to the dental surgeon for examination and emergency treatment if necessary.

During rehabilitation

- Enable Susan Hunter to carry out daily oral hygiene procedures, including brushing teeth with a fluoride toothpaste.
- Liaise with occupational therapist concerning toothbrush adaptations if necessary.
- If Susan Hunter has dentures, encourage her to wear them and arrange for dental surgeon to adjust them if necessary.
- Refer to the dental surgeon to provide basic dental care to enable Susan Hunter to eat, speak and socialise.

On discharge

The dental surgeon should:

- ensure ongoing dental care with a general dental practitioner or community dental officer
- consider that further treatment may involve more complex treatment to the patient's natural teeth and a possible need to remake dentures
- confirm the establishment and maintenance of appropriate preventive regimes.

REFERENCES

Billings, R.J., Brown, L.R. and Kaster, A.G. (1985) Contemporary treatment strategies for root surface dental caries. *Gerodontics*, **1**, 20–27.

Bush, L.A., Horenkamp, N., Morley, J.E. and Spiro, A. (1996) D-E-N-T-A-L: a rapid self-administered screening instrument to promote referrals for further evaluation in older adults. *Journal of the American Geriatrics Society*, **44**, 979–981.

Dental Practice Board (1999) *Registrations: GDS Quarterly Statistics*, Dental Data Services, Eastbourne.

Department of Health [DoH] (1994) *An Oral Health Strategy for England*, HMSO, London.

DoH (2000) *NHS Plan*, HMSO, London.

Dimitroulis, G. and Avery, B.S. (1998) Oral Cancer – *A synopsis of pathology and management*, Wright, Butterworth-Heinemann, Oxford.

Harrison, A. (1986) A simple dental marking system. *British Dental Journal*, **160**, 89–91.

Jenkins, W.M.M. (1989) The prevention and control of chronic periodontal disease. In: *The Prevention of Dental Disease* (ed. Murray, J.J.), Oxford Medical Publications, Oxford.

Johnson, N.W. and Warnakulasuriya, K.A.A.S. (1993) Epidemiology and aetiology of oral cancer in the United Kingdom. *Community Dental Health*, **10**(1), 13–29.

Kelly, M. *et al.* (2000) *Adult Dental Health Survey: Oral health in the United Kingdom 1998*, The Stationery Office, London.

Lester, V., Ashley, F.P. and Gibbons, D.E. (1998) Reported dental attendance and perceived barriers to care in frail and functionally dependent older adults. *British Dental Journal*, **184**, 285–289.

Levine, R.S. (1996) *The Scientific Basis of Dental Health Education*, 4th edn, Health Education Authority, London.

Murray, J.J., Rugg-Gunn, A.J. and Jenkins, G.N. (1991) *Fluorides in Caries Prevention*, Butterworth-Heinemann, Oxford.

Palmer, R.M. and Floyd, P.D. (1995) Periodontology: a clinical approach, 3: Non-surgical treatment and maintenance. *British Dental Journal*, 178, 263–268.

Smith, J.M. and Sheiham, A. (1979) How dental conditions handicap the elderly. *Community Dentistry and Oral Epidemiology*, 7, 305–310.

Smith, J.M. and Sheiham, A. (1980) Dental treatment needs and demands of an elderly population in England. *Community Dentistry and Oral Epidemiology*, 8, 360–364.

Steele, J.G., Sheiham, A., Marcenes, W. and Walls, A.W.G. (1998) *National Diet and Nutrition Survey: People aged 65 years and over*, Volume 2: Report of the oral health survey, The Stationery Office, London.

PART C: PHARMACEUTICAL CARE FOR THE OLDER PATIENT – FIONA BEVAN

WHY IS PHARMACEUTICAL CARE NEEDED?

Drug therapy is possibly the most common intervention in the medical treatment of elderly people (Hasan, 1998). Drug consumption increases with increasing age and predictions of expansion in the elderly population suggest that drug therapy will become an ever more important public health issue. Research evidence continues to demonstrate the benefits of continuing drug treatments into old age and, in some cases, the pharmaceutical industry is targeting new drugs at problems commonly associated with the elderly, e.g. stroke treatment and prevention, and Alzheimer's disease.

The majority of elderly people are cared for in the community with admission to hospital only when they have an acute illness. Multiple pathologies often result in an array of drugs being prescribed, needing increased support from health-care professionals. Strong communication and team work are needed if the key health professionals (GPs, community nurses, pharmacists, dieticians and so on) are to achieve maximum benefit for the patient. In some cases this will mean establishing and building new links between professionals and including patients in the team.

While elderly patients are most likely to be taking different medications, they are also among the most vulnerable to potential problems. These include adverse reactions to drugs, interactions between drugs, and difficulties in adhering to prescribed regimens.

In addition to (and sometimes instead of) prescribed medicines, patients also take non-prescription medicines, commonly known as over-the-counter (OTC) medicines. Such medicines may be purchased from pharmacies or from other outlets such as drugstores and supermarkets. Commonly taken products include laxatives, painkillers, indigestion remedies and cold and flu remedies.

It is well known that patients sometimes share medicines (both prescribed and over the counter drugs) or 'lend' them to others. People are often influenced by well-meaning friends and relatives who 'advise' them based on their own experiences. This practice should be warned against at every opportunity because of the potential for adverse drug reactions and interactions. If people need advice on medicines they should consult their pharmacist or GP. Establishing exactly what patients are taking can sometimes be a difficult and complicated process, especially if a patient has not kept his or her medication separate from another person living in the same house. It has been known for a person, on admission to hospital, to be prescribed both their own and their spouse's medication due to them being mixed in the same container.

There is clearly a need for collaboration between health and social care workers to help patients get the best from their medicines. Pharmacists' roles have changed considerably over recent years with the aim of providing expert advice on all aspects of medicines management to patients and their carers, doctors and other health professionals. Hospital pharmacists can identify problems prior to discharge and liaise with community colleagues to provide continuity of care. In the community, pharmacists are asked for information and advice on a range of health and lifestyle matters including nutrition, smoking cessation, joint problems, foot problems, incontinence and many others. Referral to and from other health professionals can be used effectively to maximise the use of expertise. Advice to team members, such as nurses and physiotherapists, who are now able to prescribe from a limited list will be increasingly important.

WHAT IS PHARMACEUTICAL CARE?

The term 'pharmaceutical care' encompasses a philosophy of practice whereby the pharmacist works closely together with patients and doctors (prescribers) (Canaday and Yarborough, 1994). The goals of pharmaceutical care are to achieve drug therapy that is effective in treating the condition/s and to minimise problems such as side-effects. The term 'medicines management' is more commonly used and describes actions to achieve effective drug therapy, in terms of therapeutic outcomes and best use of resources. Other health-care workers, together with carers and relatives, have a key role in monitoring medicine use.

Table 20.1 The key issues in pharmaceutical care for the older patient

- Compliance/adherence with treatment
- Adverse drug reactions (side-effects)
- Medication review including follow-up after hospital discharge
- Physical/sensory problems (failing eyesight, poor manual dexterity, memory loss, confusion)

Each of the issues in Table 20.1 will be addressed in turn, with suggestions of possible methods of problem resolution.

Compliance/adherence

'Compliance' in this context might be defined as the extent to which a person does/does not follow the instructions to take medicines as intended by the prescriber. The term 'adherence' now tends to be used, since it is considered to be less judgemental/paternalistic. Primary non-compliance is where the patient does not have the prescription dispensed and research suggests this occurs with 15 per cent of patients (Beardon *et al.*, 1993). Secondary non-compliance is most common, where the patient has the prescription dispensed but does not adhere to the doctor's instructions. Research on factors influencing patients' adherence to prescribed medication has been extensive (Cramer, 1989; Larrat *et al.*, 1990; Donovan and Blake, 1992; Matsuyama *et al.*, 1993), yet has failed to produce a coherent effective strategy for improvement. Variables, including age, gender, ethnicity and educational level, have been explored.

More recent work has focused on patients' views and feelings about medicines and indicates that those with negative or mixed views about medication generally might be less likely to adhere to treatment (Britten, 1994). This behavioural approach may prove more fruitful in identifying possible strategies because it is likely that patients' underlying beliefs and attitudes are the fundamental determinants of adherence. In one study the most common reason for not taking medication was 'I thought it was not needed' (Wallsten, 1995).

Health professionals may believe that simply giving more information to patients will automatically bring about a change in behaviour. There is evidence that written 'reminder' charts can help (Raynor *et al.*, 1993). Patient information leaflets can also be valuable (Gibbs *et al.*, 1990). Since January 1999 a European Directive makes it compulsory for all new medicines to carry a patient information leaflet, which must comply with a set format. Specific information about particular diseases and conditions can help to improve understanding (Cantrill and Cass, 1989; Dawes and Cantrill, 1990; Gibbs *et al.*, 1990). Patients' interpretation of label instructions has been shown to vary (Holt *et al.*, 1992) and it is helpful for all members of the interdisciplinary team to reinforce the information. Prescribers should be encouraged to state the exact dose on the prescription, even when the patient has had the medicine before, so that the label is explicit. Phrases such as 'to be taken as directed' or 'take as before' are unhelpful.

In many chronic conditions the patient will need to take medication for many years. Yet perceived benefits may not be clear, unless troublesome symptoms are felt to be improved when the medication is taken. It is vital that the pharmacist reinforces to the patient why they are taking each medicine and what the potential outcome could be if they miss it. In cases where non-compliance is suspected it is helpful to discuss potential reasons with the patient as misunderstandings can be acted on.

Many patients take their medicines out of the original containers and mix them all together in one container to make it 'easier to carry around'. This practice is dangerous as there are no instructions to follow and patients can get confused as to which tablet is which. In addition it makes it impossible for doctors or pharmacists to identify medication.

ADVERSE DRUG REACTIONS (SIDE-EFFECTS)

'Iatrogenic disease' is the name that is given to diseases caused by treatment – in this case, by drug therapy. Research studies suggest that 5 per cent of hospital admissions may occur as a result of adverse drug reactions. Studies of patients already in hospital show that the percentage of elderly patients with iatrogenic problems is even higher. Elderly patients are unfortunately particularly vulnerable to the adverse effects of drug therapy. This is partly due to multiple pathologies requiring multiple drug treatment, increasing the possibility of interactions occurring between different medicines leading to adverse effects. In addition the ageing process itself leads to changes in the body's systems so that there is increasing sensitivity to the effects of some drugs. Finally, the body's mechanisms for metabolising and eliminating drugs is reduced in old age, so that some drugs, even at normal doses, accumulate in the body.

Even when dose calculations include these factors, patients may make their own alterations either to make the regime 'easier' or because of side-effects. In some cases where the condition itself is symptomless (e.g. hypertension), the drug therapy may make the patient feel worse through side-effects. Such circumstances mean patients' reluctance to adhere to the prescribed regimen becomes understandable.

Particular drug groups are well known to be associated with problems in elderly patients:

- diuretics ('water tablets')
- non-steroidal anti-inflammatories, e.g. aspirin, ibuprofen (rheumatic and arthritic conditions)
- hypnotics ('sleeping tablets').

Drug interactions sometimes happen when a drug is added to existing medication. Non-prescription drugs bought by the patient can sometimes adversely interact with prescribed medicines.

Some drugs can cause or contribute to urinary incontinence (e.g. fast-acting diuretics). Others may cause constipation, occasionally resulting in overflow faecal incontinence (see also Chapter 20D).

All those involved in the care of older people need to be aware of the problems of adverse drug reactions and to watch out for any signs or symptoms that might be related to drug therapy, and report them accordingly. It is particularly important to identify drug-related side-effects, as often patients end up taking unnecessary new medication to treat the side-effects of the first and expose the patient to potentially more side-effects.

MEDICATION REVIEW

Some 75 per cent of prescribing by general practitioners is for repeat medication. Periodic review of medicines is an important mechanism for ensuring that inappropriate medicines, or those that are no longer needed, are stopped. Review should include monitoring for adverse drug reactions and drug interactions, and identify any problems the patient is having with medicines.

Pharmacists throughout the UK are increasingly involved in a number of schemes to review repeat medication. Many GP practices now employ pharmacists who are involved in reviewing repeat prescriptions, improving prescribing in nursing homes and liaising with hospitals about discharge planning (Mason, 2000). These pharmacists can identify problems such as probable drug-induced side-effects, non-compliance, medicines that are no longer indicated or medicines that need close monitoring in elderly patients. They are often easier to access than busy GPs and can be particularly helpful to patients and carers with specific concerns about medication as they also have access to full patient records.

FOLLOW-UP AFTER HOSPITAL DISCHARGE

During a stay in hospital, there are often changes to a patient's medication, with dose alterations, addition of new medicines and/or deletion of previous therapy. Unfortunately all sorts of problems can happen when the patient is discharged. Many hospitals currently give only seven days' supply of medication to take home, but this is changing with the advent of patient pack dispensing (easy to follow calendar packs) and soon it should be common practice to give 28 days' supply. Communication problems can result in a delay in the patients' GP being told by letter about medication changes, resulting in inappropriate prescribing. Hospital pharmacists have developed several ways to avoid these problems including patient counselling prior to discharge, liaison with carers to ensure medication compliance and immediate communication with the GP and community pharmacists to arrange follow up. One study has shown that when the pharmaceutical needs of the patient were assessed by the hospital pharmacist and communicated to the GP, community pharmacist and carers fewer unnecessary changes to discharge medication occurred (Cannon, 1999). The importance of early discharge letters/faxes cannot be over-emphasised. Sending a copy of information about the medication to the patient's regular community pharmacy could be invaluable. This enables the pharmacist to have advance notice so that drugs can be ordered if necessary and, in some cases, may be delivered to the patient's home. The pharmacist can liaise with the GP to ensure that repeat prescriptions are timely. Patients are sometimes not clear about what they should do with stocks of medicines they took previously. They may run out of supplies of their 'new' medicines and revert to taking what they have at home. They may even take both. Pre-discharge counselling by hospital pharmacists can help to avoid this and alert carers to check medication after discharge from hospital. Talking with the local community pharmacist (who may have received a discharge checklist from the hospital pharmacist) can help to sort out any problems. Most community pharmacists now have computerised patient medication records (PSusan) and are in a good position to identify previous medication.

PHYSICAL/SENSORY AND LANGUAGE PROBLEMS

Basic problems can sometimes occur, which may seem obvious but are often missed. Simply getting the medicine container open can be a real struggle for some patients. Pharmacists routinely use child-resistant closures on all medicines to help reduce accidental poisoning in children, but will use ordinary caps on request. Special winged caps may be available to help those with arthritic hands – ask at the local pharmacy.

Loose tablets in bottles are becoming less common with the move towards individual patient packs. Foil and blister packs are common and patients need to be shown how to press tablets out of the latter type. This may seem obvious, but some patients try to push tablets out through the transparent plastic and give up when this cannot be done. Research suggests that elderly patients have more problems with blister packs compared to standard tablet bottles (Horner *et al.*, 1989).

Some pharmacy computers can produce large print for labels – ask if this facility is available at your local pharmacy. Braille labels may also be available with standard medication instructions. Why not ask your local pharmacist to find out what facilities are available? You could suggest that patients/carers do this too.

Labels in minority languages are more of a problem, as the range of dialects is almost limitless, some not having a written version. Manufacturers' information is gradually being produced in majority languages, and local initiatives are beginning to address labelling and specific information.

ADMINISTRATION OF MEDICINES

Where an elderly patient has difficulty in remembering to take their medicines, or problems of sight or dexterity, the most practical approach is for someone else to administer them. This practice has gone on for years, with relatives, partners, carers and even home helps involved. Those involved in administering medicines can ask the pharmacist to clarify anything they are unsure about. Simple dosage charts can be useful, with a space to tick when a dose has been given. There is no reason why administering medicines in this way need cause problems. Most carers are conscientious and scrupulous in checking that the correct amount has been given. Many social services departments now contract with local pharmacists to provide basic training about medicines for care staff and this approach is to be encouraged.

Reminder charts can be helpful if poor memory is a problem. Special dosage packs are available where the day or week's medicines doses are packed into small compartments by the patient or pharmacist, e.g. Redidos and Dosett. Most pharmacies operate one or more systems and it is worth asking the local pharmacy to find out more about the different types available. At the moment they are not prescribable on the NHS, but they are not expensive and the pharmacist can advise on local schemes for funding if available. Monitored dosage systems, such as Nomad and Manrex, are increasingly being used in the community, for example, in sheltered housing complexes.

Non-prescription (over-the-counter) medicines

As more medicines are transferred from the POM (prescription only medicines) category to P (pharmacy only sale), a wider selection of treatments is becoming available to buy over the counter.

As more potent medicines can be purchased it becomes even more important to encourage elderly people to check first before buying. If the same pharmacy is used the pharmacist will be familiar with their prescribed medicines and will be able to check the PMR (patient medication record). In this way the possibility of interactions and adverse effects will be reduced.

WORKING TOGETHER

Elderly people have many needs relating to their medication. Improved communication between professionals providing health and social care can help to resolve medication problems. To get started, get to know the local community pharmacist/s providing care for your patients, as you have a common goal in pharmaceutical care.

Legal requirements mean that the community pharmacist has to be physically present during the hours the pharmacy is open. The requirement applies to the supervision of dispensing and sales of 'pharmacy only' medicines. This means pharmacists cannot easily leave their premises to attend meetings or visit patients, unless they have another pharmacist to cover for them. However, meeting in the pharmacy is always an option. On the other hand, this means that the pharmacist is easily accessible and can readily be found in the pharmacy.

Your local GP practice may have a pharmacist on site who would be happy to advise team members on specific patients. In addition, if a patient has recently been discharged from hospital, the hospital pharmacy will be in a position to help sort out problems with discharge medication.

Why not make contact, especially if you have particular patient medication problems you need sorting out? Talk to the pharmacist about referring patients – this is a two-way street. The pharmacist might wish to refer a patient to the nurse, health visitor, chiropodist, dietitian, continence adviser, physiotherapist, occupational therapist or GP, where needed. You might refer patients to the pharmacist for more in-depth information about prescribed medicines, compliance problems or non-prescription medicine choices. Each will need to be aware of what the criteria for referral are and how to make contact. Opening the communication channels could bring true team working and better patient care closer to reality.

CASE STUDY SUSAN HUNTER – THE PHARMACIST'S ROLE

On admission to hospital

Pharmacists in the majority of acute hospitals aim to review medication of each patient within 24 hours of admission. This would involve assessing the current hospital prescription chart and establishing a true drug history. As Susan Hunter would have had varying consciousness on admission it may be that an accurate drug history was not possible. This is vital, as very often patients may miss necessary medication or the dose prescribed in hospital may be unintentionally different than usual. The pharmacist would first attempt to speak with Susan Hunter, as many elderly people are quite knowledgeable about their medication and often carry a list with them. If Susan Hunter is able to converse she may be able to explain exactly what she takes, not what the doctors think she takes. This can very often highlight compliance or concordance issues (see Chapter 13), which may have contributed to the stroke. If Susan Hunter is not able to communicate the pharmacist would contact the GP and/or a near relative or carer. It is not safe practice solely to rely on patients' own medicines brought from home. They may not all be the current prescription (people hoard medicines) or the patient may not be taking what it says on the label.

Once a correct drug history is established the pharmacist would assess Susan Hunter's medication to check that it is still appropriate and that the doses are optimal. Susan Hunter would probably be taking an oral hypoglycaemic for her diabetes. In the acute stage of stroke Susan Hunter will probably not be eating, which means that her blood sugar may be lower than usual. The need and dose for the oral hypoglycaemic should be reviewed on a daily basis, based on blood sugar measurements. There are a number of oral hypoglycaemics available and the pharmacist should consider if Susan Hunter is prescribed the most appropriate one for her age and condition.

After a stroke many patients are unable to swallow properly and this can lead to problems and confusion with administering medicines. Not all medicines would be clinically necessary in the first 24–48 hours and the pharmacist would discuss with the doctors those that are most necessary. If the patient is not able to swallow, then administration of liquid medication through a nasogastric tube is usually the best alternative as many medicines are not available in injection form. However, in some cases, the parenteral route may be needed for speed but care should be taken with doses, as oral doses are usually far higher than the equivalent injection. The pharmacist will advise dose adjustments where necessary. The rectal route is another alternative and the pharmacist will advise on availability of dosage forms and appropriateness, depending on the patient's condition.

The pharmacist would also discuss with Susan Hunter, the nurses, doctors and therapists if analgesia is required for her arthritis and advise on an appropriate choice. Simple paracetamol would be less likely to cause side-effects but this may not be enough. Other alternatives would be discussed with reference to the kind and location of pain and the aim of minimising potential adverse effects.

Once an infarct had been confirmed the pharmacist would ensure that low dose aspirin is prescribed to help prevent further infarcts, provided there are no contraindications, e.g. true allergy or *active* gastrointestinal bleed.

Rehabilitation

The pain in her knee is obviously hampering Susan Hunter's rehabilitation. The pharmacist would review analgesia, looking at the following aspects:

- **Appropriate** – is the analgesia the most appropriate for her knee pain? It would be worth discussing with the doctor if it is inflammatory pain or not. Non-steroidal anti-inflammatory painkillers may help but they have a number of side-effects common in elderly people, particularly peptic ulceration and kidney problems. This would need to be accounted for and monitored.
- **Timing** – when is Susan Hunter's pain the worst and when does she take her analgesia? In many cases it can help if analgesia is taken about 30 minutes before physiotherapy so that it is not quite so painful. This can be discussed with the patient and physiotherapist.
- **Additional analgesia** – would Susan Hunter benefit from stronger analgesia at certain times?

Susan Hunter is also displaying signs of depression, which is common in stroke patients. The pharmacist would discuss with the doctor if anti-depressant medication would be clinically appropriate, as in many cases helping to lift the patient's mood can aid recovery. The pharmacist would advise on choice of anti-depressant as some cause more side-effects than others in elderly patients.

Discharge

Prior to discharge the pharmacist would discuss with the medical team the medication that Susan Hunter should continue and any necessary monitoring requirements that the GP should follow up, e.g. if Susan Hunter is prescribed Warfarin, who will be responsible for monitoring it Susan Hunter's discharge medication should be rationalised to aid compliance and minimise patient confusion. Susan Hunter's home situation should be taken into account with respect to times of administration. For example, if Susan Hunter requires help from carers/relatives to take medication, but this is only available once or twice a day, then the pharmacist would advise changing the prescribed medication where possible to accommodate this.

The pharmacist would counsel Susan Hunter and/or her relatives on any medication that should continue. They would explain what each is for and any specific side-effects to look out for. The pharmacist would assess how the patient could take her medication and if any medication aids are required. Susan Hunter has visual problems, so if she is to self-medicate then larger writing on the labels may be necessary or a reliable system worked out tailored to her needs. If there are any special needs this would be communicated to the community pharmacist, e.g. dosette box. The pharmacist would arrange discharge medication and ensure that the family had a copy of the discharge medication, which would be given to the community pharmacist.

REFERENCES

Beardon, P.H.G., McGilchrist, M.M., McKendrick, A.D., McDevitt, D.G. and MacDonald, T.M. (1993) Primary non-compliance with prescribed medication. *British Medical Journal*, **307**, 846–848.

Britten, N. (1994) Patients' ideas about medicines: a qualitative study in a general practice population. *British Journal of General Practitioners*, **44**, 465–468.

Canaday, B.R. and Yarborough, P.D. (1994) Documenting pharmaceutical care: creating a standard. *Annals of Pharmacotherapy*, **28**, 1292–1296.

Cannon, J. (1999) Pharmaceutical care provision to elderly patients: an assessment of its impact on compliance and discharge medication changes. *European Hospital Pharmacolgy Journal*, **5**(3), 102–105.

Cantrill, J. and Cass, Y. (1989) Diabetic patients' knowledge of hypertension. *Pharmacology Journal*, **243**, Suppl. R22.

Cramer, J.A. (1989) How often is medication taken as prescribed? *Journal of the American Medical Association*, **261**, 3273–3277.

Dawes, C. and Cantrill, J.A. (1990) An information booklet for patients with diabetes and hypertension. *Pharmocology Journal*, **245**, Supp R26.

Donovan, J.L. and Blake, D.R. (1992) Patient non-compliance: deviance or reasoned decision-making? *Social Sciences and Medicine*, **34**, 507–513.

Gibbs, S., Waters, W.E. and George, C.F. (1990) Prescription information leaflets – a national survey. *Jouranal of the Royal Society of Medicine*, **83**, 292–297.

Hasan, M. (1998) Prescribing for elderly patients: the differences in approach. *Prescribers Journal*, **38**(4), 205–210.

Holt, G.A., Dorcheus, L. Hall, E. L., Beck, D., Ellis, E. and Hough, J. (1992) Patient interpretation of label instructions. *American Pharmacy*, **NS32**, 242–246.

Horner, R., Lochery, P.M. and Sayegh, A. (1989) Is there a compliance problem with elderly people using blister packs? *Pharmacology Journal*, **243**, Suppl. R26.

Larrat, E.P., Taubman, A.H. and Willey, C. (1990) Compliance problems in the ambulatory population. *American Pharmacy*, **NS30**, 82–87.

Mason, P. (2000) A career as a practice pharmacist. *Pharmacology Journal*, **264**, 149–150.

Matsuyama, J.R., Mason, B.J. and Jue, S.G. (1993) Pharmacists' interventions using an electronic medication-event monitoring device. *Annals of Pharmacotherapy*, **27**, 851–854.

Raynor, D.K., Booth, T.G. and Blenkinsopp, A. (1993) Effects of computer-generated reminder charts on patients' compliance with drug regimens. *British Medical Journal*, **306**, 1158–1161.

Wallsten, S.M., Sullivan, R.J. Jr, Hanlon, J.T., Blazer, D.G., Tyrey, M.J. and Westland, R. (1995) Medication taking behaviours in the high and low functioning elderly: McArthur field studies of successful ageing. *Annals of Pharmacotheraphy*, **29**, 359–363.

PART D: CONTINENCE PROMOTION IN OLD AGE – JILL MANTLE

INTRODUCTION

Continence of urine and faeces is fundamental to quality of life, and to the sociological, psychological and physical well-being of the individual. Therefore, it deserves very high priority at every stage in the planning of an older person's rehabilitation. The quality and reliability of continence frequently controls the balance between success or failure in rehabilitation, because it is of such crucial importance to morale and to social integration. Incontinence has been defined as the involuntary or inappropriate passing of urine and/or faeces that has an impact on social functioning or hygiene (DoH, 2000). It carries a social stigma and causes great anxiety, shame, depression and loss of self-esteem; it may differ in emphasis between cultures and is expensive. Frequently, it results in sufferers withdrawing from society and positively avoiding social contact (Grimley et al., 1993), often the person is fearful that they may smell offensive and/or that they may stain or soil the soft furnishings of others. Nothing demoralises an older person or demotivates them from physical activity and effort more than perceiving that it may cause them to have 'an accident' and disgrace themselves in company. Further, incontinence causes physical discomfort and predisposes to infections and bedsores. In addition, older people with urgency (urinary or faecal) are at risk of falling and sustaining a fracture as they hurry to reach the toilet in time (Stevenson et al., 1998; Brown et al., 2000). It also has adverse effects on carers, which can result in the sufferer being ostracised, neglected or even abused. It has been suggested that incontinence is a major factor in sufferers and carers reaching crisis point, with consequent referral to residential care and its attendant cost implications for the individual and/or the state (Continence Foundation, 2000a).

Continence in a patient is an indicator of positive prognosis and should be actively promoted. Where continence is disturbed, the matter must be critically addressed. It is often the case for older people that little or no specific attention is given to the reason for any continence problems or whether there is a cure. It is assumed that such problems are due to age and therefore irremediable; sadly older people and their carers rarely challenge this assumption or expect improvement. Rehabilitation of the older patient has tended to concentrate on trying to regain and/or increase independence in such physical activities as eating, dressing and walking, while just containing or coping with urinary and faecal leakage, often in very unsatisfactory and undignified ways. However, the primary and community care teams will find patients very motivated to contribute ideas and co-operate in rehabilitation plans, which include aspects designed to overcome problems with continence.

The ability to be continent is a construct of many factors:

- the ability to recognise and react to the need to empty the bladder and/or bowel both day and night

- the ability to store urine and faeces temporarily and to 'hold on' reliably and for long enough to select and reach an acceptable place to void without leakage
- sufficient balance, mobility and strength to get to an appropriate place/position and manage clothing/aids, ideally without help
- the ability to void effectively and attend to own hygiene
- the ability to return to the status quo.

Independence in toiletting is priceless; needing the help of another is problematic in terms of convenience as well as psychologically. For example, most public facilities are single sex, which excludes an accompanying spouse; some people find that voiding is inhibited by the presence of another; the conventions of certain ethnic groups preclude one partner assisting the other in such intimate matters (see Chapter 3). Regrettably much misery is caused in hospitals, residential and nursing homes where an inadequate staff to patient/resident ratio results in people, who need assistance of any sort to void, being required to 'hold on' for unreasonable lengths of time. The distress this must cause can only be imagined.

Continence of urine and faeces is a largely unappreciated faculty until things start to go wrong. Incontinence is not a disease but a symptom, indicating that there is some underlying problem. It takes very little to threaten and disturb continence, and the cause of the leakage may have absolutely nothing directly to do with any disease process, but be due to stress, depression, not knowing where the toilet is, having to wait in a long queue for a vacant toilet or for a commode to be brought. Medication can precipitate incontinence, e.g. sleeping tablets, as may some foods, and drinks containing caffeine, e.g. tea and coffee. Some people try reducing their fluid intake to reduce urine leakage and become dehydrated. The result is very concentrated urine, which irritates the bladder and tends to increase leakage. The provision of high toilet seats certainly aids getting on and off the toilet, but almost inevitably changes the trunk to thigh angle adversely (Chiarelli and Markwell, 1992), predisposing to constipation. Training and the co-operation of all rehabilitation team members in identifying and addressing such matters in an informed and considered way is essential.

In simple terms the most common causes of incontinence are:

- irritable bladder, e.g. urinary tract infection/cystitis, too much caffeine
- weak urethral sphincter and pelvic floor muscles, leading to urinary leakage with effort, e.g. cough, sneeze – called genuine stress incontinence
- an overactive bladder that contracts, giving a strong sense of urgency, and may empty without voluntary initiation or warning (often on movement) – called urge incontinence; urge and stress incontinence may occur together
- difficulty in emptying the bladder due to a blockage of the urethra, e.g. caused by an enlarged prostate gland in men, resulting in a dribbling overflow incontinence
- damage to the anal sphincter muscles, e.g. from a third-degree tear in childbirth

- disorders affecting the nervous system, e.g. stroke, multiple sclerosis, Parkinson's disease, diabetes, resulting in a variety of motor and sensory deficits in the control of bladder and bowel function, ranging from emptying without warning to difficulty in emptying
- constipation and other bowel problems, e.g. mega-colon, impacted faeces (common in inactive and/or institutionalised elderly people), irritable bowel syndrome
- diarrhoea from any cause
- any hindrance to reaching the toilet, such as physical disability or frailty, stairs, heavy doors, pain, confusion and poor signposting.

For some people the leakage is minimal and/or infrequent, e.g. only when they have a bad cough; for others it occurs often and/or is severe. The prevalence of incontinence tends to rise for adults with age and is more common in women (Table 20.2). With increasing life expectancy for both sexes, it becomes ever more important to educate the public regarding continence from an early age; prevention is so much better than cure. Frequency and the urgent need to pass urine correlates with the risk of falling, and possible fracture, in old age (Brown, 2000). The inclusion of such assessments in a comprehensive falls assessment, and access to relevant specialist help, should be an integral component of falls clinics (see Chapter 15).

Table 20.2 Prevalence of incontinence in older and institutionalised people

	Percentage incontinent
Urinary incontinence	
Women living at home, over 65	10–20%
Men living at home, over 60	7–10%
Either sex living in an institution:	
Residential home	25%
Nursing home	40%
Hospital – long stay	50–70%
Faecal incontinence	
Men and women at home	
65–84 years	3–5%
85+ years	15%
Men and women in an institution:	
Residential home	10%
Nursing home	30%
Hospital – long stay	60%

(Royal College of Physicians, 1995)

People need to be encouraged to value continence and seek investigation/explanation for any disturbance of their usual patterns. Increasingly over recent years, continence advisers (mostly nurses) have been appointed in localities and their role has been developing (Rhodes and Parker, 1993), but has varied from place to place. As there is a substantial range of clinically effective treatments for most types of urinary and faecal incontinence, it is important that these are made accessible to all. Cure or significant improvement is usually possible, even for many older people. According to the Association for Continence Advice (1993), 'Continence for all should be the initial aim' and 'Where this proves impossible the highest standards of care and management should enable social continence'. See also the Charter for Continence (Table 20.3).

Table 20.3 Charter for Continence

The Charter for Continence presents the specific needs and rights of people with bladder or bowel problems. It outlines the resources available and the standards of care that can be expected.

As a person with bladder or bowel problems you have the right to:

- Be treated with sensitivity and understanding
- Become continent if achievable
- Receive a thorough individual assessment of your condition by a doctor or nurse knowledgeable in this aspect of care
- Request specialist advice about continence care
- Be provided with a clear explanation of your diagnosis
- Participate in a full discussion of treatment options, their advantages and disadvantages
- Be provided with full, impartial information on the range of products available and how to obtain them
- Expect products to have clear instructions for use
- Receive regular reviews of treatment and be given the opportunity to change treatments if your condition has changed
- Be made aware of any treatments or products as they become available
- Be provided with a personal contact point able to give you on-going advice and support.

(Developed by: The Continence Foundation, IconTact, Association of Continence Advisors [ACA], the RCN Continence Care Forum, the Enuresis Resource and Information Centre [ERIC], the Spinal Injuries Association and the Multiple Sclerosis Society. Produced by an educational grant from Bard Limited, March 1995.)

In March 2000 an important new government-sponsored document was published by the DoH, entitled *Good Practice in Continence Services* (DoH, 2000). These guidelines recommend that continence services provided for each area's resident population should be organised as **an integrated continence service**, managed by a director who is either a specialist continence nurse or specialist physiotherapist. The plan is for public education, prevention, identification of sufferers, and initial assessment and treatment to be the responsibility of the Primary Care Groups (PCGs) and Primary Care Trusts (PCTs). The director will be responsible for developing and maintaining care pathways to and from primary care and local specialist services, e.g. medical and surgical specialists (including a physician for older people), and specialist investigation and treatment facilities. In addition, as a third tier, there will be specific referral arrangements with national or regional specialist units. Those concerned about the quality of care of the frail elderly will welcome the statement in the DOH document (2000) that 'many older people will live in continuing or long stay accommodation and they should have the same access to services as those living in their own homes'.

In addition there is a requirement to ensure 'users and carers are involved in all aspects of the service'. The National Service Framework for Older People (see Chapter 6) sets a milestone of 2004 for the establishment of a properly integrated continence service for older people.

Therefore relevant staff (especially doctors, nurses, physiotherapists and occupational therapists) must be thoroughly knowledgeable regarding the possible effects on continence of certain pathologies, medicaments and changes in environment. There should be corporate responsibility within the rehabilitation team for anticipating and avoiding problems where possible, or at least recognising difficulties speedily. Key primary health-care members need to be trained to make an initial continence assessment to an agreed format as an integrated component of the holistic consideration of the patient's rehabilitation needs. Where necessary, this assessment should then form the entry point to an efficiently managed integrated continence service so that the patient receives treatment, reassessment and/or referral to appropriate specialist services.

ASSESSMENT BY THE PRIMARY HEALTH-CARE TEAM

The initial assessment should be by a trained assessor to a standardised evidence-based protocol agreed with the area Continence Services. The new government guidelines, *Good Practice in Continence Services* (DoH, 2000), lists ten key components of the initial continence assessment:

- review of symptoms and their effect on quality of life
- assessment of desire for treatment alternatives
- examination of abdomen for palpable mass or bladder retention
- examination of perineum to identify prolapse and excoriation, and assess pelvic floor contraction
- rectal examination to exclude faecal impaction (not to be carried out on children)
- urinalysis to exclude infection
- assessment of manual dexterity
- assessment of the environment, e.g. accessibility of toilet facilities
- use of an 'Activities of Daily Living' diary
- identification of conditions that may exacerbate incontinence, e.g. a chronic cough.

Great empathy, sensitivity and superior communication skills are required when listening and enquiring about continence problems from patients and/or carers. How this is done and the language used often determines whether the outcome is positive or negative. The language used will preferably be the patient's first language, clearly spoken and audible to the patient. An interpreter may be required. If a hearing aid is used by the patient, it is important to check that it is being worn and is working (see Chapter 20F). Privacy is crucial for discussion and examination, and patients should have the option of being assessed with or without their carer present. Sometimes there is flat denial that a problem exists.

There is always a danger that well-informed professionals, particularly in the community setting, will assume their clients have already tried all the simple remedies; for example drinking sufficient and eating appropriately to avoid constipation and ensuing faecal impaction induced by inactivity. Have they discussed with the pharmacists (see Chapter 20C) the possibility that some medications can cause 'slow transit time' as a side-effect or with the dietician (Chapter 20A) that malnourishment may result in reduced strength, so affecting manoeuverability? Helping both patient and carer to understand the problems is crucial.

The objective of the initial assessment in the primary care setting is to form a clear picture and establish a working diagnosis that allows immediate remedial action to be taken and/or identifies those sufferers who require immediate referral for a specialist consultation, investigation or treatment. In any event there must be clearly defined criteria for reassessment, review and, when appropriate, discharge. For example, where certain first line interventions have been tried but have failed to produce significant improvement in 8–12 weeks, referral to a specialist should be reconsidered.

In the past, there has been failure on the part of health-care professionals (particularly in hospitals and residential care) to consider the effect of the normal taboos of society in relation to toiletting. For some individuals, a unisex toilet, toilets without doors, voiding in company (particularly emptying the bowels) or no realistic means of washing and drying hands may be sufficient to inhibit voluntary voiding. Some women have been brought up never to sit on the toilet seat when voiding, except in their own homes, for fear of infection: hovering just above the toilet seat to void predisposes to residual urine and infection (Moore and Richmond, 1989). Others have a horror of sharing the use of a toilet with a stranger or using a soiled toilet. Those readers who think this unduly fastidious would do well to reflect on the reasons for staff toilets invariably being separate from those of patients (see also Chapter 5).

TREATMENT

The new government guidelines (DoH, 2000) list ten treatments suitable for use in the primary care setting:

- advice to patients and carers on healthy living – especially diet and drinking appropriate fluids
- bladder and bowel training regimes
- bladder training/timed voiding/prompted voiding for urge incontinence
- improving quality and access to toilet facilities and improving mobility
- pelvic floor exercises, particularly for women during and after pregnancy, to prevent or cure stress incontinence, for patients with urge incontinence and for men with post-prostatectomy problems
- pelvic floor and anal sphincter exercises to improve faecal continence
- provision of pads, aids such as enuresis alarms and other supplies
- reviewing existing medication

- managing faecal impaction
- medication – anti-cholinergics for detrusor overactivity, anti-diuretic hormone for nocturnal enuresis.

From the older person's point of view, it is important that both they and their carers know that drinking very little is *not* the answer to urinary leakage, but may actually worsen the problem by resulting in the urine being concentrated and irritating to the bladder. Some people find reducing their caffeine intake very beneficial. Similarly an appropriate, appetising diet (See Chapter 20a), and ensuring that false teeth are in place to chew food (see Chapter 20b), are essential to digestion and strength, as well as the avoidance of constipation. As is described earlier in this chapter, expert dietary advice is available within the NHS and this should be called upon more readily. Medication can assist the relief of constipation and anti-diarrhoeants may be appropriate for loose stools. An anal plug has been devised and is being tested.

Where possible, several alternative solutions should be suggested for continence problems to allow for the individual and carer to choose according to their perception of what is or is not acceptable and manageable. The whole issue needs discussing in some detail. For example, a commode may be acceptable, to save struggling all the way to the toilet, but the prospect of opening one's bowels on one in the sitting room may not be. Such feelings may be overcome or may prove strong enough to inhibit defecation and cause constipation. Simple grab rails and home adaptations, e.g. arranging for the toilet door to open outwards rather than inwards may be all that is needed. Where the problem does not improve with simple measures, referral to local specialists should be considered, e.g. for urodynamic investigations, colposcopy, ultrasound scanning, further medication, biofeedback or neuromuscular stimulation of the pelvic floor musculature, surgery or training in intermittent self-catheterisation. Occasionally quite radical options may be worthy of consideration, for example, for the heavily dependent patient, it may be reasonable to consider an in-dwelling catheter for the carer's sake, even when urinary continence is substantially intact.

MANAGEMENT OF INTRACTABLE INCONTINENCE

The objective of such management is to gain 'social continence', i.e. to organise or contain voiding in a way that is acceptable and practical to the patient and anyone else who has to be involved. It should enable the patient to live life as fully as they are able and interact socially without fear of embarrassment, accidents or odour. Each patient's sensitivities must be accommodated and their dignity preserved as far as is humanly possible.

PRODUCT PROVISION

There is an increasing range of products available, including disposable and reusable bedding, pads and body garments and collecting devices, e.g. male and female urinals, penile sheaths, catheters and drainage bags; however quality and price, and patients' personal needs and preferences vary. As patients become better informed it is inevitable that there will be an increasing demand for choice (see also Chapter 5). Some independent, scientific evaluation of products is being carried out by the Continence Product Evaluation Network, which is funded by the Medical Services Agency. Recently published results include *Reusable Female Urinals* (Medical Services Agency, 1999a) and *All-in-one Disposable Bodyworn Pads for Heavy Incontinence* (Medical Services Agency, 1999b).

CASE STUDY SUSAN HUNTER – CONTINENCE PROMOTION

Susan Hunter was referred by the nursing staff for assessment of her continuing urinary incontinence. While Susan Hunter had regained faecal continence, the staff were unclear whether her problem was due to the central neurological damage or local bladder problems. Susan Hunter's daughter-in-law remembered that she had reported an occasional problem with stress incontinence when she coughed, which she had accepted was just a problem of age, childbirth and lifting her husband.

Susan Hunter had considerable physical problems and required support to transfer to the toilet and manage her clothing. She was dependent on nursing staff responding quickly to her needs. A full physical assessment was carried out and a review of fluid and nutritional intake with the nursing staff and dietitian was undertaken. The occupational therapist undertook to review the ward toilet environment to make sure it met Susan Hunter's needs and all the team worked towards achieving urinary continence. Anti-cholinergics were prescribed to decrease detrusor overactivity. By working together and making slight environmental changes a level of social continence was achieved to allow Susan Hunter home.

Products should only be supplied to sufferers by the Continence Service after assessment by an appropriately trained assessor. The availability of over-the-counter products allows the assessment route to be circumvented, but denies proper appraisal of causes and subsequent treatment. The following factors need to be considered in collaboration with the patient and carer: the choice of product(s) that are most appropriate and acceptable; delivery or collection of supplies; storage of supplies; hygienic disposal of disposable products; laundry of soiled clothing, bedding and reusable products; regular reassessment and monitoring of patient needs and satisfaction.

The cost of product provision and allied services needed to support a patient with long-term incontinence is borne by the relevant Health Authority, except for private (paying) patients in hospitals and residential care. Each Health Authority has discretion regarding eligibility as well as type, quality and quantity of products to be provided. There is also variation between authorities as to whether and by whom products must be collected, and the arrangements regarding disposal and laundry.

Professionals, patients and carers, who experience difficulty in obtaining help, information and/or advice on any continence matter should contact the Continence Foundation. The Continence Foundation was established in 1992 with three key purposes – advice, awareness and advocacy. It has produced an excellent Continence Resource Pack (Continence Foundation, 2000b) and has up-to-date databases on local continence services throughout the UK and all continence products available on the UK market. It produces a range of publications for public and professional enquirers, contributes to a wide range of national initiatives to inform and raise awareness, campaigns for improved policies and funding for continence services, and has a telephone Helpline (for number see below) for the public and professionals.

References

Association for Continence Advice (1993) *Guidelines for Continence Care*, Association for Continence Advice, London.

Brown, J. (2000) Urinary Incontinence: does it increase risk for falls and fractures? *Journal of American Geriatric Society*, 48(7).

Chiarelli, P. and Markwell, S.(1992) *Let's Get Things Moving,* Health Books, Gore & Osment, Woollahra, Australia. Obtainable from Neen Healthcare, Old Pharmacy Yard, Church St, Dereham NR19 1DJ.

Continence Foundation (1995) *Commissioning Comprehensive Services: Guidance for purchasers*, obtainable from Continence Foundation, 307 Hatton Square, 16 Baldwins Gardens, London EC1N 7RJ.

Continence Foundation (2000a) *Making the Case for Investment in an Integrated Continence Service*, obtainable from Continence Foundation, 307 Hatton Square, 16 Baldwins Gardens, London EC1N 7RJ.

Continence Foundation (2000b) *Continence Resource Pack*, obtainable from Continence Foundation, 307 Hafton Square, 16 Baldwins Gardens, London EC1N 7RJ.

Department of Health [DoH] (2000) *Good Practice in Continence Services*, obtainable from DoH, P0 Box 777, London SE1 6XH or website address www.gov.uk/continenceservices.htm

Grimley, A., Milson, I., Molander, U., Wiklund, I. and Ekeland, P. (1993) The influence of urinary incontinence on the quality of life of elderly women. *Age and Ageing*, **22**, 88–89.

Medical Services Agency (1999a) *Reusable Female Urinals: An evaluation*. Copies obtainable from Medical Services Agency, Business Services, 9th Floor, Hannibal House, Elephant and Castle, London SE1 6TQ.

Medical Services Agency (1999b) *All-in-one Disposable Pads for Heavy Incontinence: An evaluation*. Copies obtainable from Medical Services Agency, Business Services, 9th Floor, Hannibal House, Elephant and Castle, London SE1 6TQ.

Moore, K.H. and Richmond, D. (1989) Crouching over the toilet seat: prevalence, and effect on micturition. *Neurourology and Urodynamics*, 8(4), 422–424.

Rhodes, P. and Parker, G. (1993) *The Role of Continence Advisers in England and Wales*, Social Policy Research Unit, York.

Stevenson, B., Brown, J.S., Vittinghoff, E., Wyman, J.F., Nerett, M.C., Ensrud, K.E. (1998) Falls risk factors in an acute-care setting: a retrospective study. *Canadian Journal of Nursing Resources*, 30(1), 97–1, 11.

FURTHER READING

Abrams, P., Khoury, S. and Wein, A. (eds) (1999) *Incontinence, 1st International Consultation on Incontinence*, World Health Organisation and International Union Against Cancer, Plymbridge Distributors, Plymouth.

Barrett, J.A. (1993) *Faecal Incontinence and Related Problems in the Older Adult*, Edward Arnold, London.

Bennett, G.C.J. and Ebrahim, S. (1995) *The Essentials of Health Care in Old Age*, 2nd edn, Edward Arnold, London.

Cardozo, L. and Stakin, D. (eds) (2001) *Textbook of Female Urology and Urogynaecology*, Isis Medical Media, Oxford.

Chiarelli, P. (1992) *Women's Waterworks*, Health Books, Gore & Osment, Woollahra, Australia. Obtainable from Neen Healthcare, Old Pharmacy Yard, Church St, Dereham NR19 1DJ.

Polden, M. and Mantle, J. (1990) *Physiotherapy in Obstetrics and Gynaecology*, Butterworth-Heinemann, Oxford.

Royal College of Physicians (1995) *Incontinence Causes, Management and Provision of Services*, Report of a working party, Royal College of Physicians, London.

Sanderson, J. (1991) *An Agenda for Action on Continence Services*, Community Services Division, Department of Health, London.

Sapsford, R., Bullock-Saxton, J. and Markwell, S. (eds) (1998) *Women's Health*, W.B. Saunders, London.

Tobin, G.W. (1992) *Incontinence in the Elderly*, Edward Arnold, London.

USEFUL ADDRESSES

The Continence Product Evaluation Network, 5th Floor, South Wing, St Pancras Hospital, St Pancras Way, London NW1 OPE.

Continence Foundation, 307 Hatton Square, 16 Baldwins Gardens, London EC1N 7RJ, Tel 020 7404 6875, Fax 020 7404 8678. Telephone Helpline for the public and professionals: 9.30 to 4.30 Monday to Friday on 020 7831 9831.

PART E: THE OPTOMETRIST'S CONTRIBUTION TO VISUAL REHABILITATION – NORMAN F. BUTTON

INTRODUCTION

The importance of a normally functioning visual field to normal daily living for successful rehabilitation is considered. The author provides detail of incidence and management of the common visual problems in old age, and the need to prevent deterioration in visual acuity through early detection and management of the systemic diseases that may cause blindness. It concludes with consideration of the visual impairments and their management in the case study.

The profession of optometry was established by the Opticians Act 1958, although unregulated provision of spectacles as a form of optical rehabilitation is documented by Bacon as far back as 1268. Optometrists form a large independent sector of the Primary Eyecare Service. The graduate profession of optometry currently numbers approximately 8,000 practitioners with some 4,000 dispensing opticians also providing eyecare services in approximately 6,000 practices, regulated by the General Optical Council. Any member of the team may refer a patient to an optomotrist who can visit the patient in hospital or in their own home.

The profession currently provides 15.2 million eye examinations annually (7.1 million privately and 8.1 million through the General Ophthalmic Services), resulting in some 13 million spectacle dispensings. Five per cent of eye examinations now result in contact lens fittings, leading to 76 million pairs of contact lenses being dispensed annually. Optometrists carry out much of the routine refraction work previously undertaken by ophthalmologists and with current trends in shared-care development they may soon take over a significant part of the therapeutic workload in diabetes, glaucoma and anterior eye disease.

Medical statistics clearly indicate the increasing incidence of eye disease with age, with the incidence increasing from 9 per cent in the sixth decade to some 80 per cent in the eighth decade. Although the incidence of individual eye diseases is usually low by comparison with many systemic diseases, the insidious nature of many such diseases means that they may be well established, causing irreversible damage, before they are diagnosed. The number of persons in the UK with a registerable visual impairment is currently over 1 million. By the year 2020 this will have increased to more than 1.3 million (Esperjesi, 1998).

In children, visual impairment, because of the pivotal role vision normally plays in information acquisition, may result in an increased risk of delayed general development, especially if concurrent sensory or motor impairments exist, e.g. Rett syndrome (Saunders et al., 1995). The main causes of visual impairment in children are albinism, congenital cataract, idiopathic nystagmus and hereditary macular degenerations (Evans, 1995), all of which continue into adulthood and old age.

With up to 5 per cent of children having strabismus (squint) and 10 per cent amblyopia (lazy-eye), both of which have a good prognosis if treated early, rehabilitation of childrens' vision problems is an important optometric contribution to visual health. This is particularly so when correction of these problems at an early age may open up vocational opportunities that may otherwise be lost. The key factor is early diagnosis and intervention in the form of visual training or provision of optical aids. This ensures that appropriate advice may be given on environmental adaptations and support organisations that may be involved at an early stage if necessary.

In developed countries, the four major causes of visual impairment in adults are ARMD (age-related macular degeneration), diabetes mellitus, glaucoma and hereditary retinal degenerations. These result in a blindness prevalence of 0.3 per cent and accounts for some 10 per cent of the world's blind population. Approximately 20 per cent of the conditions are either preventable or treatable. In developing countries, the major causes of blindness are cataract, trachoma, glaucoma, onchocerciasis and xerophthalmia. These result in a blindness prevalence of 1.4 per cent and account for 90 per cent of the world's blind population. Approximately 75 per cent of the conditions are either preventable or treatable (Dickinson, 1998), with many of these conditions being contracted in childhood and persisting to adulthood.

DEGREES OF VISUAL IMPAIRMENT

There are many different definitions of visual impairment used throughout the world. In the UK two levels are used, 'blind' and 'partially sighted'. The statutory definition in the National Insurance Act 1948 (reviewed 1959) is that the person is 'so blind as to be unable to perform any work for which eyesight is essential'.

This translates to a visual acuity:

- of less than 3/60 Snellen; or
- of better than 3/60 but less than 6/60 with a very contracted visual field (except if the defect is long-standing and hence is subject to adaptation); or
- 6/60 or better with a very contracted field especially the lower area.

There is no statutory definition of 'partially sighted', but a person may be registered if they are 'substantially and permanently handicapped by defective vision caused by congenital defect, injury or illness'.

This translates to a visual acuity:

- of 3/60 to 6/60 with full fields; or
- 6/24 with moderate field contraction; or
- 6/18 or better with severe field contraction.

The importance of a normally functioning visual field is clear in both definitions as vital to normal daily living visual function; consequently attention must be paid to this when any form of visual rehabilitation is being considered.

Contrast sensitivity, the ability to see objects in poor contrast, e.g. pavement kerbs or newsprint, is not currently included in the definition of visual impairment. Research shows that a reduction in this function is as visually disabling as visual field loss and may be more disabling than loss of central visual acuity. Contrast sensitivity is of particular concern for various daily living tasks such as reading and has been shown to be a better predictor of mobility performance than central visual acuity.

Although low vision rehabilitation forms part of all British optometric training, there is little encouragement to apply this training in practice since there is no spectacle voucher scheme to cover even simple LVA dispensing. Consequently, most of the provision is through optometrists working in the Hospital Eye Service. The role of the optometrist is to assess the visual function and to prescribe suitable optical and non-optical aids. There are many community-based schemes where trained social workers and carers provide the day-to-day support for visually impaired people. Social workers for the blind are employed by the RNIB and may be based in local authority departments to provide a local service.

Rumney (1992) audited a series of low vision patients and found that 20 per cent were unable to benefit from an optical aid but required referral for rehabilitation assistance. Of the remainder, 69 per cent required the provision of a simple hand-held magnifier of less than 4X magnification. This is relatively cheap to provide as a hand or stand magnifier, but appropriate training is vital if the aid is not to be discarded. This is even more important for the 31 per cent who require more sophisticated aids such as spectacle mounted telescopes and magnifiers. These are normally only supplied to well-motivated patients who have demonstrated their adaptability to use simple aids. The important factor in the provision of vision aids is that they must be prescribed to suit the patient's daily living requirements, e.g. reading at home, prices in shops, VDU, TV and social interaction. To this end it is important that the vision care team involves not only optometrists but also occupational therapists, social workers and mobility officers.

VISUAL REHABILITATION: MAIN POINTS FOR POTENTIAL REFERRAL

- Look at the patient's eyes for signs of opacity/squint/nystagmus or unusual head posture.
- Observe for signs of visual neglect, clumsiness, unsteady gait.
- Listen carefully to the patient as they describe visual problems.
- Ensure all patients have regular eye examinations (including blind and partially sighted).
- Ensure that you:
  - are aware of what aids and services are available for the patient, e.g. talking books and local newspapers, etc.
  - know what aids the patient has
  - know what the aids are to be used for
  - check that the aids are being used appropriately
  - check that the aids are in good condition and working properly;
  - check that aids are being reviewed regularly and updated as necessary.
  This ensures optimal visual function for the patient.

CASE STUDY	SUSAN HUNTER – THE OPTOMETRIST'S CONTRIBUTION

To evaluate the effect of the stroke on Susan Hunter's visual function; this may have diagnostic and prognostic significance and also a bearing on rehabilitation:

- central visual acuity
- visual field integrity
- oculomotor function (extra and intraocular muscles)
- perceptual.

All four features may have a disabling effect on Susan Hunter. Poor central visual acuity may restrict various aspects of the patient's lifestyle, such as reading, handling money etc., while visual field damage may seriously affect the patient's ability to function in the normal environment such as in traffic or on stairs. If oculomotor function is affected Susan Hunter may suffer from strabismus with attendant insuperable diplopia. Perceptual problems may give rise to visual agnosia and disorientations, such as judging distance and relative position correctly. The optometrist would normally deal with these problems in the order shown.

The first step would be ensuring that central vision is unaffected, by means of a standard refraction using objective and subjective means. Ready access, at short notice, to an optometrist also means that the progress or regression of the condition can be determined. Suitable spectacles may be provided and changed as required.

A visual field test would be carried out to ensure that the visual pathway is intact and that Susan Hunter has fully functioning visual fields, which ensure that there is no compromise in her social vision, i.e. reading, in traffic etc. Hemianopic field loss can impair reading by interfering with tracking eye movement to the right, causing the person to lose their place on the line, or to the left causing difficulty in refixating each line start position. The use of simple card masks may be suggested in such cases. The use of reflecting spectacles may also be suggested in cases of homonymous hemianopia, accompanied by suitable training and lighting advice. These may be either as mirrors or as Fresnel partial-aperture refracting prism systems. Visual field expanders, a Galilean telescope reversed, may also be prescribed as an addition to the patient's spectacles. The person may also be trained in eccentric viewing techniques, where the eye is directed to such a position that the image falls on a functioning part of the retina.

Oculomotor problems may result from CVA and may manifest as acquired nystagmus with attendant oscillopsia, manifest incomitant strabismus and diplopia or reduced or abolished accommodative (focusing) power, causing near vision to blur and reading to become difficult. In nystagmus, training in finding the 'null zone' by adopting a modified head posture, where image oscillation is minimised, may be given. In manifest strabismus the application of prismatic lenses may alleviate the diplopia and appropriate application of extra positive power lenses may ameliorate the loss of accommodative power.

Perceptual problems such as the Pulfrich effect, which may result from cerebral injury, are difficult to identify and treat and the optometrist, having ruled out optical, visual field and oculomotor problems, would generally refer such problems for full psychological assessment.

Having determined the effect of the CVA on all aspects of Susan Hunter's visual system the optometrist would then be in a position to give her and her family appropriate advice on the 'lifestyle' changes and visual aids, which may become necessary.

REFERENCES

Dickinson, C. (1998) *Low Vision: Principles and Practice*, Butterworths, Oxford, Chapter 1, pp. 3–16.

Esperjesi, F. (1998) Low vision Part One: terminology and incidence. *Optician*, **215**, 14–18.

Evans, B. (1995) *Causes of Blindness and Partial Sight in England and Wales 1990–1991. Studies on medical and population subjects No. 57*, HMSO, London.

Rumney, N. (1992) An optometric approach to low visual services. *British Journal of Visual Impairment*, **10**, 89–91.

Saunders, K.J., McCulloch, D.L. and Kerr, A.M. (1995) Visual function in Rett syndrome. *Developmental Medicine and Child Neurology*, **37**, 496–504.

PART F: HEARING IN OLD AGE – TALI MENDELSOHN

Total or profound deafness destoys normal communications, robs people of their confidence and imprisons them in a cocoon of silence. A man can be blind but not isolated, lose his limbs but retain his confidence – but the chilling consequence of loss of hearing is alienation and insecurity. Cut off from the hearing community, a deafened person is deprived not only of communication but often of the will to bridge the chasm to the rest of mankind . . . Blindness evokes sympathy, while deafness provokes irritation.

Lord Jack Ashley (1992)

HEARING LOSS AND OLD AGE

One in seven people in the UK have some loss of hearing – that is 8.7 million people (Davis, 1995) There are many causes of hearing loss but by far the most common is ageing. Two-thirds of people over 60 years old have some degree of hearing loss or deafness (Davis, 1995).

Poor vision isolates a person from objects in their environment, but poor hearing distances them from people and human communication. Hearing loss has an adverse effect on functional status, quality of life and emotional, behavioural and social well-being (Soucek and Michaels, 1990; Hetu *et al.*, 1993; Kricos, 1995) This is especially true in older people who may also have mobility, visual and other problems, and rely on hearing to maintain contact with people around them.

Presbyacusis is the term used to describe hearing loss associated with the ageing process. It is permanent and cannot be corrected by medical or surgical intervention and is sometimes, but not always, related to high blood pressure or general atherosclerosis. Age-related hearing loss is most commonly noticed at around 60 years of age (Figure 20.1), but a premature onset may be associated with otitis media in childhood and with prolonged exposure to extreme levels of noise.

In presbyacusis, the progressive atrophy of hair cells and auditory fibres in the inner ear causes a sensori-neural hearing loss that begins and progresses for no apparent reason with advancing years. The result is an ability to hear or detect speech, but difficulty understanding its meaning. Hearing loss occurs first and more markedly in the high frequencies, reducing or eliminating the perception of consonants, which carry much of the meaning of speech. Low frequency hearing is not affected initially, allowing vowel sounds to be heard. People with presbyacusis therefore report difficulty hearing in background noise or group situations, may be unable to hear birds singing or bells ringing and may find that people around them 'mumble'. As presbyacusis develops, the hearing loss worsens and all frequencies may be affected. General age-related slowing of reaction time makes matters no easier.

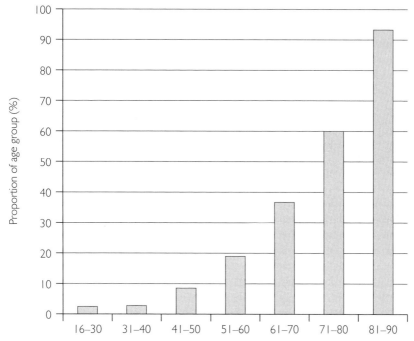

Figure 20.1 How prevalence of hearing loss increases with age
(*Davis, 1995*)

HOW THE TEAM CAN HELP

Identifying a hearing loss

The multidisciplinary team can assist significantly by being aware of the possibility and consequences of hearing loss. Since a hearing problem is an invisible disability, people are often at pains to deny the problem, attempt to ignore it or hide it from others. MP Tony Benn, interviewed on *One in Seven*, August 1998, said, 'The problem with deafness as I've come to realise is that it's the one disability nobody notices. People often think you're not listening or you're not interested.' People are much more open about admitting a visual problem, seeking help and wearing, perhaps designer, glasses.

In older people the added complication is the slow progressive nature of presbyacusis. The hearing loss can progress so slowly that people can be unaware of how much they are missing. It is after an average of *18 years* of living with hearing impairment that people feel inclined to seek help (Brooks, 1976) and this makes their adjustment to using hearing aids much more difficult. Early referral results in greater success with hearing aids and with communication, as well as less likelihood of feelings of isolation and exclusion. Below is a checklist to determine whether a referral for hearing assessment may be appropriate:

Signs of a hearing loss:

- You can hear people talking but cannot always make out what they are saying.
- In a noisy environment, you struggle to follow the conversation.
- Other people seem to mumble rather than speak clearly to you.
- People have to repeat things several times before you understand what they are saying.
- If you are talking to people in a group, it is hard to keep up with the conversation.
- You feel excluded from conversations and others wonder why you don't join in.
- Other people think your television is too loud, but you cannot hear it properly if it is turned down.
- You often have difficulty hearing on the telephone.

Referral is indicated if any of the above are acknowledged or evident.

Assisting deaf and hard of hearing people

If the person has a hearing aid, make sure he or she is using it. It should be switched on, have batteries that work and be used at the correct volume. Hearing aids function best at a distance of 1–2m.

If patients are known to have a hearing loss and attend clinics regularly, recording this on their case notes will allow arrangements to be made for them to be called appropriately for their consultation or treatment.

Hearing loss affects individuals and their family, friends and colleagues. Information about how to help compensate for the hearing problem needs to be shared as openly as possible. Embarrassment prevents many people from communicating with those who have hearing disabilities. Sharing information can be very helpful in reducing this problem. Such information (and help on many other related topics) is available from the Royal National Institute for Deaf People (RNID) (see Useful information).

The ways in which we speak to someone who has a hearing loss will influence his or her ability to communicate with us. The following guidelines are appropriate whether or not a person uses a hearing aid.

CASE STUDY SUSAN HUNTER – HEARING PROMOTION

Susan Hunter is 81 years old and has mobility and health problems, which necessitate contact with a number of health professionals. Her family visits frequently and has noticed that she does not always respond appropriately in conversation. Observations that she is 'becoming detached', maybe due to a hearing loss that has yet to be identified. A hearing aid may make visits more enjoyable for both Susan Hunter and her family, and may make her contact with the health-care team and carers easier and more productive.

Your communication:

- Try to ensure that you have the person's attention before you begin to speak and that they are facing you.
- Look at the person and do not turn away while you are talking to them.
- Sit so that your face is well lit and not in shadow. Don't cover your face or mouth.
- Use facial expressions, body language and gestures to complement your spoken messages and clarify what you are saying.
- Slow your speech down slightly but maintain the rhythm and normal pattern of speech. This makes it easier to follow what is being said.
- Do not shout!
- If necessary repeat or rephrase a sentence that has not been heard or understood. As a last resort, you could write down words or symbols to help the person.
- If the person uses a non-verbal communication system (such as Makaton), try to learn a few signs/symbols to assist the person's understanding of what you are trying to say.
- Give the person plenty of time to communicate. Be patient!

The environment:

- A good acoustic setting is one with smaller dimensions and soft furnishings. Therefore a lounge will be an easier setting than an open clinic or treatment room because echoes and distortions are reduced.
- Good lighting is important to assist lip reading.
- Wherever possible, reduction of background noise in places such as busy clinics and waiting rooms will be of great benefit. Unwanted sounds will be dampened by the introduction of a tablecloth, carpet, double-glazing and curtains.
- The fewer people present, the easier it is to follow conversation. If a room is unavoidably crowded, communication will be easier if the person with a hearing loss has his or her back to a wall. Sound will approach from fewer directions so identification of the sound source is simplified.

HEARING SERVICES: ASSESSMENT AND ASSISTANCE

At present, a visit to the general practitioner is the first step in accessing NHS help for a suspected hearing loss. GP referral is required for a consultation with an ear, nose and throat (ENT) specialist and/or audiologist.

If the person is over 60 years old and the GP is sure that no related medical conditions or ear abnormalities exist, the GP may refer the person directly to an audiology department. The primary aim of this referral method is that the ENT department is bypassed, thus reducing waiting times. The Audit Commission (2000) recommends that all Health Authorities should ensure that GP direct referral schemes are in place in their area.

Good working relationships and cross-referral between audiology and ENT are essential to ensure thorough audiological and medical investigation and treatment wherever necessary.

Whichever way a referral occurs, a hearing assessment will be carried out by the audiologist and a decision will be made regarding further treatment. This may include any (or all) of the following.

Amplification

While hearing aids do not restore or provide normal hearing, they may be indicated in order to help the person hear more effectively . One or two hearing aids may be required and impressions will be taken of the ears so that moulds may be made for the individual. When the hearing aid is issued, further tests should be carried out to ensure the amplification provided by the hearing aid is the best match for the individual's hearing loss. Management and use of the hearing aid will be explained. A follow-up appointment should be provided for progress and satisfaction to be assessed and any necessary changes to be made.

Once a person has an NHS hearing aid, they may self-refer to audiology for reassessments as required, but they should have access to local free battery and maintenance services at open-access clinics (i.e. no appointment required).

Some NHS audiology departments offer a domicillary/home visit service for housebound people. This should include all aspects of the service from initial assessment to hearing aid fitting and repair appointments.

The NHS provides hearing aids to more than 80 per cent of hearing aid users in the UK (Institute for Hearing Research, 1999) and the majority of the aids provided at present use 1970s technology. However, in January 2000, the government initiated a programme in England to introduce advanced technology hearing aids and other general improvements in audiology services into the NHS. John Hutton, Minister of State for Health (2000) said, 'We have to ensure that that technology [digital hearing aids] is available to NHS patients who use audiology services in local trusts and we intend to do so . . . in a major modernisation of hearing aid services.' The two-year programme will include 20 NHS audiology centres and will then be rolled out to other audiology departments. This signals an awareness of the importance of better quality hearing aids for improved quality of life for deaf and hard of hearing people.

Advanced audiological tests

Further testing may be indicated for diagnostic purposes. These may include site of lesion tests and tests of vestibular function.

Aural rehabilitation/hearing therapy

This service may include assistance with hearing and/or hearing aids, counselling for adjustment to hearing loss, communication skills, tinnitus therapy, management of hearing-related balance disorders and advice, and information about aids to daily living, such as those for television and telephones.

Referral to other professionals or service providers

Various referrals may be indicated, particularly to occupational therapy for advice on manipulation of aids by those with disabilities (Chapter 16). Audiology departments should have strong links with their local social services departments (Chapter 19). Social services are responsible for provision of assistive listening devices for deaf and hard of hearing people. These aids to daily living are television and telephone aids, text phones, communicators, doorbell systems, alarm and alerting devices. Part Three of the Disability Discrimination Act (DfEE, 1999) requires reasonable adjustments to be made for disabled people, and this includes all service provision to people who are deaf and hard of hearing. Assistive devices may therefore be required in medical clinics as well as all locations used for provision of services.

SUMMARY

Hearing impairment may lead to social isolation and decreased quality of life for older people. To counteract this, medical and/or audiological intervention, aural rehabilitation and a wide range of technological solutions may be indicated. However, the most significant benefit is provided by people's awareness of hearing impairment and their knowledge of how to communicate with those who have a hearing loss. This allows for more effective communication, independence and quality of life of older people with hearing loss.

REFERENCES

Ashley, Lord J. (1992) *Acts of Defiance*, Reinhardt Books, London.
Audit Commission (2000) *Fully Equipped: The provision of equipment to older or disabled people by the NHS and social services in England and Wales*, HMSO, London.
Brooks, D.N. (1976) The use of hearing aids by the hearing impaired. In: *Disorders of Audiological Function II* (ed. Stephens, S.D.G.), Academic Press, London.
Davis, A. (1995) *Hearing in Adults*, Whurr, London.
Department for Education and Employment [DfEE] (1999) Part Three of the *Disability Discrimination Act (1995) Discrimination in other areas: Goods facilities and services*, Section 21: Duty of Providers of Services to Make Adjustments, HMSO, London.

Hetu, R., Jones, L. and Getty, L. (1993) The impact of acquired hearing impairment on intimate relationships: Implications for rehabilitation. *Audiology*, **32**, 363–381.

Hutton, J. (1 February 2000) Oral Answer, Column 905–906. *Parliamentary Debate (Hansard)*, HMSO, London.

Institute for Hearing Research (1999) *ENT Survey*, Medical Research Council, London.

Kricos, P.B. (1995) Characteristics of the aged population. In: *Hearing Care for the Older Adult: Audiological rehabilitation* (eds Kricos, P.B. and Lesner, S.A.), Butterworth-Heinemann, Boston, MA.

Richards, A. and Gleeson, M. (1999) Recent advances: otolaryngology. *British Medical Journal*, **319**, 1110–1113.

Soucek, S. and Michaels, L. (1990) *Hearing Loss in the Elderly*, Springer, London.

USEFUL INFORMATION

Royal National Institute for Deaf People (RNID) Helpline
PO Box 16464, London EC1Y 8TT
Tel: 0808 808 0123
Textphone: 0808 808 9000
Fax: 020 7296 8199
E-mail: helpline@rnid.org.uk

OVERVIEW AND FUTURE OF THE
REHABILITATION OF OLDER PEOPLE

Amanda J. Squires

AIMS OF THE CHAPTER

This book has highlighted the ongoing and fundamental changes that are occurring in both health and social care in the UK. The focus has been on the consequences – both opportunity and threat – to all members of the interdisciplinary team involved in the rehabilitation of the older person. The team is described as consisting of the professionals and paid and unpaid carers all centring their attention on the key member – the service user.

This chapter aims to summarise the key issues and suggest strategies for the future that will facilitate successful integration of policies, services and disciplines shown to distinguish the effective team from the rest. The chapter emphasises that a patient-centred partnership in assessment, goal setting, implementation and monitoring of a treatment plan will maximise cost-effectiveness. For success, an understanding of the traditional and emerging components of the team is essential, together with accurate, comprehensive and shared documentation. The author describes the numeric, economic and political power being shown by current and upcoming generations of older people (Vincent, 1999), who comprise the largest group of users of the NHS and will increasingly focus their attention on quality of health and social care. The author concludes by suggesting that rehabilitation of older people requires different attitudes, an expanded evidence base and access to a wide range of competent skills.

BACKGROUND

The history of rehabilitation of older people in the UK has evolved from the care of the poor by religious institutions, poor law provision in the Middle Ages and the eventual realisation in the mid twentieth century that, for some, rehabilitation, rather than just care, was an option. The demographic changes in the latter half of the twentieth century have resulted in not only escalating numbers of older people both indigenous and ethnic minority, but also their attendant health and social problems; their need for functional ability to remain independent; their rising expectations; and the shortage of both formal and informal carers to meet these needs.

REFORM OF HEALTH AND SOCIAL CARE

Like many national health systems, the NHS responded to the mismatch between supply and demand by instituting reform in 1990. It was hoped that the resulting market culture would improve efficiency and at the same time raise standards (Department of Health [DoH], 1989a). The negative connotation of a market in public health care and the increasing importance of primary care in coordination of the expanded health-care provision outside of the hospital, led to further reform (NHS Executive, 1997), which detailed that:

- Primary Care Trusts (PCTs) were given responsibility for commissioning secondary care
- Health Improvement Programmes (HimP) would meet the needs of the local population in partnership with all local interests, ensuring that those with continuing health and social care needs get access to more integrated services through Joint Investment Plans (JIPs)
- evidence based standards would be set by a National Institute for Clinical Excellence (NICE), including the production of National Service Frameworks (NSFs) for major care areas and disease groups, with that for Older People being among the first tranche
- a 'clinical governance' framework to make service quality both the responsibility of NHS organisations and individual professionals would be monitored by a Commission for Health Improvement (CHI).

The NHS Plan (DoH, 2000) is described as a plan for investment and reform to provide a health service fit for the twenty-first century and includes proposals for investment in structures, development of staff, integration between agencies and expansion of clinical roles.

At the same time, complementary reform of social care has also been ongoing. The White Paper, *Caring for People* (DoH, 1989b), set in motion a series of changes which, while giving local authorities the lead role in community care, shifted their priorities to:

- targeting support on those most eligible
- using the independent sector as much as possible
- introducing new rights to assessment.

This resulted in much loss of low-level preventive or rehabilitative provision. The result of the assessment is a 'statement of need', developed with and agreed by the user and any carer. The ensuing package of care can be set up by care managers using their departments' allocated budgets and making use of local, perhaps non-traditional, services or informal supports. Formal arrangements for care will increasingly be made by older people themselves, some using direct payment money to purchase their own care, while others use their savings. The 1997 NHS reform proposals have been reinforced in a number of areas by more detailed guidance. This includes a consultative document *Partnership in Action* (NHS Executive, 1998), which proposes three ways of facilitating partnerships between the NHS and Local Authority Social Services or social work departments:

- pooled budgets
- delegation to a lead commissioning agency, and
- integrated provider organisations.

Further changes in 2001 (DoH, 2001a) required the reduction in bureaucratic layers, development of a strategic plan and joint management of health and social care.

The policy agenda therefore emphasises joint working, joint delivery and joint financing. For some working in Social Services, there is concern that their particular contribution to the holistic support of older people will be marginalised. Utilising social models of ability and valuing concepts such as choice, independence and autonomy, social workers have been able to offer a certain independence from the hospital and NHS systems. At best they have conceived of themselves as being able to represent older people's point of view in face of a more unified health edifice and have advocated on their behalf. In particular they have managed difficulties around social relationships, including conflict between family members, service users who are reluctant to engage with services and been able to sustain relationships with those whose mental capacity is frail.

STAKEHOLDER EXPECTATIONS

For a partnership to be successful, the needs of the three stakeholder groups (user, provider and (perhaps joint) commissioner) must be identified, understood and met. Mutual satisfaction will depend on equal partnership, reciprocal education, common assessment of need, shared information, mutual understanding, agreed values and clear specifications. To avoid complacency and a static culture when expectations are known to be forever changing, ongoing review of standards will facilitate the ultimate goal of a service pursuing continuous quality improvement (CQI).

Services for older people have to date been largely exempt from expressed and rising public expectations. This has been due to the cohort effect of the user group, many remembering the pre-NHS days and eternally 'grateful' for what they receive. Newer cohorts are, and will be increasingly, different. The potential size of this group of newly/early retired users, who have much to give, little to lose, available resources and a lifetime of contacts and experience on which to call is an influence seriously underestimated by the service. Having lost the opportunity for efficient proactive partnership, the service will ultimately respond in a costly reactive way. How these individuals are identified and their contribution used will provide a productive opportunity for the proactive – and a serious threat to the reactive.

Ethnic minority elders

Historically, Britain has always included a variety of ethnic minority groups within its population so that many different races and cultures are represented in the older population with specific health and social profiles, which may result in different rehabilitation needs. A multi-cultural workforce that reflects the cultural make-up of the local population is advantageous in understanding culture specific issues.

Carers

Rehabilitation is largely conceived of as a professional task involving the patient and expert, while carers consider themselves as lay people, able to provide ordinary, common-sense support. It is clear, however, that many carers learn and exercise highly developed skills and that professionals often invoke their active participation in the rehabilitation process. Carers can also contribute their skills to the repertoire of the professional through their experience in solving practical problems. Relatives and informal carers continue to constitute the mainstay of community and long-term care. The importance of the enabling role of health and social services in providing adequate training, support, advice and relief cannot be over-stressed.

The White Paper *Caring for People* (DoH, 1989b) placed as the second most important objective of community care policy the need 'to ensure that service providers make practical support for carers a high priority'. *The NHS Plan* (DoH, 2000) is more specific and acknowledges that its plans for developing rehabilitation services will necessitate support for carers, and legislation (Carers (Recognition and Services) Act 1996) now gives carers the right to be consulted and assessed for their own needs as a potential carer.

Among a number of initiatives, Carers' Centres offer a resource that may provide support, professional or voluntary advice, information or activities. Such centres will increasingly provide access via the Internet to the latest information, confidently challenging professionals from an informed base. One key task for professionals is to introduce carers to such local networks and ensure resources to enable them to participate if it is their wish.

HEALTH AND HEALTH CARE OF OLDER PEOPLE

Not only is the number of older people increasing with 20 per cent of the population currently over 60, compared with 7.5 per cent at the beginning of the century and expected to rise to 24.3 per cent by 2021, but the elderly population is itself ageing with those aged 75 and over projected to account for 8 per cent of the total population by 2021.

The *OPCS Disability Survey* (Martin *et al.*, 1988) identifies an approximate doubling of the prevalence of disability with each successive decade over the age of 50 years. Forty-one per cent of those aged 70–79 were found to have some level of disability, with 4 per cent in the severest category with a major concentration of disability during the three years prior to death (Guralnik *et al.*, 1991, 1993). Mainstream services (including acute care) should be planned on the basis that episodes of illness increasingly go hand in hand with short-term, medium-term and long-term disability as day-to-day practice reflects the ageing of populations.

The number of older people with complex problems who live in the community is also increasing. Many of these people live alone and informal care is problematic, because the main carer is often elderly, and social expectations and traditions around family support are changing. Against this background, national policy for both health and social services has been to move away from institutional care to integrated services, which enable vulnerable people to be supported in the community. *The National Service Framework (NSF) for Older People* (DoH, 2001b) emphasises a new cohort of older people – those with learning disabilities who have now begun to survive into old age, bringing with them their own special needs.

Health and social care for older people

The principles of health care for older people are based on the existence of good health in older people; the possibility of multiple pathology; the need for accurate and comprehensive assessment; and effective and timely team work by specialists to implement care plans at a pace compatible with the capacity of the older person to respond; and the involvement of older people and their carers in health promotion.

Settings

The settings in which activity may take place to meet the needs and aim of rehabilitation are expanding and include inpatient or outpatient treatment at a hospital, at a day hospital, health centre, the person's own home, day centre, care home, sheltered housing, prison, intermediate care unit, hospice or facility for those who are homeless. Each of these may present different challenges to practitioners in terms of the delivery of efficient, effective and safe care or treatments, as well as the need for assessing the risks associated with treating people in different settings.

As an example, the drive to establish and expand 'intermediate care' is a concept with the intention of accelerating the discharge of older people from acute hospital beds. In some cases admission may be diverted from an acute facility that risks disadvantaging their access to mainstream diagnostic and treatment facilities. Similarly, a proposal in the NHS Plan (DoH, 2000) to use private sector nursing homes for rehabilitation of older people will only succeed where provision is part of an integrated service. The principles of different space, equipment, philosophy and specialist personnel requirements that have evolved over many years in the NHS will need to be transferred.

The challenge to the team is to deliver efficient, effective and equitable treatment in whichever setting is required. To do so it must take into account the effect that the setting has on both the older person and the staff involved, as well as other people with whom the older person comes into contact. Each setting has strengths and weaknesses that affect service delivery and present challenges to the team in their delivery of care. An awareness of the social and psychological impacts of the different settings, the staff and capital resources, the role and purpose of the 'unit' in which treatment is provided, and the role and workload of staff contributing to the interdisciplinary team, will allow the team to deliver treatment to the best of its ability.

While rehabilitation has historically been led by secondary care, the NHS Plan (DoH, 2000) states that Primary Care Groups/Trusts will set up Intensive

Rehabilitation Services to help older patients regain health/independence after illness/surgery. They are also charged with establishing recuperation facilities in nursing homes, one-stop services and integrated home care teams. In addition, there are also proposals to establish Care Trusts, which will provide integrated health and social care (already in place in Northern Ireland), with some of these in place by the end of 2001. For success, all of these developments will need to be part of a larger, revitalised, integrated specialist service for older people (covering acute general hospital care and rehabilitation), which otherwise may risk disadvantaging their access to mainstream diagnostic and treatment facilities. Rehabilitation of the older person after illness must also be perceived and evaluated in the context of such a comprehensive service.

Discharge

Henwood (1994) describes discharge as follows:

> ... *a discharge from hospital is an admission – or transfer – to community care; and an admission to hospital is a transfer from the community. It is crucial, therefore, to recognise that actions and decisions made at any point in a care episode can have consequences for other parts of the health and social care system.*

The NHS and Community Care Act 1990 placed certain responsibilities upon Local Authorities of direct relevance to hospital discharge. In particular, at the level of individuals, it passed responsibility and finance to Social Services departments for the funding of residential and nursing home care for those it considered eligible on grounds of need and resources. Social Services, therefore, have devised their own assessment criteria and 'banding' systems to allocate financial support.

Two main effects on Social Services can be observed. First, their available funding is becoming increasingly restricted. Once a person is eligible for and admitted to residential or nursing home care, the cost to the local authority is considerable and largely non-negotiable. Furthermore, even if a high level of community care services can be set in place – the cost is also high. The second effect is that much attention becomes focused on patrolling the entry into Social Services care and funding: low-level needs may be not met until a crisis develops. Any help is scaled down and may be withdrawn too quickly. Where possible care is charged for and income from service users is maximised.

Commentary on the implementation of the NHS and Community Care Act 1990 has noted the limiting of the process of care management to a narrow focus on assessment as a means of controlling resources (Bradley and Manthorpe, 1997). Fewer people now receive domiciliary support, but those who do receive it at higher levels (Harding, 1999).

In hospitals there are continuing and accelerating pressures to reduce the length of inpatient stay, but, clearly, successful earlier discharge from hospital can only be achieved if patients can manage to function in their own homes or supported accommodation. Focused and timely rehabilitation is of crucial importance and will reduce unnecessary residential and nursing home placements (Millard, 1999), acknowledged to place an unsustainable demand on Social Services and other resources that could be aimed at primary prevention (Audit Commission, 1997).

REHABILITATION

Baker *et al.* (1997) defines rehabilitation as:

> ... *an enabling process in which societies, communities, agencies and professionals meet the social, psychological, physical and economic needs of the disabled person through knowledge, skill, respect, understanding and agreement. The rehabilitative process includes an assessment of where the individual, community and carer(s) are, where they wish to be, and the contributions each must make to achieve ambitions and meet needs.*

It is therefore a process to which specialist staff provide specialist interventions within their professional and legal remit (for example medicine, nursing, physiotherapy, occupational therapy and podiatry) as part of a comprehensive plan. In addition, all members of the team, including the patient or service user and carers, carry out the routine practice of different skills and endurance activities, maintaining continuity of progress, on aspects for which they have been trained. Rehabilitation does not therefore only occur when specialist staff are present, just as nutrition does not occur only at mealtimes.

The King's Fund (Sinclair and Dickinson, 1998) points to the fact that effective rehabilitation is achieved by the coordination of complex interventions addressing multiple risk factors, involving multiple professional disciplines and multiple phases of rehabilitation. Multidisciplinary implies many different groups of professionals. Interdisciplinary infers professionals working together and this inter-dependent approach is held to be the key to successful and meaningful rehabilitation, differentiating the specialist service from those to which multiple disciplines merely contribute.

The basic structure of rehabilitation is based on the interdisciplinary team of people who:

- work together towards common goals with each patient/user
- involve and educate the patient and family
- have relevant knowledge and skills
- can help patients resolve most of the common problems.

The process is cyclical, incorporating assessment, goal setting, interventions, reassessment and review, all directed at a measurable outcome.

The skills required for effective team working can be learned and developed to ensure that the sum of the parts of the team is greater than the whole. Above all team work involves trust, knowledge and effective communication skills. Team working is most valuable when members have to work together with a common purpose to achieve a consistent quality of service with the resources available. A well-managed team will work effectively and efficiently ensuring that resources (mainly costly professional time) are used appropriately. There will be transfer and sharing of skills to ensure people's needs are met and provider and service user time is not wasted. In the continually changing health and social care sector effective and flexible team working will be essential in sharing the workload to meet deadlines and in providing support to team members.

Ethical considerations

Traditional values within health and social care are being challenged by social changes. Practitioners, already working autonomously as a result of the unique multi-pathology and multi-dimensional social influences on older people, will increasingly have to address the basis of their decisions. Professional codes of ethics provide guidelines for such decision-making, and the issues – seldom taught in basic training – need to be considered and debated by teams of practitioners.

The process of ethical rehabilitation is therefore based on an interdisciplinary assessment that includes the views of the user and carer; goal setting that meets user and carer needs; intervention in which the user and carer are active participants; and review, which includes evidence of achievements identified by the user and opportunities for progress. By pursuing such best practice, the rights of users and autonomy of providers can maximise the potential of rehabilitation.

COMPONENTS OF THE REHABILITATION TEAM

What emerges is the existence of a number of teams along the patient's pathway of care. Although some professionals may be members of more than one team, each team has its specialist contribution to make, along with responsibility for timely and informed handover to the next team to ensure efficient and effective care. The development of nurse and therapist consultant roles offer almost limitless opportunities for personal and service development, working across professional and organisational boundaries to progress clinical governance. Such consultants, of whichever discipline, demonstrate expert practice, undertake research and service development, ensure education and training supports practice development, and provide supervision and leadership.

Before rehabilitation can take place a full interdisciplinary assessment should be performed (Audit Commission, 2000). Remediable conditions should be treated before the final rehabilitation plan is prepared for discussion with the patient and carer. The general 'core' services for assessment and rehabilitation of older people are complemented by a number of other services, which play an important role in certain circumstances. All have general and specific roles, audit and review requirements, responsibility for ensuring routine rehabilitation is continued and joint responsibility for the allocation of an appropriate key worker for individual patients and supervision of support staff. The key components and their core tasks are as follows:

- **Patients and their carers** are partners in the assessment process, actively implement agreed treatment plans, and take part in the audit and review of their care. They will increasingly supervise provision of their social care.

- **Doctors** are responsible for the medical management of the patient, diagnosis of disease, instigation of drug regimens, ensuring that autonomous colleagues are notified regarding the need for any specialist assessments and coordination of the ensuing team.
- **Nurses** are responsible for providing basic care and enhancing the patient's functional ability, ensuring that the appropriate screening tests are carried out, and facilitating team communication. Being available 24 hours a day, 7 days a week, nurses have a key role in consistent implementation of appropriate parts of the patient's care plan. The nurse has a specialist role in areas of tissue viability and pain management.
- **Physiotherapists** are the movement specialists within the rehabilitation team, their key role being to identify and address impairments responsible for disorders in movement and balance, and to manage the consequences of residual impairments, in order to increase activity and participation.
- **Occupational therapists** focus on occupational performance and its restoration, development and improvement through the use of selected occupation. Clients' homes are usually the venue for assessment and intervention, and as such are more realistic.
- **Speech and language therapists** concentrate on communication disorders to identify impairment, and maximise activity and participation in communicative interaction. Integral swallowing assessments will provide essential information on people's ability to understand and communicate their nutritional needs and problems with eating and drinking.
- **Podiatrists** note and treat the lifetime of trauma to feet, foot symptoms of other disorders such as diabetes and rheumatoid arthritis and, along with other team members, identify the presence of and attempt to rectify wearing of unsuitable shoes, all of which may affect mobility.
- **Social workers** focus on assessment of social care needs, choice, carer support, and the coordination and financing of packages of social care to enable people to live as independently as possible

The core services for rehabilitation of the older patient are complemented by a number of others, in particular:

- **Nutritionists and dietitians** aim to aid recovery, maintain health and help the older patient adapt to changed dietary intake, necessited by swallowing difficulties following stroke. The impact of illness and disability on nutritional status and the effects of this on the ability to recover from illness are of special concern for older people.
- **Dentists** consider oral health for social as well as nutritional benefit, and promote and maintain health. The reduction in the number of functional natural teeth and the reduced effectiveness of dentures may result in altered food choices, which in turn can lead to alterations in nutrient intake and nutritional status with consequences for recovery.
- **Pharmacists** provide prescription advice and awareness of side-effects and prescription adherence. Multiple pathologies in older people often result in an array of drugs being prescribed to a group who are the most vulnerable

to potential problems. These include adverse reactions to drugs, interactions between drugs, and difficulties in adhering to prescribed regimens.

• **Continence Advisers** diagnose, treat and reassess problems of continence, which are frequently the cause of admission to hospital or institutional care and a barrier to discharge. Continence of urine and faeces is fundamental to quality of life and to sociological, psychological and physical well-being of the individual. The quality and reliability of continence frequently controls the balance between success or failure in rehabilitation, because it is of such crucial importance to morale and social integration.

• **Optometrists** diagnose and compensate for eye disease, the incidence of which increases from 9 per cent in the sixth decade to some 80 per cent in the eighth decade. Vision is vital to normal daily living, particularly the ability to see objects in poor contrast, e.g. pavement kerbs, found to be a predictor of mobility performance.

• **Audiologists** diagnose and provide compensation where possible for the two-thirds of people over 60 years who have some degree of hearing loss or deafness. This has an adverse effect on functional status, quality of life, and emotional, behavioural and social well-being. This is especially important for older people who may also have mobility, visual and other problems, and rely on hearing to maintain contact with people around them.

The complexity of the specialist input to rehabilitation led the author to develop a model to demonstrate the integration opportunities, avoidance of duplication, as well as responsibilities of the various components (Figure 21.1).

TEAM WORK

Not all rehabilitation staff will be natural team members or leaders, although they may have the necessary client based skills. In a career in rehabilitation, especially with older people, these interpersonal skills are essential and can be acquired where there is a genuine desire to learn.

Teams that are in total harmony and avoid conflict will not work effectively. The team will be working in a closed system and encouraging 'group think' (Ovretviet, 1994), rather than lateral and innovative thinking. Inter-disciplinary teams can bring together different perspectives and skills in a coordinated manner to provide for the needs of the individual user. Conflict and differences are to be expected and need to be handled positively for the good of the user and the creativity of the team.

Team-working skills should be a fundamental component of basic training for all disciplines, particularly where continuous policy change affects consistent team membership, with teams needing to form and work together in increasingly shorter time spans. The formation, development and outcome of teams will no longer be optional, but will need planning and evaluation.

To help the interdisciplinary team continue to develop, a number of questions are posed in the following section for their consideration.

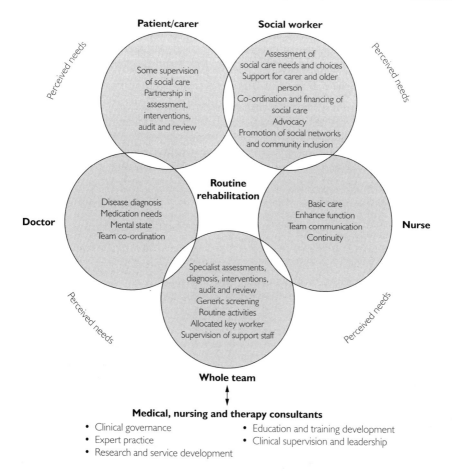

Figure 21.1 Responsibilities and integration of the interdisciplinary health-care team

ASSESSMENT, GOALS, OUTCOMES AND PATHWAYS

The personalised rehabilitation process includes interdisciplinary assessment and reviews using standardised measures where possible; problem identification using disease specific measures where relevant; goal setting using goal attainment scales; and clinical interventions based on evidence based practice.

Interdisciplinary assessment is the key to the formulation of shared goals and consistent treatment plans acceptable to the older person and his or her carer. The danger of gaps and duplications occurring when a number of people are involved can be avoided by use of key workers and accurate and timely communication. The outcome of the process will be increasingly sought by all stakeholders, but is disconcertingly complex and must be appropriate to the work of all members of the team.

Outcome refers to the effectiveness of the rehabilitation interventions in achieving the expected goal. The key is that the goal is agreed by all participants. Thus outcome measures are used to assess the relative change within the rehabilitation process.

Within the holistic approach of interdisciplinary team working with older people there will be a plethora of assessment tools and outcome measures used. A consistent approach from the different team members, crucially including carers, is essential for success, and may require informed debate to agree the approach to be used.

Having agreed the goals with the patient and carer, an intervention plan will be agreed by members of the team with a role to play. Changes may be necessary should new problems arise and as progress occurs.

Mental health

Mental health problems may be identified by any member of the team and all should be aware of the common issues that surround the mental well-being of older people. Physical ability and mental health are interlinked and assessment findings should be used to enhance the treatment plan and its implementation. The effect of mental illnesses on carers and their own mental health should also be included in the assessment, and support facilitated.

Memory and motivation are important components for rehabilitation. It appears that older people are less likely to be accurate about what they have done than what they have thought of doing. The effects are quite subtle but can have very real practical consequences, for example for medication. Poor motivation may be linked to any of the following – fear, pain, anxiety, depression, irrational health belief, an awareness of the inability to function as before, and disbelief in the optimism of the team. Successful goal negotiation is a highly skilled competence for professionals.

Pathways

Integrated care pathways (ICP) are being developed as part of the response to calls for evidence based, equitable and outcome oriented care. A care pathway determines locally agreed interdisciplinary practice, based on guidelines and evidence where available, for a specific patient/client group. It forms all or part of the clinical record; documents the care given; and facilitates the evaluation of outcomes for continuous quality improvement (Swage, 2000). Systematic recording within the pathway system facilitates audit of variances from which to learn. Pathways are essential in specialities such as rehabilitation of older people, where interdisciplinary input is paramount in providing care to people with problems resulting from multiple pathology. Where inter-professional pathways are team developed and owned, team work and collaboration will be enhanced.

EMERGING THEMES

The preceding chapters have considered the rehabilitation of the older person from a number of perspectives. The key emerging themes noted by the editors that readers may wish to consider with their own teams are skills, commitment, screening, specialisation, governance, outcomes, conflict, new elders and development.

Skills

The core and expanded members of the interdisciplinary team bring an amazing array of skills. The descriptions of their work will do much to educate their colleagues and enhance rehabilitation of the older person. Much of the content will be new to some readers. If we are to provide an efficient and comprehensive service, knowledge of the skills available, criteria for access and referral requirements must be more widely known and actively used.

- Can the team take further steps to ensure wider knowledge and active use of the skills available within the extended interdisciplinary team?
- Have the skills of the team been audited and a development plan identified to ensure the sharing of these skills and that they are not reliant on one person?

CASE STUDY SUSAN HUNTER – MULTIDISCIPLINARY REHABILITATION

To give a practical example of the complexity of the multidisciplinary rehabilitation process and ways of mapping the use of outcome indicators with older people, a case study of an older person, Susan Hunter, has been addressed in the preceding chapters, with each author including their contribution to comprehensive care. The emerging lessons are as follows:

- That coordination and integration of the team is essential to ensure that all of the patient's relevant problems are identified and managed.
- Each discipline brings a different knowledge base and focus that can be shared with key workers. The summative result provides greater depth and improved quality of treatment and outcome.
- Different disciplines have more specialist input at differents stages of the patient's journey from acute hospital admission, through rehabilitation and return to the community and vice versa.
- All members of the rehabilitative team recognise the need to involve the carers (if they and the patient wish the involvement).
- The culture of rehabilitation is about enabling people to do things for themselves and not to create dependence.

Commitment

The commitment by all the disciplines included in this book is encouraging, particularly when much work with older people has to date often been met with a passive and negative acceptance by some health and social care providers and much of the population at large. Political attitudes towards older people vary between priority, as consistent voters, and targets, slowing hospital throughput. Despite the social stigma, the committed have kept going. As older people are already the largest users of health care and social care, their rehabilitation will emerge as a cost-effective solution. The explosion of enthusiasm that committed practitioners could create with additional psychological, financial and physical resource can only be imagined.

- What steps can the team take to influence improved psychological, financial and physical resources both locally and nationally?
- How is the commitment to rehabilitative services for older people measured locally?

Screening

Despite older people being the largest users of health care, not all will need the services of the specialist rehabilitation team. The local strategy must ensure that those who do require the input of the team, or its individual members, can access it. Contributors have indicated simple 'top-to-toe' generic screening tests that can be used by any practitioner to indicate appropriate referral routes. Referral will not necessarily result in an intervention, but at least the specialist will have cost-effectively reviewed those with a potential need.

- Is a comprehensive screening tool used that identifies the need for specialist health and social care intervention?
- Do we need to review the comprehensive generic screening tool to cost-effectively match specialist treatment with need?

Specialisation

Where specialist input is required, there can be no doubt that a comprehensive specialist team provides the most cost-effective response – whatever the speciality. For rehabilitation of older people, the unique features are the breadth of skill required, the depth of experience and the interpersonal skills for active team working. The integration of geriatric medicine with acute care has probably been of more benefit to the latter. Single purpose wards have been shown to provide the best results due to a different philosophy of care.

- What steps can an integrated team make to apply the proven philosophy of care of older people to improve its overall results?
- What audit activity identifies effective service delivery of the integrated team?

Governance

Maintaining a successful team of autonomous, often crusading, individuals from different agencies requires continuous attention. The two key themes of clinical governance are the progressive improvement of services and the provision of systematic evidence of quality of service. These form a useful frame of reference for such work, with development of communication, team-building and leadership skills being an essential component.

- Are changes to the current framework for clinical governance and personal development needed to maximise functioning of the interdisciplinary team?
- How do you measure the performance of the interdisciplinary team?

Outcomes

Outcome refers to the effectiveness of the rehabilitation interventions in achieving the expected goal (Bowling, 1997). The key is that the goal has to be agreed by all participants. Thus outcome measures are used to assess the relative change within the rehabilitation process. When interdisciplinary working is considered, outcome measures become complex but will be increasingly sought by commissioners as proof of success of investment. The emphasis on cost-effectiveness, outcome measurement and evidence based practice since 1990 has resulted in a range of methods to measure clinical outcomes and allow qualitative performance indicators to be identified.

• Is the sophistication of outcome measures used by the team sufficient to meet the quantitative and qualitative clinical, financial and political needs of stakeholders?
• Do the outcome measures used measure what they are supposed to measure?

Conflict

Central policy is driving reform of health care. While individual themes may appear rational, application in a multi-agency interdisciplinary context may prove otherwise. For example, teams might reflect on their position for each of the following:

• At a policy level, moving and handling encourages dependence while NHS legislation promotes independence.
• Social care is now largely means tested, causing confusion to users and friction between providers of health and social care as users, quite naturally, seek the cheapest option.
• Promoting healthy lifestyles and exercise is costly when local leisure services are required to generate income for local authorities.
• At an interdisciplinary level and based on evidence, physiotherapists and occupational therapists will encourage the team to approach a stroke patient from the affected side to improve restoration of function while speech and language therapists will encourage approach from the unaffected side to maximise communication.
• At a practical level, the provision of high toilet seats aids getting on and off the toilet but almost inevitably changes the trunk to thigh angle adversely predisposing to constipation.
• Prescription of certain medications to facilitate rehabilitation may cause a decrease in salivation, affecting denture wearing, mastication, swallowing, nutritional intake and the nutritional status necessary for rehabilitation.
• While pathways aim to reduce variation, responsiveness to individual needs is being promoted.

A team with no conflict may make little progress and become complacent. A team with too much risks being destroyed. The size of teams will also affect the level of conflict. Interdisciplinary teams can bring together different perspectives and skills in a coordinated manner to provide for the prioritised needs of the individual user.

- How well does the interdisciplinary team welcome and manage conflict?

New elders

Practitioners need to be aware of cohort differences among current and future generations of older people. Herzlinger (1997) draws attention to the knowledgeable, energetic, financially secure, health-promoting health activists. Such individuals are undertaking or commissioning database searches on their health topic of interest. Their aim is to confront providers on a more equal, and in some cases superior, knowledge basis. Carers are also becoming increasingly assertive in their service demands, which many find easier to make on behalf of a third party.

- How does the team cope with rejection of informed best practice by increasingly assertive and expert service users and their carers?

Development

Now that the principles of specialist interdisciplinary team working in rehabilitation of older people has been established, maintenance and development will be largely dependent on continuing personal and team development. The following provide suggestions for local, national, single and interdisciplinary/ multi-agency programmes that will be particularly useful for the development of consultant roles.

- **Personal development** should include team-building, team-working, leadership, communication, supervision, negotiation and change management skills.
- **Team development** should include quality theory, ethics, risk management, minority issues, performance management, user enablement, research, skill mix, skill sharing and substitution, assessment tools and outcome measures, communication systems, record keeping, family dynamics, discharge procedures, provision of equipment and evidence based practice.

Particular attention will need to be paid to new ways of working and the implication of new venues. The team should become actively involved in undergraduate and postgraduate education of all disciplines. Smaller departments having episodic contact with the core team may feel isolated and excluded from its work and social activities, and opportunities for reciprocal involvement should be actively pursued – and responded to.

Above all, improving the knowledge base of all professions of the work of their colleagues will do much to break down barriers frequently based on false perceptions and facilitate cost-effective provision.

SUMMARY

What is clear from the contributions to this book is that all the key services involved are jointly addressing the functional problems of older people in a variety of ways, and often against social and professional prejudice. For all these services, assessment, goal setting and treatment planning in conjunction with formal and informal carers are essential. The agreed plan of treatment must be personalised, consistently implemented and regularly reviewed. The contributors to the older person's care plan need to work in a coordinated way to achieve effectiveness, efficiency and value for the older person and their carers. Each service has its outcome measures – but for the individual user, their outcome view is the most important, and evaluation of service quality should be from that perspective. Teams will therefore need to work towards shared, person-centred goals and outcome measures.

As community based rehabilitation of older people develops, the coordination of services will become even more important and the GP, community nurse and care manager will play pivotal roles. All those involved will need to have an understanding of the contributions available, criteria for referral and ensuing process so as to be able to make appropriate referrals, and to ensure consistent information is presented to the potential user. The sharing of appropriate skills will enable a more cost-effective approach by qualified staff, so long as access to expert help is available. More use will need to be made of trained support workers to carry out appropriate routine work under supervision. A generic approach will enable implementation of such care delegated by a number of disciplines, but has a number of problems that need to be overcome for success such as accountability, supervision and training. Carers will also have an expanding role, and their training, empowerment and support will become more important as the numbers and felt needs of older people increase.

Providers, both traditional and non-traditional, will be commissioned for variable periods and will need to quickly integrate, and be made to feel welcome, early in the contract period. Accurate documentation is essential and will be needed to ensure effective handover between departing and arriving providers.

The Health Service Ombudsman regularly reports that complaints about the service are mainly about lack of, or inconsistency of, information and staff attitudes. Addressing this in community based care will set even bigger challenges. An understanding of the work of the key disciplines involved will address the former, and the 'good practice' examples within this book encouraging effectiveness, efficiency and enthusiasm should address the latter.

There can be no doubt about the continuing drive for cost-effective, high quality, responsive, seamless health and social care, intended to focus on more flexible community based care and multi-agency prevention strategies. Those planning services for future generations of older people will need to be aware of cohort differences. They will age in better health than their predecessors, although the divide between prosperity and poverty affecting their health will be apparent.

The delivery of care will be demanded in a style more conducive to the user than convenient to the provider. The drive for accountability will affect providers and commissioners alike. Evidence based access criteria, validated assessment tools, rationale for the choice of pathways of care, audit of processes, comparison of outcomes, subsequent change as part of a learning culture and confirmation of staff competence will be the expected norm, and confirmed through regular internal and external reviews. Such information on the various services will be sought and compared by funders, potential users and staff respectively seeking to commission, use and work in areas of excellence. Commissioners and providers will seek quantitative evidence, and while potential users may initially employ softer quality measures as proxy for competence, they too will gradually share quantitative measures. As part of this drive for 'contracts of care', users too will be expected to take greater responsibility. Not meeting evidence based access criteria, non-adherence to a programme, non-attendance at an appointment and so on, may be objective grounds for discharge from the programme.

Professional providers will also undergo change. The 'job for life' expectation has ended, and so a range of skills will need to be developed to meet innovative requirements for time-limited and part-time contracts. New approaches to training for all staff, both professionals and others, will require constant revision to keep pace with the times.

Rehabilitation will take place within many settings for user convenience, not just the specialist centre. This multiplication of venues will have its own consequences for staffing levels, assistance, supervision, development, professional fragmentation, loss of clinical leadership, continuity, equipment and travel. With it come opportunities for recognition of greater responsibility, enhanced clinical autonomy and innovative ways of working.

Current and future generations of older people are already showing their numeric, economic and political power (Vincent, 1999). As the largest users of the NHS, the writing is on the wall for a similar assertiveness in health care. What is apparent is that rehabilitation of older people requires different attitudes, an expanded evidence base and access to a wide range of competent skills. These are integral in a successful interdisciplinary team.

REFERENCES

Audit Commission (1997) *The Coming of Age: Improving care services for older people*, Audit Commission, London.

Audit Commission (2000) *The Way To Go Home. Rehabilitation and remedial services for older people*, The Stationery Office, London.

Baker, M., Fardell, J. *et al.* (1997) *Disability and Rehabilitation: Survey of education needs of health and social service professionals*, Disability and Rehabilitation Open Learning Project.

Bowling, A. (1997) *Research Methods in Health*, Open University Press, Buckingham.

Bradley, G. and Manthorpe, J. (1997) *Financial Assessment: A practitioners' guide*, Venture Press, Birmingham.

Department of Health [DoH] (1989a) *Working for Patients*, HMSO, London.

DoH (1989b) *Caring for People*, HMSO, London.

DoH (2000) *The NHS Plan*, The Stationery Office, London.

DoH (2001a) *Shifting the Balance of Power within the NHS*, The Stationery Office, London.

DoH (2001b) *The National Service Framework for Older People*, The Stationery Office, London. www.doh.gov.uk/nsf/olderpeople.htm

Guralnik, J.M., LaCroix, A.Z., Branch, L.G., Kasl, S.V. and Wallace, R.V. (1991) Morbidity and disability in older persons in the years prior to death. *American Journal of Public Health*, **81**(4), 443–447.

Guralnik, J.M., LaCroix, A.Z., Abbott, R.D., Berkman, L.F., Satterfield, S., Evans, D.A. and Wallace, R.B. (1993). Maintaining mobility in late life. I. Demographic characteristics and chronic conditions. *American Journal of Epidemiology*, **137**(8), 845–857.

Harding, T. (1999) Enabling older people to live in their own homes. In: *With Respect to Old Age* (ed. Sutherland, S.), Research Volume 3, Chapter 3, The Stationery Office, London.

Henwood, M. (1994) *Hospital Discharge Workbook: A manual on hospital discharge practice*, Department of Health, London.

Herzlinger, R. (1997) Market Driven Healthcare, Addison Wesley, New York.

Manthorpe, J. and Bradley, G. (2000) Care management across the threshold. In: *Working on the Fault Line* (eds Bradley, G. and Manthorpe, J.), Venture Press, Birmingham.

Martin, J., Meltzer, H. and Elliot, D. (1988) *OPCS Surveys of Disability in Great Britain*, Report 1, HMSO, London.

Millard, P. (1999) *Nursing Home Placements for Older People in England and Wales. A national audit 1995–1998*, Department of Geriatric Medicine, St George's Hospital Medical School, London.

NHS Executive (1997) *The New NHS: Modern and dependable*, NHS Executive, London.

NHS Executive (1998) *Partnership in Action: New opportunities for joint working between health and social services*, NHS Executive, London.

Ovretveit, J. (1994) *Coordinating Community Care – Multidisciplinary teams and care management*, Open University Press, Buckingham.

Sinclair, A. and Dickinson, E. (1998) *Effective Practice in Rehabilitation: The evidence of systematic reviews*, King's Fund Publishing and the Audit Commission, London.

Swage, T. (2000) *Clinical Governance in Healthcare Practice*, Butterworth-Heinemann, Oxford.

Vincent, J.A. (1999) *Politics, Power and Old Age*, Open University Press, Buckingham.

APPENDICES

Appendix I

ARGYLL & CLYDE ACUTE HOSPITALS NHS TRUST

DAY HOSPITAL PATIENT DATA SHEET

HOSPITAL: ....   CONSULTANT: ....   NAMED NURSE: ....

Surname:	Forename:	Age:	Unit Number:
Address:	Telephone number:	Male/female:	DOB:
		Marital status:	Occupation:
Next of kin:	Relationship:	Second contact person:	Relationship:
Address:	Telephone number:	Address:	Telephone number:
Religion:	Church:	Family:	Key worker:
Lives alone/with:			
GP:	Address:	Telephone number:	District nurse:
Reason for referral:			
Past medical history		Known allergies	

Appendix I

ARGYLL & CLYDE ACUTE HOSPITALS NHS TRUST

_____ DAY HOSPITAL

PRIMARY NURSE: _____

PATIENT PROBLEM AND ACTION LIST

DATE	NO.	PROBLEM	Med	Nur	OT	SLT	PT	Dt	SW	Oth
	1									
	2									
	3									
	4									
	5									
	6									
	7									
	8									
	9									
	10									

PATIENT GOALS

DATE	NO.	GOAL	REVIEWED	ACHIEVED
	1			
	2			
	3			
	4			
	5			
	6			
	7			
	8			
	9			
	10			

Med Medical	Nur Nursing	OT Occupational therapy	PT Physiotherapy	SW Social work
SLT Speech & language therapy		Dt Dietetics	Ch Chiropody	Oth Other

PATIENT'S NAME: _____   HOSPITAL NUMBER: _____   DATE OF BIRTH: _____

Appendix II

ARGYLL & CLYDE ACUTE NHS TRUST

AMTS (Abbreviated Mental Test Score)
Each Question Scores 1 Mark

	DATE	DATE
1. Age		
2. Time (to nearest hour)		
3. Address for recall at end of test – 42 West Street (patient repeats to ensure it has been heard correctly)		
4. Year		
5. Name of hospital		
6. Recognition of two persons (e.g. Doctor, Nurse)		
7. Date of birth		
8. First year of First World War		
9. Name of present monarch		
10. Count backwards, twenty to one		

SCORE

8–9	Mild impairment
5–7	Moderate impairment
<5	Severe dementia

_____ DAY HOSPITAL

GERIATRIC DEPRESSION SCORE

		TICK RESPONSE	
1.	Are you basically satisfied with your life?	Yes	No
2.	Have you dropped many of your activities and interests?	No	Yes
3.	Do you feel that your life is empty?	No	Yes
4.	Do you often get bored?	No	Yes
5.	Are you in good spirits most of the time?	Yes	No
6.	Are you afraid that something bad is going to happen to you?	No	Yes
7.	Do you feel happy most of the time?	Yes	No
8.	Do you often feel helpless?	No	Yes
9.	Do you prefer to stay at home rather than going out and doing new things?	No	Yes
10.	Do you feel you have more problems with memory than most?	No	Yes
11.	Do you think that it is wonderful to be alive now?	Yes	No
12.	Do you feel pretty worthless the way you are now?	No	Yes
13.	Do you feel full of energy?	Yes	No
14.	Do you feel that your situation is hopeless?	No	Yes
15.	Do you think that most people are better off than you are?	No	Yes

TOTAL   Second column

Scores greater than 5 indicate probable depression

PATIENT'S NAME _____   Hospital number _____   Date of Birth ____ / ____ /

Appendix II

ARGYLL & CLYDE ACUTE HOSPITALS NHS TRUST

Patient's name: _____ Hospital number: _____ Date of birth: ____ / ____ / ____   DAY HOSPITAL

Address: _____ Telephone number: _____

Postcode: _____ GP: _____

MEDICAL PROBLEM LIST

DATE	NO.	ACTIVE	INACTIVE

DRUG SENSITIVITIES

MEDICATION

STARTED		FINISHED

Appendix III

DAY HOSPITAL NURSING ASSESSMENTS

EATING AND DRINKING

Diet consistency, swallowing, choking, time taken, aids required, etc.
Liquid intake, appetite, dentures, likes/dislikes

PERSONAL CARE AND DRESSING

Skin: Bath/shower/bathing service/awaiting aids. Requires prompting. Safe and able to sponge down. Dress upper and lower body. Fastenings, underwear. Suitability of clothing, etc.

BARTHEL ADL INDEX

AD/DC

FEEDING
2 = Independent (may use aid)
1 = Requires help (cutting/spreading, etc.)
0 = Dependent

☐

GROOMING
1 = Independent (wash face, hands, clean teeth, do hair, put on make-up, etc.)
0 = Dependent

☐

DRESSING
2 = Independent (including buttons, zips, laces)
1 = Requires help (but does half)
0 = Dependent

☐

BATHING
1 = Independent (able to wash and dry body)
0 = But not necessarily in/out bath)
      Dependent

☐

Appendix III

NAME : .... UNIT NUMBER : .... WARD : ....

ELIMINATING

BOWELS:
2 = Continent
1 = Occasional accident
0 = Incontinent
☐

BLADDER:
2 = Continent (including managing catheter)
1 = Occasional accident
0 = Incontinent
☐

TOILET USE:
2 = Independent (may use toilet seat/rails)
1 = Needs help
0 = Dependent
☐

Normal frequency; reach toilet in time; cope with pads/clothing; night frequency; constipation; change; level of personal hygiene; incontinence; stress/urgency; etc.
Toilet: List equipment required and in situ/awaited.

MOBILITY

TRANSFER:
Also wheelchair
3 = Independent
2 = Minimal help (verbal/physical)
1 = Major help (but sits)
0 = Dependent
☐

WALKING:
3 = Independent (may use aid)
2 = Help of one person (verbal or physical)
1 = Wheelchair dependent
0 = Dependent
☐

STAIRS:
2 = Independent
1 = Needs help (verbal or physical)
0 = Unable
☐

Pain, falls, immobility, type of aid, etc. On stairs – number of steps, rails required.
In community: walks safely in/out house, in street, manages public transport/car.

D / C

DATE OF ASSESSMENT : _____

TOTAL BARTHEL INDEX SCORE

A /D

☐ ☐

Appendix III

SLEEPING

Sleep pattern; medication/other

COMMUNICATION

Make self understood; understand others; hearing; eyesight; summon help.
Communication aids – gesture; diary. Use telephone. Able to read/write.

CONTROLLING BODY TEMPERATURE

EXPRESSING SEXUALITY

BREATHING

Smoker; breathless on exertion/climbing stairs.

EMOTIONAL ASPECTS

Mood, lability, adjustment to limitations, social interaction.

LEISURE ACTIVITIES

NAME : ....   UNIT NUMBER : ....   WARD : ....

Appendix III

LEARNING & KNOWLEDGE NEEDS

MEDICATION: Compliance; ability to self medicate; dossett box.

Memory: problem-solving; orientation to time and place; safety judgement, full meal, etc.)
Insight; concentration; ability to self-medicate, compliance.
Laundry, etc.

HOUSING

Type: Bungalow/semi/terraced/flat/maisonette/sheltered/owned/rented

Lives alone/lives with

Bedroom downstairs/upstairs

Bathroom downstairs/upstairs

Lift or stairs – flights   Inside/outside

Comments

MAINTAINING A SAFE ENVIRONMENT

Alert alarm; use telephone.   Safety in kitchen (hot drink, cook snack).

Home-making ability – household tasks, shopping, money management.

EXISTING SERVICES	MON	TUE	WED	THU	FRI	SAT	SUN
HOME-HELP							
MEALS-ON-WHEELS							
DISTRICT NURSE							
BATHING SERVICE							
DAY HOSPITAL							
DAY CENTRE							
HOME SUPPORT							
OTHER							

DATE OF ASSESSMENT : _____

SIGNED: _____

Appendix IV

 ARGYLL AND CLYDE ACUTE HOSPITALS NHS TRUST
_____ **DAY HOSPITAL**

MULTIDISCIPLINARY DISCHARGE SUMMARY

GENERAL PRACTITIONER   Dr ....

....

....

COMMUNITY NURSE   ....

REASON FOR REFERRAL

NURSING REPORT

LAST BP   WEIGHT   BM   URINE

Signed: Date:

PHYSIOTHERAPY REPORT

Signed: Date:

OCCUPATIONAL THERAPY

Signed: Date:

SOCIAL WORK INVOLVEMEMT   Social worker:

Home help .... Meals on wheels .... Home support ....

Day care at ....
....

INDEX